The Science and Art of Healing

The Science and Art of Healing

Ralph Twentyman
M.B., B.Chir., F.F.Hom.
late Consultant Physician Royal London Homoeopathic Hospital
late Editor *British Homoeopathic Journal*

Floris Books

First published in volume form in 1989 by Floris Books

British Library Cataloguing in Publication Data

Twentyman, Ralph
The science and art of healing.
1. Medicine. Homoeopathy
I. Title
615.5'32

ISBN 0–86315–095–0

Printed in Great Britain
by Billing & Sons Ltd, Worcester

Contents

Acknowledgements

I am most grateful to the Editor of the *British Homoeopathic Journal* for permission to make use of various papers which have previously appeared in that Journal and also to the Trustees of the New Atlantis Foundation for their permission to use the lecture 'The Nature of Man approached through the philosophy of Randolf Steiner.'

I am very indebted to Owen Barfield who gave a lot of his time and effort during the preparation of this book to clarifying obscurities and to encouraging the author to bring it to its completion. These efforts culminated in his writing the most helpful Introduction.

Finally, it must be obvious that over many decades I have been fortunate in having many friends, colleagues and teachers whose personal help and wisdom have contributed most of what may be of value in this book.

Ralph Twentyman

Foreword

In England when someone is referred to as 'the doctor', it means he is a doctor of medicine, unless there has been something in the context to indicate the contrary. I have sometimes regretted this; for after all the word really means 'teacher'. In France or Germany, and perhaps in America, it may even denote a doctor of science or philosophy or perhaps literature. But since reading this book I have found myself wondering whether there may not after all be a profound wisdom underlying our convention, whether in fact it is *only* a doctor of medicine who can hope to acquire that probing insight into the universal nature of things that the word *wisdom* — which is what we look for in a teacher — connotes.

Insight incidentally is one of the words I have watched growing steadily more fashionable among thoughtful people during the last fifty years or so, just as *reason* grew more and more fashionable during the eighteenth century. But I doubt whether many of them have stopped to consider what it signifies. I suggest it is the capacity to perceive the particular phenomenon not simply as one unit of a numerical aggregate but as part of a whole whose nature its own nature manifests; and that as such it is allied to imagination. Is it perhaps in the realm of medicine more than anywhere else that the researcher and the practitioner alike are compelled to think in that way? Confronted with a particular symptom, whether a pain or a pustule, a good doctor must, in the long run, go beyond seeking its 'cause' in another symptom and look as well for its 'source' in the whole patient and his life-history as an entelechy. Substitute phenomenon for symptom, and the same is true of a good scientist.

Ralph Twentyman is not simply a doctor; he is a homoeopathic doctor. And it is especially the homoeopathic stream in medicine that has been leading in the direction I have indicated. But he is also an exceptionally well-read, indeed a learned man, one with a mind capable of surveying the ages. Familiarity with the fundamental principles of physiology, biology and zoology and some knowledge of recent developments therein are perhaps no more than we should expect in an author who takes it on himself to write a book focused *imprimis* on sickness and the healing of it. Here we find in addition the like familiarity not only with the sister province of psychology, but also with such 'humanist' realms as history, notably the history of ideas, reaching back as far as mythology. Hence the distinctive quality of the book. For its author the proper study of the art of healing begins, not with Harvey and Hahnemann but with Aesculapius and Apollo. Moreover the light that such a long-drawn perspective can shed is brought to bear on his matter, not in separate inserted paragraphs, but *currente calamo*. He has the Goethean knack of awareness in the act of perception of the hidden provenance of what is being perceived.

The chapters that follow are assembled from a variety of sources, some earlier and some later. Several of them were addressed to a limited, professionally qualified audience and include therefore highly technical, even clinical, observations and analyses. But whether their appeal is ostensibly so limited, or is aimed rather at the philosophically awake portion of the laity, the reader has the same unusual experience. It is one for which I have difficulty in finding the right words — that of travelling on a kind of shuttle-service between the particular and the general, or rather the narrow and the wide. I could illustrate with plenty of examples, but this is an Introduction, not a review, and I leave him to encounter them for himself.

Additionally to its centripetal focus on homoeopathy the book has in it one unifying theme of much wider significance. It is a theme that is heard at intervals in many, or perhaps most of his chapters, but which is most firmly and explicitly sounded in Chapter 6 'The problem of potentization'. The validity, or not, of the theory of potentization is the *casus belli* between those physicians who accept homoeopathy and those allopathic, or orthodox, practitioners who reject it out of hand. It involves the assumption that certain herbal and mineral remedies depend for their effectiveness on being diluted so drastically that no physical molecule of the original substance remains in the final solution. Those who reject that assumption do so upon the contrary assumption that there are no forces operative in nature other than physical ones. The conflict therefore raises the whole issue of philosophical reductionism, and this is something of which the author is very much aware. It is also something that gives his book a special relevance at the time of writing. Organicism (or holism) and environmentalism seem both to be attracting more and more attention from the general public; both of them are concerned with the relation between man and nature, and both are suspicious of a tacitly reductionist presupposition that that relation is exclusively technological. But while this is reassuring, as far as it goes, it is unfortunately the case that the remedies publicly advocated for our perilous *malaise* are themselves generally based on that same presupposition. They are themselves essentially technological, inasmuch as they assume that any measures taken to protect our health or our environment must be based on that Cartesian dichotomy between mind and matter, which has produced what Coleridge long ago called the 'outness' of nature. They are themselves therefore mechanical or manipulative rather than organic. Would-be healers of the sickness of a cancerously urbanizing world must first learn to heal themselves.

That will not happen until they are brought to perceive not only that man is part of nature and not its enemy, but also that his 'partness' is not (as the very word 'environment' presumes) that of one physical object among other physical objects, but rather that of a flower on its stalk, and that it would be equally true to hold that nature is a part of man. That perception in its turn depends on the discovery that the 'outness' of nature is not one of the eternal verities, but an historical and psychological phenomenon peculiar to the age in which we live.

It is here that the author's many para-clinical gifts and qualifications, to which I have referred, are important. They have enabled him to lace his exposition with penetrating glimpses into the past history of thinking itself, into the evolution of consciousness, — and, with that, of what we call 'nature' — as thinking has gradually developed from a communal and natural process into the personally determined intellection it has now become. He is familiar not only with the Goethean critique of scientific methodology and the restrictions imposed on it by the scientific revolution, but also with the cosmological teachings of Rudolf Steiner and the researches of some of his followers. Consequently when his mental scalpel is applied to distinguish between, let us say, homoeopathic medicine and anthroposophical medicine, or between the (admittedly valuable) holism or organicism of the Soil Association and biodynamic methods in agriculture, there is no nit-picking of details. Rather there is a profound understanding of the difference between genuine holism and the nescient uneasiness that sometimes usurps its name.

A contrast is often insisted on between the theoretical and the practical approach to problems. It is a stupid one. If theory without practice breeds impotent pedantry, practice without theory breeds reckless blundering. I can think of few better examples of a fruitful marriage between the two than *The Science and Art of Healing*.

Owen Barfield
Forest Row, Sussex
January 1989

PART I

1. Retrospect and prospect

Disease has always been part of the human experience. Man has an inherent tendency to fall ill and to unfold a balancing, healing activity from within himself, sometimes spontaneously and sometimes in response to various outside influences, whether substantial or ritual and procedural. To be ill is an experience which befalls us, but also it is a deed, an expression of our deepest being. It belongs to our biography, and no account of human illness would be complete without seeing it in relation to the individual and his unique destiny and life-story. It is as important as any of the other major events of life. This biographical aspect of human illness of course sets it apart from disease as it may manifest itself in the natural kingdoms.

Man is perplexed by the experience of illness and seeks explanations of it according to the consciousness and prevailing ideas of the time. In the Book of Job we can hear how Job seeks for a cause of his disease and misfortune. He knows that he has not transgressed against the Law, therefore why is he suffering? His friends tell him that he must have sinned, else he would not be in this predicament. He does not know of course that a sort of wager between God and Satan has been agreed and that he is being sorely tried not by God but by the Devil. Eventually he challenges God to explain himself and, as Jung has pointed out, the answer is not an explanation of God's justice but an assertion of his omnipotence. Illness as judgment on sin is a profound motif which runs throughout history and, even into our over-intellectual and scientific age, it runs as an under-current to the discussions on the current epidemic of AIDS. Indeed thoughts of this nature are not infrequently openly voiced. Almost everyone faced with sudden unexpected serious illness will ask 'Why has this happened to me?' Inside this question is the search for meaning in contrast to the type of answer given by scientific knowledge. This scientific knowledge leads to the picture of a statistical, chance-ridden world, accident-prone and bereft of all meaning. Such explanations invade our most individual existence. Our medical, biological, characterological destinies are conceived as determined by the chance meeting of sperm and ovum with the consequent chance-determined genetic make up. Man must rebel against this vision of meaninglessness, must aim at finding, releasing, creating the meaning even in disease.

The anthropologists have brought to our attention a whole range of magical concepts and practices preceding the religious view of disease as punishment for transgression. Discarnate entities, such as ancestors or elemental beings, were discerned as invading or interfering in the life and health of individuals. Sometimes these disturbing factors were manipulated by a magician. Only another magician could combat such activities. Or for instance, the soul leaving the body in sleep might get lost or ensnared and again a magician would be needed to find the lost soul and entice or lead it back again. Ceremonial ritual practices still survive, no doubt in decadent form, in many parts of the world. Ellenberger has described and discussed these and shown how similar ideas of disease and healing are found today in the various psychologies of the unconscious. Once such phenomena were felt and experienced as immediate reality; today they become theory, abstract ideas and only in dire crisis do they again assume real reality.

All these cultish healing practices passed through a metamorphosis in the temple medicine of Greece and this again can be seen as a stage in the ancestry of our modern psychotherapeutics. Healing in Greece was experienced as the Epiphany of the god Asklepios. Asklepios manifested in the healing process. This could come about in the temples, the Asklepieions, during the temple sleep in which the god appeared to the patient. Careful preparation preceded the ritual sleep in the Abaton. But side by side with this temple medicine there existed secular physicians of whom Hippocrates (fifth, fourth century BC) is best remembered. These physicians belonged to the family of the Asklepiadae, tracing their origin to Asklepios. In their family inheritance ran the blood of Asklepios and so even in these secular healings the god manifested. It is worth noting that probably many more patients today visit Lourdes and other shrines than visited Epidauros, Cos, Pergamon and other Asklepieions in antiquity.

In the secular schools of Greek medicine there arose, in mutual relationship with Greek philosophy and natural science, a search for natural causes of natural phenomena, disease being conceived as belonging to nature. With what sorts of idea was this attempt made? The paradox that first appears between two Greek views, the one that healing is a manifestation of the God and the other that nature heals, is to some extent resolvable. We are confused because our experience and concept of nature is very different from that of the Greeks. For them nature was still a divine goddess, the mother of us all. For us nature has been reduced to a machine which natural science studies with cold intellectual and dissecting faculties. As Gutkind expresses it, we have risen above nature. But for the Greek, nature was living and from her womb gave birth to all creatures including ourselves. She therefore with wisdom infinitely greater than our own cared for us. If she gave us fevers or diarrhoeas, these were to be understood as her healing efforts, not to be suppressed but even aided. Diarrhoea was to get rid of poison, therefore treat it with some plant which would promote diarrhoea.

We can easily see that such ideas underlie current 'natural therapies'. The question is whether we can today honestly regard man as part of nature, as in his day the youthful Goethe still could.

There is another strand in the legacy of Greek medicine. The world was conceived by different natural philosophers to have originated from water, or air, or fire, or in the atomism of Leucippus and Democritos (460–360 BC) from earth. These views became systemized by Empedocles (504–443 BC) into a double polarity of fire and water and of air and earth. These were the four elements. Internally in our physiology they had their correspondences in the four humours: yellow bile and phlegm, and blood and black bile. The harmonious balance of these four humours was health; whilst their disbalance or dyscrazia, arising from excess or plethora of one of the humours, or of course from a deficiency, was disease. This enabled one to characterize diseases and to choose remedies whose characteristics could help to restore the balance. A plethora of blood led to the universal practice of blood letting. The four temperaments, choleric, sanguine, phlegmatic and melancholic (black bile), were also based on these four humours. The pathology based on these concepts only finally disappeared in the middle of the nineteenth century. The notions of balance and disbalance still play their part in both professional and lay thinking.

Historically, we find this idea of illness as disbalance first formulated by the Pythagorean Alcmaeon of Croton (c. 500 BC). For him health was Isonomie, equality before the law among these humours; and illness Monarkie, the dominance of one of them. This conception was taken from the observed struggle of factions in politics. This reminds us that earlier in Babylonia and Egypt both social disorder and pestilences were looked upon as earthly reflections of disorder in the heavens. To this idea Shakespeare gave expression in Ulysses' speech in *Troilus and Cressida*:

> . . . but when the planets
> In evil mixture to disorder wander,
> What plagues and what portents, what mutiny,
> What raging of the sea, shaking of earth,
> Commotion in the winds, frights, changes, horrors,
> Divert and crack, rend and deracinate
> The unity and married calm of states
> Quite from their fixure.

In Babylonia the starry heavens were understood as the script in which were written the deeds of gods. Now in Greece in the humours and the elements we come into the earthly realms, and in the dyscrazia of the humours we approach a natural explanation of disease. The elements and humours were permeable by the quintessential ether which already partook of a 'heavenly nature'. Life could emanate from the ether into the humours.

Thus there came about the change from a spiritual and religious conception of disease and healing to a dawning scientific one. For two thousand years the Greek ideas of medicine, systematized by the great Galen of Pergamon (AD 138–201) and passing east to the Academy of Gondishapur from whence the Arabs brought it back to the west via Spain and Sicily, dominated medicine.

But it is not quite so simple. When we look at this double polarity of the four humours, we cannot help asking, what can hold them in balance? Only nature, acting as the *Vis medicatrix naturae*, as it has come down to us in the Latin. The divine nature in whose womb the ancients still were, has to be invoked or else the god Asklepios must restore the lost balance. The holding of and restoring of the balance does not arise from within but from the divine in which man felt himself. The ego was not yet born.

In the early Christian centuries the cult of Asklepios was one of the most important rivals to the growing Church. During those centuries there was a succession of devastating epidemics throughout the Roman world. Whole cities were wiped out and the population reduced to a small remnant by, probably, malaria, typhus, small-pox, measles and perhaps other diseases too. The physicians were powerless to control these scourges and the population flocked to various mystic sects. Theologians argued as to whether Asklepios or Christ was the true healer. Gradually the attributes of Asklepios were assimilated to the figure of Christ and even the face of Asklepios became the model for many figures of Christ. What had been sought outwardly must now be sought inwardly. The figure of Christ as the healer and saviour must now be sought inwardly. Nature became of less importance, inner spirituality of intense importance. The science of medicine declined in the West, its traditions being preserved to some extent in the monasteries. It was in the East in Gondishapur, and later in Baghdad and other Islamic universities, that Greek science and medicine were mainly preserved and cultivated, until via Spain and Sicily they fertilized the development of medicine in the early Renaissance from 1200 onwards. But the Christian centuries had brought about the beginnings of individual self-consciousness and a realization of the importance of illness on the path of individual development. That this incipient self-consciousness, this Ego, had an inner capacity for restoring the balance through its own spiritual growth and metamorphosis must also have become a dawning realization. An inevitable confrontation between the Greek legacy transmitted through the Arabs and the early dawning of a Christ-orientated medicine had to come about. The one regarded disease more as fate, destiny, suffering; the other as opportunity.

In the strange figure of Paracelsus (1493–1541) this Christianized concept of disease and healing came to expression. From the more strictly medical or organic side Paracelsus emphasized the threefold constitution of the human organism. Sal, Mercurius and Sulphur were the three alchemical substances or processes co-operating in the human organism. Sal and Sulphur stand as polarities to each other whilst Mercurius mediates between them. Today we can relate Sal to the processes in the nerves and senses, Sulphur to the metabolic processes and Mercurius to the rhythmic processes. These last as balancing and mediating functions bear the healing processes, now within us. Of course these alchemical terms must not be confused with the modern chemical usages.

But the question still arises, can the rhythmic system by itself maintain and restore the balance between the two opposing poles? Is this an automatic self-regulating process or does a superior wisdom have to act in and through this 'mercurial' element as nature did for the ancient Greeks? For Paracelsus nature was still full of wisdom and the physician must school himself in nature and learn her wisdom. But for Paracelsus God is also the healer who can cure without the medicaments which the physician uses, though these too are provided by God. Christ can heal through the soul.

Paracelsus lived at the beginning of the sixteenth century when the modern world was being born. He died only two years before the publication in 1543 of Copernicus' new model of the universe and of Vesalius' great work on human anatomy. These two books, the one on the corpse of the solar system, the other on the corpse of man, provided the basis on which modern science has been constructed.

Paracelsus' medicine was heartfelt; the heart's feeling, passionate and exuberant, for another human soul in suffering, throbs through his work. Jacobi compares it with a Gothic cathedral or a Bach fugue. It stands in complete contrast to the works of Hippocrates and the Greeks. There it is nature or Asklepios who can heal; the physician calmly watches and acts out of the inherited clairvoyant instinct. It was a medicine of the belly, of the unconscious empathy and wisdom.

Out of the organic unity of soul and body which we still find in Paracelsus there developed modern chemistry on the one hand and on the other a more hidden current of psychological knowledge. We could also say that the sharp division between an objective world of extension and motion bereft of all other qualities of colour, tone, taste, smell, beauty and ugliness and so on, on the one hand, and on the other the subjective mental world to which these qualities had been banished, had not been accomplished. Man as microcosm was set within the macrocosm and they were both compounded of the quantitative and qualitative. From alchemy developed modern chemistry as from astrology comes astronomy. The soul side of this ancient science of alchemy has been brought to light again particularly in the work of C. G. Jung. This division into two parts of these old traditions was initiated by Galileo (1564–1642) who distinguished between the primary qualities of mass, extension and movement and the secondary qualities which came to mean everything else which we experience, the colours, tones, smells, tastes and so on we have mentioned. On this basis it was possible to build the modern ideas of mechanism and the whole scientific revolution. Descartes (1596–1650) developed this theme philosophically, and medicine to this day is dominated by the divide between a body conceived as mechanism and a soul conceived as merely subjective.

The mechanical view is based on the sense of touch, of push and pull. Other sense experiences such as colour and tone have first to be translated into concepts assuming an imagined experience of the sense of touch in order that they can be handled mechanically. Colours become either particles or vibrations and tones vibrations. Colour and tone are lost to the world and re-invented in our subjectivity. Out of this has developed the body-soul riddle and the isolated estrangement of modern man imprisoned within the witch's cottage of his skull, alone with his utterly subjective, private experience. This experience is divorced from the outer objective world constructed by science. The consequence of all this is that Nature has become mere mechanism, purged of that wisdom she possessed so powerfully for the Greeks and for Paracelsus as well. We have however to admit that Nature was becoming more and more ghost-like all that time and the final stripping from her of all qualitative attributes and so-called occult qualities was little more than taking mere threadbare trappings from her ghost.

Since interest was focused on the spatial we find an ever-increasing study of the structure of the body becoming the foundation of medicine. The changes in structure discoverable in the corpses of those dying of diseases led first to observations of the organs such as liver and lung, a discipline known as morbid anatomy, founded by Morgagni (1682–1771).

When the microscope became available the studies turned to the tissues (Bichat 1771–1802) whose interweaving was discerned in the organs. These tissues derive from the embryonic layers or leaves, the ecto-, meso-, and endoderms. There is in them a tendency to two-dimensionality, a vegetative note, from which the organs developed by progressive in-turnings, invaginations, giving rise to animal forms.

With yet more powerful microscopes attention focused on the cells, regarded as the building stones of the organism. To start with, the seat of disease was regarded as the organs, then it was the tissues and then the cells. All disease for Rudolf Virchow (1821–1902) has its seat in the cells. Now in this century with electron microscopes and other new techniques attention has shifted to the intracellular components, genes and molecules, and the search goes on. But the further it goes in this compulsive drive to the ever smaller unit, purged more and more of any content accessible to direct human perception, the less does it have human meaning for us. We can measure, calculate, correlate findings; knowledge increases but understanding vanishes.

If we compare for a moment our body with a house we can raise some questions which may help us. In a house made of bricks or other materials we do not live in the bricks. We live in the spaces called rooms. The actual building materials could be very varied without making a great difference to the rooms. Of course if they crumble, get dry rot and so on it will be detrimental to the room, but we would not search primarily in the stuff of the walls to grasp the character of the house. It would be the shape and size of the empty spaces that would interest us and only secondarily the soundness of the bricks, walls, windows, etc. But science goes on as if only the bricks, the cells, etc. of our bodies are important.

Now whilst this mainstream medical progress was becoming more and more deterministic and mechanical another stream began to take shape. Out of medieval and clerical concepts of mental disease in which possession by devils played a considerable part there emerged towards the end of the eighteenth century a secular study of bizarre behavioural phenomena. Mesmer (1734–1815) was the pioneer and by means of what today would be called hypnotism, but which he called magnetism, he produced phenomena rivalling those of the exorcising priests. It is true that he was as a child of the Enlightenment concerned to get rid of the superstitions of devils, exorcisms and the rest of mumbo-jumbo and to substitute the equally superstitious idea of animal magnetism. But it sounded more enlightened. An epidemic of magnetic circles spread over Europe. Nevertheless it led to gradually increasing awareness and study of the phenomena of hypnotism and of all the bizarre symptoms associated with hysteria. These phenomena are very hard to reconcile with an anatomical and mechanistic view of the organism. Awareness of 'unconscious' soul life gradually grew throughout the nineteenth century. Eduard von Hartmann's great work *The Philosophy of the Unconscious* appeared in 1868 and medically many physicians throughout the century had begun to appreciate the dynamic reality of unconscious mental phenomena, forgotten memories and the like as well as the importance of repressed sexual problems. Freud's name has of course been associated with this movement as its pioneer, but there were many others before him.

There has therefore come about an inner split in medicine between the objectively orientated mechanistic physiology and pathology and the subjectively orientated psychology in which even the unconscious is conceived purely as soul phenomenon. This is the natural outcome of the scientific revolution and its separation of primary from secondary qualities. We can characterize the outcome of the split as follows:

bodies without souls and souls without bodies.

Now we must retrace our steps a little and consider the figure of Samuel Hahnemann (1755–1843) who at the beginning of the nineteenth century introduced his new art of healing known as homoeopathy. It is not easy to discover the essential core of this revolutionary idea and method. It has been customary from Hahnemann himself onwards to define the revolution in terms of treating disease by likes instead of opposites. When the Hippocratic writings recommend treating diarrhoea with Veratrum, which itself brings about diarrhoea, it is treating like with like.

When in these same writings a plethora of blood should be opposed by a blood letting or remedy to oppose it, this is treating by opposites. So is giving opium, which constipates, for diarrhoea. But, as we have seen, it was understood in Greece that the symptom, diarrhoea for example, was the expression of the healing power of nature and that nature was full of wisdom. By Hahnemann's time this relationship to nature, of child to mother was no longer viable. For Hahnemann it was the disease, conceived as dynamic Idea, which came to expression in the symptoms. The disease was known through its actions just as a human person is known through his actions and gestures. These actions of the disease are the totality of symptoms. The disease is an idea, real and dynamic in the sense of a Goethean idea. For Hahnemann it is only knowable in its expression in which it so to speak incarnates. It is that which gives unity to the plurality of symptoms. Now Hahnemann finds that medicinal substances given to healthy individuals also produce symptoms, produce a medicinal disease and that this new disease will negate and banish the similar natural disease. We could take a further step and say that the 'Idea' of the remedial plant, for instance, which is the unity of the plant in nature is also the 'Idea' of the disease. The idea which manifests in, say, the Pulsatilla, the wind flower, comes to a higher manifestation in the whole drug-picture, as it is called, of Pulsatilla or in the symptom complex of which Pulsatilla can be both cause and remedy. But the human realm is not the realm of nature and the manifestation of the Pulsatilla idea in man is a higher metamorphosis in a realm above nature. Hahnemann recognized that nature unaided cannot heal; she overdoes or underdoes it. Either the deeper individuality of the patient, which Groddeck much later called the It, or the higher intuition of the physician, consciously or unconsciously, must guide the healing process. To work with these metamorphoses calls for an artistic mode of perception to supplement the scientific. Therefore Hahnemann rightly changed his original subtitle from a 'new science of healing' to a 'new art of healing'.

The essentials however from our present point of view of Hahnemann's method are first the observation of disease on the human scale and the resolute avoidance of reductionism. Disease is not primarily a disorder of molecules, cells or any other abstraction. Disease has meaning as a human phenomenon on the human scale. Secondly we notice that there are local or bodily and mental symptoms in all cases though, as Hahnemann most importantly emphasized, there is a spectrum of disease. At one pole some diseases are one-sidedly local or bodily with almost no discernible mental changes; at the other pole are the so-called mental diseases when the manifest symptoms are all mental and the local disorders scarcely discoverable. This cuts through the sharp body-soul division and replaces it with a spectrum of illness. Thirdly, healing must involve a change in consciousness as well as a change in somatic symptoms. Something unconscious or forgotten must be recalled or something be allowed to sink into forgetfulness which is 'sticking in the gullet'.

The further elucidation of these themes is undertaken in other sections but they all involve a more artistic mode of observation and activity than is current today.

We are therefore suggesting that following on the religiously orientated medicine of early times and the scientifically disciplined medicine from Greek times on, there began with Hahnemann an impulse for the artistically inspired healing of the future.

The arguments concerning treatments by like or opposite, the traditional ground for distinguishing homoeopathy from orthodox medicine, are no longer valid today. The uses of the Similia, the like, in Hippocrates and Hahnemann are utterly different from each other, as we have shown. They cannot be treated as identical. Further modern orthodox therapeutics with modern chemical products are in fact based, almost entirely, on the 'Similia' principle. Molecules similar to others involved in the disease pathways are introduced to block or antagonize them, in a manner akin to Hahnemann's giving a new disease to block the natural one. The distinction is today between the reductionist model of disease on the molecular scale as against Hahnemann's conception of disease as human on the human scale. Nor can the range of desensitizations in allergic disorders or immunizations be ranged directly with or against Hahnemann's idea. They constitute another whole field of phenomena. These problems are more fully discussed in Chapter 5.

It has come about since Hahnemann's time, and increasingly as the scientific study of disease has grown, that the homoeopathic school has been pushed into the position of opposition to all mechanistic or materialistic tendencies. It has been lumped with Vitalism in confrontation with Mechanism. But Hahnemann's treatment of one-sided diseases, local as opposed to mental, points to a potential resolution also of these problems. Mechanism and death are interiorized in man. We owe our awake consciousness not to vital processes but to death processes within us. Mechanism and Vitalism are not two alternatives but two poles of a spectrum. We carry the skeleton about with us, we use it, death is our daily companion and we must make use of the mechanistic discoveries of our time by incorporating them within the more comprehensive picture of man. Nature has been killed and become dead, abstract mechanism; the realm of law-determined necessity is not the whole but one limiting pole. Man and the world of freedom is another realm between nature and the Divine. Only God, Man and nature can constitute the whole.

Once it is realized that Man is not just part of nature it becomes obvious that nature cannot heal man. Nature has to be overcome and contradicted before it can healthily enter man's world. The great *Naturphilosoph*, contemporary of Hahnemann, Lorenz Oken (1779–1851) formulated it thus: Physiological processes in animals are pathological processes in Man. Or processes which are healthy in animals are human diseases.

The significance of Hahnemann's contribution in homoeopathy becomes clearer when we understand it as a beginning of a bridge over the great divide which opened up with what Barfield called the Cartesian guillotine. The absolute split between the objective body and the merely subjective soul which finds expression in a one-sided mechanistic medicine and equally one-sided psychodynamics begins to find a solution in the idea of the spectrum of disease. This idea has reappeared quite independently in the work of the Bahnsons.

What then have been the hindrances to greater acceptance of this Hahnemannian contribution? Hahnemann himself in asserting the human scale of observation and fighting against the tide of reductionist science laid down an embargo, a prohibition against investigation into the inner workings of the human organization, and denied the possibility of worthwhile knowledge of medicines being obtained from observation and study of them in nature. The inner realities of the human organism he rightly understood as different from processes in outer nature and inaccessible to the methods available for their investigation. The remedial potentialities of medicine, he affirmed, could only be brought to light by the study of their action on man, not by the study of their chemical content or their physiognomic signature. In consequence homoeopathy was cut off from fruitful relations with both natural science and pathology and medicine. One further factor served to complicate this isolation. Hahnemann introduced the process of potentizing remedies, by which through a process of repeated dilution and shaking, the ponderable aspect of the substance was reduced to zero and beyond. During the first decade of the nineteenth century whilst the atomic theory was being established on the basis of the weight changes during chemical reactions and the elements arranged according to their atomic weights, Hahnemann introduced the imponderable aspects in the form of the potencies. In the prevailing climate of materialism this was enough to rule it out of court. Only what could be weighed was real.

Let us take another simple example. A mirror image lacks material reality. A picture lacks reality materially; after all, it is not the chemistry of the paints that constitutes the picture which may thrill us with its beauty. These 'unrealities' can change our consciousness; the image can activate some content in the unconscious. It seems that this formal or ideal aspect of a substance can be conveyed to the media and become available for use as a sort of image. One's consciousness can be changed by a look at oneself in a mirror or by identifying with a character in a play which 'holds a mirror up to nature'. Psychotherapy performs a similar task. Only our one-sidedly materialistic picture of a man as a body makes it difficult for us to see these connections.

We have therefore a trinity of medical approaches. The basic mechanistic study of structures of the body, then the exclusively subjective psychological interpretation which can explain all illness as purposive, albeit unconscious, and the third, the homoeopathic, which potentially mediates between them.

At present these three cannot communicate with each other. There is no common concept or image of man shared between them; for science man is at best an animal, but ultimately a heap of molecules; for psychology man is a battleground of instinctive impulses and moral sanctions, in which the role of the organs is almost disregarded. Homoeopathy lacks a conception of man whose illnesses it claims to treat as a whole and lacks any conception of the relations between man and nature. It is my contention that the stream of anthroposophical medicine could be the mediator between the three, fertilizing each approach and enriching itself in the process. The trinity must become a triunity.

These distinctive medical approaches and disciplines would not then be seen as alternative or complementary but as distinctive functions within an organic whole.

2. Anatomy — the form and structure of Man

Ever since Vesalius published his textbook on human anatomy in 1543, modern medicine has been dominated by structural concepts. In this it has followed the general tendency to mechanistic ideas and explanations pioneered by Galileo, Newton and other leaders of the scientific revolution. The great work of Vesalius *De humani corporis fabrica libra septum* was based on dissections of human corpses. No concept of a living human being can be discovered in this way; the corpse is that which has been discarded by the human person who once built it, used it and has now deserted it; it has become a mere fact. Nevertheless this disciplined study of the structural aspect of the body of man has been the foundation of all that is good and bad in modern medicine. In a way modern medicine is the attempt to understand diseases as faults in the mechanical structures of the body. Technological advances have led to ever more refined studies of structure right into the cell and the intracellular contents. The modern work on heredity arises out of a geometrical concept, the double helix.

During the four centuries since Vesalius' book appeared the search for the seat of disease has moved by stages to ever smaller entities. At first it was observed how, in the corpse of someone dying from some disease, a particular organ was damaged. For instance the lungs of tuberculous patients were found to contain large cavities or the livers of old drunkards might be hardened and studded with nodules, the so-called hob-nailed liver. Morgagni pioneered this work and published his life's work in 1761 when he was nearly eighty, *De sedibus et causis morborum per anatomen indagatis libri quinque* — five books concerning the seat and causes of diseases anatomically studied. This implied that illnesses were localized, the seat of an illness was an organ or several organs.

A little later, in Napoleonic times, a French physician, Bichat, using microscopes, sought the seat of diseases not in organs but in tissues. Bichat, in spite of belonging to the Vitalist School and being much concerned to elucidate the differences between the living and the dead, sought the seat of healthy and diseased processes in anatomical structures. But he was not content to localize them in an organ. Observation taught him that similar illness could manifest in changes in different organs; therefore he sought for constituents which were common to different organs. He called these entities membranes and distinguished twenty-one of them. The organs are composed of the interweaving of these membranes or tissues and Bichat considered these membranes as the seats of the vital functions. Today we can look for the origin of these membranes in the primitive germ layers of the embryo, the so-called ectoderm, endoderm and mesoderm. These leaf-like, two-dimensional, forms are easily related to the plant-like vital functions. The three-dimensional organs, such as heart, lung, liver and so on belong to the animal order of existence. Only in animals do proper organs develop.

Soon the cell was discovered as the building stone of all the tissues and organs of the body and Virchow initiated the cellular doctrine, that all diseases are localized in the cells. He regarded disease as the reaction of cells to abnormal stimuli. During all this time chemistry had been advancing as well as physiology.

The new chemistry based on the atomic theory at first understood these atoms as if they were small solid balls whose interrelations, joining together and separating, made up the chemical processes. In this way chemistry became a study in sub-microscopic mechanics.

Physiology, the study of the living organism, became dominated by chemical ideas on the one hand and by electrical ideas on the other. Since Volta had observed that frogs' legs jerked when acted on by electrical stimuli, a tendency entered into physiology seeking in electricity the secret of life. This has led today to the crude ideas of the brain as a sort of enormously complicated computer or telephone exchange.

Even without going into details we can see how in all these ways the idea of the human body has become entirely mechanical and electrical. The concepts of Euclidean space underlie this. Life is abolished and the life of soul can find no place in all this complicated machine in which to enter. The more recent discoveries in the intracellular and subatomic worlds only continue the same tendencies. The human body is studied as a dead mechanism, a corpse, and we can only stand outside it and observe it, just as we do any bit of inorganic nature.

Against this materialistic, natural scientific movement, a counter movement came about. In the eighteenth century Mesmer appeared and unleashed on the public phenomena of dramatic and mysterious nature. Strange behaviours which had mostly, up till then, been the concern of priests and theologians and explained largely in terms of possession, became now of secular interest. The prevailing mental climate led to even these bizarre phenomena being explained by 'animal magnetism'. But out of this movement there gradually developed during the nineteenth century the psychology of the unconscious, culminating in the psychoanalytic schools and their descendants. It was largely in the study of hysteria and hypnotism that these movements originated. The phenomena studied seem to contradict the mechanical notions of the body. Hysterical paralysis and anaesthesia for instance do not follow the anatomical nerve distribution.

A situation came about when one party seemed to study bodies without souls and the other souls without bodies. The philosophic origin of this split has to be sought in Descartes and the division into primary and secondary qualities.

The question now faces us, how can we begin to understand the human body in ways which enable us to grasp the living and ensouled bodies of our actual experience. For the ancients anatomy had played a negligible role in their concepts of disease; it had been confined to the surgical treatment of accidents and fractures. The early Greek ideas of disease were holistic, balance or disbalance in the four humours. Only after the foundation of Alexandria in the fourth century BC did anatomical studies and dissections start, implying a great change in the attitude to the corpse, an overcoming of what we today would call superstitious fear of the dead body. For three hundred years those studies continued and then slowly faded away again until the Renaissance. Since then the study of anatomy and structure has become the foundation of scientific medicine and we have seen how this has proceeded from the anatomy of the gross body, to the organs filling that body, the tissues or membranes which as warp and weft build the organs, to the cells as building stones themselves now revealed as complex structures constructed from molecules whose minute anatomy or structure today becomes revealed. How then can we begin to enliven and animate again this complex machine which our bodies have become? If we do not do so the present crisis in medicine can only get worse: the split, the division between body and soul, whose origin can be discerned in antiquity but which became the methodological basis of modern science only with Galileo, Descartes and Locke, still dominates medical research.

It belongs to our present day notions that we approach all parts and functions of the human body with the same ideas. We study liver and brain, lung and kidney with the same methods and basic concepts. One sometimes thinks that for modern science we might as well walk on our heads as on our feet for any difference it would make. But artists have revealed the human body as a supreme work of art, not as simply a mechanical contrivance. Leonardo da Vinci combined precise anatomical study with supreme artistic revelations of the human form. The great artist enables us to see the hidden potentialities struggling to expression within 'the muddy vesture of decay'. The hidden laws of nature are brought to expression in great works of art, whereas in nature they remain confused and concealed.

Where, to start with, in the history of art may we be able to find the expression of those laws which underlie the building of the human form, which was formed originally in the image or likeness of God? May not the ancient prohibitions against the mutilation of the dead body have arisen, not from superstition but from the sensitive perception that this body was the artistic creation of the spirit and soul which had left it? The reverential care of the body of the dead, we suggest, is rather like the way today we enshrine works of art in galleries and museums, to be stared at.

24

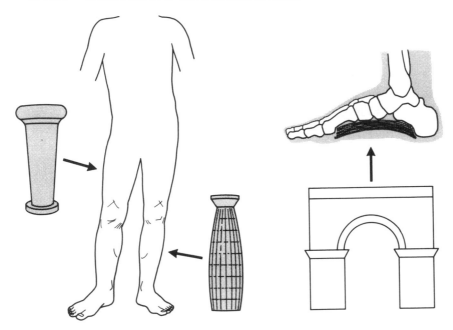

Figure 1. The form of the early Cretan column (left) corresponds to the thigh. The Greek column shows the same swelling as the calf. The later Roman arch is reflected in the arch of the foot.

If we take the human body as an artistic creation of the soul and spirit who dwelt in it, could we not look to architecture for the expression of the same creative activity? When a little baby is born it is still mostly head, the limbs are scarcely formed. As it grows the child grows down into its limbs, gradually it learns to stand upright on its feet. The growing down into the limbs we find expressed architecturally in the development from Crete to Rome. Cretan architecture in the so-called palaces, which may well have been mortuary temples, had characteristic columns which were wider at the top than the bottom. Are not these columns the outer expression of the inner forms of the thigh? As the baby grows down it first begins to form the thigh which narrows from the hip to knee. It is a Cretan column. Civilization moved from Crete to Greece and the Greek temple appeared. The columns of the Greek temple show a slight swelling so that they are narrower both at the top and bottom than in the middle. They seem to breathe in perfection of rhythmic balance. The baby grows down into its leg from knee to ankle and the calf shows this same swelling as the Greek column. The leg also has two bones which in the upper limb, in the forearm, can rotate around each other. Here we can glimpse the correlation with the rhythmic middle system of man.

Civilization moved on to Rome and came to earth, forgetting the heavenly dreams, reminiscences of babyhood. Rome, if not actually inventing, at least developed and carried everywhere the architectural arch. The arch became a basic note of Roman architecture in bridges, basilicas, baths, the circus buildings and aqueducts. The growing child at last puts his foot on to the ground, toe and heel, and the leg is supported on the keystone of the arch of the instep.

Now the child has to enter into his body. The Greek temple was the house of the God whose statue it contained. The people were outside and the altar for the sacrifices was outside the temple. The colonnades of columns were outside, inside them were the walls of the rooms, the *cella*, in which were the images of the God, and the treasury. Then this turned inside out, as we can see for instance in the Serapeum at Pergamon. The walls were outside, the columns inside, and we have the basic structure of the basilicas. Now the people could go inside.

The anatomy of the human body is based on three great body cavities which contain the organs. First there is the cavity of the head containing the brain; secondly there is the chest or thoracic cavity which contains the heart and lungs. And thirdly divided from this by a great dome of muscular and fibrous tissues, the diaphragm, there is the abdominal cavity containing the alimentary canal, the liver, kidneys, spleen and other organs. As a subdivision of this cavity there is the pelvic cavity containing the bladder and in women the uterus and ovaries. Into this pelvic cavity, during labour, the head of the baby fits almost perfectly as a ball and socket joint.

The states of consciousness related to these three cavities are quite distinct. The head is a domed cavity, inwardly quiet, but in this cave we live in a world of images. We are really in the situation of the prisoners in the cave in Plato's myth. We can only see the shadows cast on the wall, not the real actors. That they are indeed images amidst which we live in our heads can be easily experienced by a game played by school children. If we stand under a lamp looking up at it and then turn round for half a minute, when we stop turning the room appears to turn. It is of course only the image of the room that rotates. In front of this cave in which the brain floats in the cerebro-spinal fluid, there is as it were stuck on the bones and tissues of the face. It is really stuck on and if we take a skull and hold it upside down then this face appears like a turret or gatehouse crowned by a semi-circle of teeth, the castellations. Protected by this face, gatehouse, mask or persona we can remain serene within, amidst the thoughts and images.

If we return to Rome we find a remarkable building dating from the first or second Christian century, the Pantheon. On entering this temple we enter a vast dome whose roof seems to float above us. It is quiet and cool within and in the centre of the dome is a hole, through which come light and rain. It is like the open fontanelle on the top of the baby's head, through which it is still connected to heaven. The entrance to this enclosed windowless space is through a sort of Greek temple, colonnades of Greek columns, stuck on to the front of the great spherical enclosure. This temple was supposed to house statues of all the gods including the imported oriental deities. It therefore looks to the past, commemorates the past even as our own heads do.

The dome was taken up, in a higher development, in Constantinople, in the

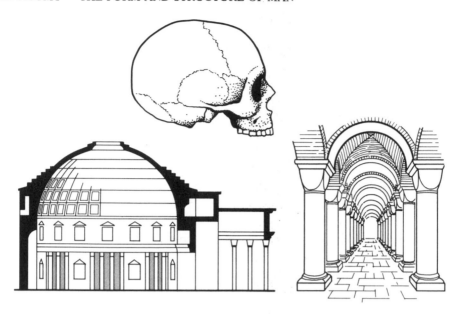

Figure 2. The dome of the skull compared with the early Christian dome of the Pantheon in Rome and the rounded arch of a Romanesque crypt.

great church of Hagia Sophia. Inside it became a glowing world of divine images in the mosaics on the walls. In the overwhelming majesty of the liturgy and rituals a world of truly divine images burst forth. But this divine imagery did not penetrate into the world outside the church.

In the West there gradually emerged the architecture of the Romanesque, in this country known to us as Norman. One finds oneself within massive walls with only narrow windows. These walls were once coloured and adorned with frescoes. The inner meditative contemplation of monks and priests accompanied the ritual of the Mass, protected by these massive walls from the outside world. And in the crypts more rites were performed around the corpses of the saints. One is in caves, harking back to those antediluvian caves with their wall paintings and to Egyptian crypts and Mithraic temples.

These considerations are brought forward to try to discover the life which proceeds within the vaulted caves of our skulls, those veritable images of death. It is a life in images, sensory images and the reflections we call thoughts. The head itself and the brain were built by the still living thoughts during foetal and childhood life. The skull and brain have now become almost dead corpses, images of the forces that built them; one could almost say ruins. Yet for this reason they can offer resistance, like a mirror, so that we can become conscious of the activity we unfold in thinking. We wake up in this thinking activity. The Romanesque church does represent the whole body but in the style of the head. Therefore we experience mainly a sense of massive statics and quiet stillness.

A quite different feeling rises in us in a Gothic cathedral. The walls are opened up and become glorious stained glass through which the sunlight penetrates dappling the inside with coloured patterns. The great shafts soar upwards branching into the ribbed vaulting overhead. As one gazes up the nave to the east one is led rhythmically from column to column in steady procession forwards. The whole building becomes filled with the great congregations which unite in shared ecstatic wonder as they witness the miracle of the Mass. No longer do we feel the contemplative meditative life of monks but the rising communal devotion of the people. And outside, the flying buttresses bring the gigantic dynamics of these buildings to visibility. Have we not moved from the cave into the forest glade, celebrating again with the Gothic tribes under the trees? The sun filters through the leaves as it does through the stained glass windows.

We have moved into the chest, the thorax, containing the heart and lungs, the culmination of all the rhythmic processes in man. The lungs themselves are trees, the bronchial trees are the trunk and branches and the alveoli of the lungs are the leaves. The heart is the altar in the midst of the forest grove and here the divinity manifests.

It is the life of our feelings that we discover rising and falling on the great rhythms of our breath and pulse. These feelings are not so awake as is our thinking; they are comparable more to dreams. The age of these great cathedrals was the age of the exalted feelings of the Grail romances and the troubadours and the Crusades. We all tend to live through these again as we grow up to adolescence and learn to harmonize our rhythmic processes.

Descending below the great dome of the diaphragm which separates the chest from the abdomen we enter an entirely new world. Now eating and digesting, all the processes of metabolism come to ascendency. In a sense we can say that real things happen, in digestion we destroy what we eat. In the head we awake in a world of images whereas in the processes of metabolism we enter into real transformations of substance but in doing so we lose our consciousness. We do not consciously follow what happens in digestion and metabolism. In architecture we enter the world of the Baroque. In these churches decoration and display reach heights of absurdity but we enter in the paintings of saints and angels into a very substantial world. The heavenly story has here become truly flesh. We now not only walk on earth, we become earthy. Till then we had participated in a dream world of longings and romance, now this lost world only reaches us in the dynamically powerful paintings on the vaulted roofs of these buildings; they are dramatic and move our wills. At the same time the modern picture-frame theatre comes into existence, the audience becomes interested in itself and looks on at the play in detachment. The churches themselves come to resemble opera houses and the congregation even assemble in their own boxes to be witnesses of the drama at the altar on the stage. The economic life of merchants, of the bourgeoisie, becomes dominant and natural science, characterized by Nietzsche as the will to power of

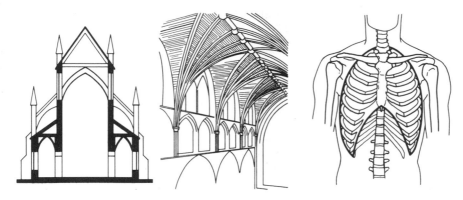

Figure 3. The thorax and the Gothic style.

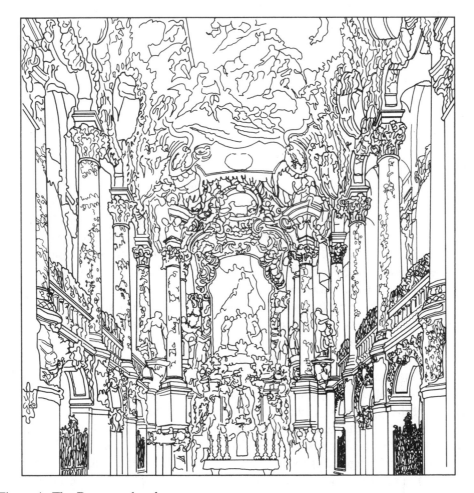

Figure 4. The Baroque church.

the bourgeois class, takes over the life of learning. This science is not concerned with truth but with technology: 'Does it work?'

As youths and maidens grow into their metabolism and limbs, these limbs become powerful and frequently autonomous in vandalism. The life of sex now bursts forth often in exaggerated ugliness.

We have attempted to sketch the basic anatomy of man so that we can relate this image of the gods to our experience. Of course, what we have looked at as structures, architecture, is only a small part of our living bodies, basically just the solid parts. At the most, this can express only one of the four ancient Greek humours or elements, the earth element. But some eighty-odd per cent of our weight is fluid not solid and through this fluid man, in constant ebb and flow and in continuous diverse circulations, there also stream currents of air taken in through the lungs. Thus there are also a fluid man and an airy man and we sometimes even get distended with fluid and airy tumours. Finally there must be remembered the warmth man. Not only do different organs and regions of the body have different temperatures but we sometimes find local warmth or coldness. Cold feet are common and even though the blood may be pulsing freely through the feet, they feel icy cold both internally and to external touch. Equally, in others, the feet may be hot so that their owners push them out of the bed clothes or on to cold areas of the sheets. In inflammations local areas of warmth come about. We can imagine away the solid or earthy man, the fluid man and the airy man and picture a warmth man of varying patterns of warmth in ever-changing movement.

Water is properly in continuous inner and outer movement. When stationary or stagnant it dies. When we study the movements of water as Schwenk has done, we see that it is the expression of countless surfaces, veils, or films which weave in and through each other. Its proper nature is two-dimensional and we can see this when a drop of ink or milk falls into a tumbler of water. The drop expands into weaving veils which reveal the nature of the fluid element to us. When water becomes three-dimensional it becomes ice. We also notice when watching streams flow and tumble over rocks how forms develop which stay as it were static and permanent whilst the water flows ever changing through them. The relative permanence of the forms, the eddies, waves or vortices, does not imply the permanence of the substance. The typical forms of plants, in particular, are the forms which develop in the flow of water and all the membranes and tissues in our bodies are the expression of the fluid man within us. We can imagine that obstructions to the flow of the fluid may produce as vortices and turbulences those knots which become organs. These membranes of the fluid element are sensitive to all tones and colours. Precious stones show how sensitively the fluid, out of which these forms developed, responded to the minutest trace of mineral colouring. And the water-colour artist discovers and works with the dynamic gestures of the colours working in the watery film on the paper.

Colour and tone exemplify the working of all that we know as psyche or soul working into and on to these living and ever-flowing currents of the watery man which are also sensitively open to all the more substantial influences. Like to a photographic plate or to a mirror these films respond selflessly to what plays upon them.

We must return to the solid anatomy and take up the contrast between the head and the rest of the body, a contrast focused in the symbol of the skull and crossbones. At the beginning of the nineteenth century much controversy raged over how many vertebrae were fused and metamorphosed in the skull. Goethe and Lorenz Oken were amongst those involved in these heated arguments. The idea was that a number of vertebrae became fused and the canal, which in the spine contains the spinal cord of the nervous system, became expanded to become the cranial cavity containing the brain. The ribs corresponding to these cranial vertebrae became the jaws. In this way the head was conceived as the continuation of the trunk. But in spite of the feeling we can have that some true intuition is trying to come to expression, in these attempts they proved inadequate. They took no notice, for instance, of the fact that the bones of the dome of the skull come into existence as membrane bones, not from cartilage — as do the vertebrae and bones of the trunk and limbs.

Karl König wrestled with this problem and suggested the following solution. The head represents the whole rest of the body. If one imagines a man kneeling, then to begin with, one can see his lower limbs as repeated in the lower jaw, the mandible. The hip joint becomes the temporo-mandibular joint in which the jaw moves on the skull. The thigh becomes the ramus of the jaw leading down to the angle of the jaw, which becomes the knee, and the lower jaw the leg. The chin becomes the heel and we must imagine the feet rotated so that the toes become the teeth. The number of the first teeth is the same as the number of our toes and when we shed these teeth, and cut off our toes, we find the number of our second teeth in the bones of the tarsus.

We have then a man kneeling and facing backwards. This orientation seems significant; we remember the past in our heads. And when we consider the cervical, neck region of the spinal cord we find the crossing of the left and right, the so-called decussation of the pyramids, which accounts for the left side of the body being reflected in the right side of the brain and vice versa. We could almost say the head has been turned round 180° to look backwards. We must now imagine this kneeling man arching over backwards, an act best performed by those hyperflexible acrobatic snake women sometimes seen at circuses. The foetus is in the womb arched forwards, the foetal position. Now we must imagine the kneeling man arched backwards so that this abdominal wall and the front of the chest arch over, becoming the vault of his skull. The umbilicus becomes the fontanelle and the division between abdominal and thoracic wall is repeated in the change from the hair covered head to the forehead. Even the ribs may show on the furrowed brow of the anxiety ridden. At the top of the chest we find the clavicles, the collar

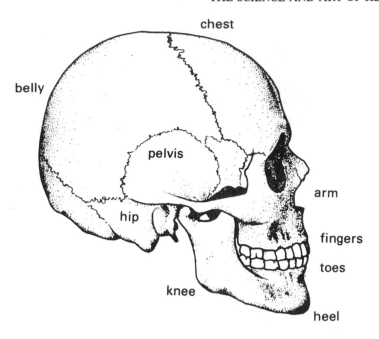

Figure 5. The human skull seen as transformation of the body.

bones, which we now find in the eye brows and the bony ridge over the eyes. The eyes themselves fit into the sockets lying between the collar bones in front and the shoulder blades behind. In the arching over they now come to look what we call forwards, but is for the kneeling man backwards. The arms now come to form the upper jaws, the maxillae, the elbow is in the cheek bone and we find the shoulder blades in the so-called sphenoid bone with its greater and lesser wings, to which the maxilla is joined. The head of the kneeling man is cut off, his whole body has become his new head. The spine of this kneeling man has in the backward arching become compressed into the basi-occiput and basi-sphenoid bones, they form the foundation of the skull. Within this cavity floats the brain in cerebro-spinal fluid. It is an embryo, a larval form. Poppelbaum indicated how this larva, looking even rather like a grub-like larva from under a stone, would like to become a bird or butterfly. Then it could pump up the hemispheres into wings, but it has sacrificed this organic metamorphosis and with the sacrificed forces we can soar on the wings of thought.

Jaworski showed how our lungs are birds internalized or birds are externalized lungs and we now rediscover them in the head. We can also rediscover the uterus which, externalized, swims in the oceans as octopus, squid and cuttlefish and is rediscoverable in the head and face, the lips and tongues being the tentacles. We have already suggested how the baby in the uterus finds its correspondence in the brain within the skull. We can indeed find the animal phyla internalized as the

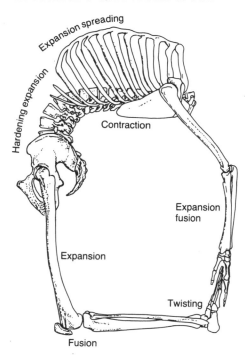

Expansion spreading

Hardening expansion

Contraction

Expansion
fusion

Expansion

Twisting

Fusion

Figure 6. The human skeleton and its relation to the skull.

organs of our bodies. All the organs are to be found again in the head but fused and synthesized whereas in the body they are analysed and separate. We find these organs again dominating or setting the key-notes for the different animal phyla in nature. The mammals we find again in the human psyche as enfleshed emotions.

Finally, taking a look at the erect human form we can see how the legs have become given over to the forces of gravity in becoming pillars. Only the human has a straight knee, in all animals the knee is bent. The head is set free and soars balanced on the upright vertebral column. In it everything outside is reflected as images and all the inner organs are reflected as the forms of head and brain. The outer world is analysed in the differentiated sense images, the already separated inner world of the organs is synthesized again in the head. We can see this head simultaneously as lung or bird, as uterus or octopus, as liver or tortoise and so on. It is all of them in wonderful synthesis and can reflect the whole universe in cognition.

There is the great polarity of the sphere above with the brain and of the sphere below, the pelvic cavity, containing uterus and baby. Reflection and reproduction stand polarically opposed. Death processes reign in the head, bone has there its centre and citadel. Nerve cells die throughout our lives, they cannot regenerate. But here awake consciousness is born. In the uterus takes place in unconsciousness the marvel of the regeneration of the human form and flesh. In these two poles

33

the spheric form dominates and subdues the segmental. But between them stretches the segmented vertebral column like a snake and we can see these segments arising like rhythmic waves in the embryo. The nervous spinal cord extends inside the arches of these vertebrae from the base of the skull to about the bottom of the thorax. Here is the brain of the middle, rhythmic man, a consciousness akin to dreaming dwells here. Whilst in the lower pole the autonomic or sympathetic nervous system reigns in the deep instinctive unconsciousness of sleep.

In due course we shall understand that what is here described in spatial terms, in spatial structural anatomical images, must be transformed into living processes in time. We live in the processes which have created these spatial forms as images. The structures are the corpse we carry around with us as the snail carries his shell.

3.   The seven ages of Man

During this troubled twentieth century there has been an effort to understand the element of time in new ways. In the nineteenth century the idea of evolution dominated scientific thought. From focus on static forms, created and immutable, attention became riveted on the transformation of forms both in evolution and embryogenesis. Forms have to be seen in time as well as in space and this implies an act of imagination since our senses present us only with the present. At the very beginning of this century the French philosopher Henri Bergson started wrestling with the problem and it has been with us ever since. Time as duration, not merely as changed position of hands on a clock. Time has to do with an element other than space and the mechanical is not really in time at all. We only begin to come nearer to the problem of time when we observe the realm of the living. Living beings carve out, as it were, an organic, qualitatively differentiated form in time as much as they obviously do in space. To me it is important that we should begin to work at the problem of qualitative measuring sticks. Today everything must be measured. This has resulted in quantification of everything, with the consequence that those phenomena and experiences which are qualitative are denigrated and even regarded as having no reality. All our inner life, our souls, are qualitative. Emotions are qualitative. To exclude these is to exclude our very human reality and we are today in great danger of forgetting that we are the measurers and not only measurable objects.

Now a small step towards a more real experience of the qualitative differentiation of the time organism can be found in some of the ideas of Sir Patrick Geddes, ideas which were one of the gifts of his many-sided genius. Professor of Botany at Dundee, main inspirer of modern town planning movements, sociologist, author of works on the evolution of sex and biology, seminal inspirer of innumerable activities, and prolific writer of original papers on almost everything, Geddes was one of the most remarkable figures living in this century. At Dundee in his Botanical Garden he planted different plants so as to let them bring out a wonderful illustration of the phases of development of a plant. First of all there is swelling and then budding, followed by shooting and leafing, then it will go on to flowering and a new greening. Then fruiting and seeding go on to drying and resting or dying. Now different plants illustrate these different phases and by planting them accordingly he brought to wonderful expression these ages of the plant. So it went like this. For the swelling phase he had cacti, and for the budding, cabbages, and if possible he would have had palm trees with their great buds on the top of the trunk. For the shooting phase he had plants like Bryonia growing entwined amidst the hedges, followed by the leafy ones from grasses through leafy plants like the *Ranunculaceae* to leafy trees. Next the pre-eminent flowerers, lilies and roses, and all the splendid annuals burning themselves away. Renewed greening and persistence after flowering was exemplified by the evergreens and the fruiting plants with the vine as their king, the seeding plants queened by the corn, and as the drying, resting phase, the thorns.

A strange, unusual way to plant a garden, but a marvellous exercise in the sort of imaginative way of studying which we need in the realms of life, and a clear example of a qualitative measuring rod.

Turning attention to the realm of the animals I would like to contrast two especially typical but opposed groups. Two ways of animal life and form, incredibly different, present themselves when we look at the molluscs and then at the arthropods. We all have at least a superficial familiarity with the molluscs, the snails, the bivalves like the oyster, and such cephalopods as the squid, octopus and cuttlefish. In all these creatures the bodies are soft, plastic, mobile. They are not segmented and in their development they show little tendency to larval forms but mostly just grow. They are neither segmented in space nor in time. Now when we consider, say, the octopus with its tentacles and the suckers on them and, above, the great eyes and the body of the creature, we can see it as a head with lips and tongue drawn out into these grotesque tentacles. The suckers are of course metamorphoses of the vallate papillae on the tongue and the whole body incidentally tastes the surrounding water. The creature walks on its tentacles and we have the spectacle of sense organs becoming limbs. In the snail, its so-called foot is like the tongue and it can almost be said to swim forward on the surface of the slime it secretes.

At a contrasting pole to these molluscs we find the arthropods, the insects, spiders, beetles, crabs, lobsters and the rest of these jointed, segmented creatures covered in hard articulated skeletons whose bodies and limbs are segmented into sharp divisions. Mostly too we find larval forms which not only grow but metamorphose from one form into quite different ones before becoming the adult imago. The butterfly is the most perfect example of this metamorphosis, with grub, caterpillar, chrysalis, butterfly. Now these creatures turn their limbs into sense organs, antennae. It is quite reasonable to contrast the soft gelatinous 'embryonic' molluscs with the rigid, hardened arthropods. And what I want to suggest is that we can establish the difference not only in spatial anatomical terms, descriptively, but also in terms of age. The molluscs are embryonic, the arthropods old and sclerotic, so that in a similar way to Geddes' with the plants, we can begin to sketch a zoo with different animals typifying the various stages of life. In this way our qualitative experience of time grows richer.

We can also take a look at the inorganic world and the metals which play so valuable a part in our homoeopathic therapeutics. We can take a metal such as lead. It is a very old fellow, grey and dull, and if you hit it you can get only a dull thud out of it. It is heavy and aged. We can by contrast take silver, shining, making the best mirrors and the best bells, singing when you strike them. It is full of the power of reproduction, in mirror images and in photographic film; it is young, singing, joyful, contrasted with the sclerosing, aged lead. No wonder the ancients associated lead with Saturn or Chronos, Old Father Time, whilst silver was associated with the Moon and Artemis or Diana.

Perhaps now we can move on to the world of man. It is of course obvious that when we speak of the whole man we have to make the effort to see imaginatively not only the person standing before us with the interrelationships between his various organs and functions, but also the whole coming into being of this man as he now is, his conception, embryonic existence, birth, growth and development. Not only this, but also the largely unknown future and death to which he is walking. We must also realize that it is quite arbitrary to start with conception and with death, this is after all a segment of the whole. It is with the eye of imagination that we must make this whole live, though sometimes we do seem to get insights into the strange relationships between different parts of our own lives or those of others. Moreover, sometimes it seems as if some future event were calling forth some present happening, and in these realms we must look in the future for causes and not only in the past.

Because, as yet, for most of us, imagination is a bit uncertain and can very casily slip down into mere wild fancy, I have suggested these other realms where we can discipline and train ourselves. In the human world we come for the first time upon biography, but it is not possible to write biography as natural history. The inner experience of and the meeting with individual destiny belongs to the human, not to the natural kingdoms.

Before launching on to the seven ages of man themselves I must add, rather in the spirit of our consideration up to now, a few words on the human organism as we face it. We are not of the same age, in the qualitative sense I am trying to invoke, in all parts of our organisms. You will perhaps be able to agree with me in characterizing the head as old. The head sits upon our shoulders and allows itself to be carried around. It observes the world and discusses it like an old man sitting in the village watching the younger generation about its business. The agedness of the head shows, too, in the lack of vitality of the nerve tissue, with no power of cellular regeneration, static and fixed in its position, 'sicklied o'er with the pale cast of thought'. There is much death process in our brains and more note should be taken that our consciousness becomes most awake where vitality is lower and death intensified. Consciousness does not appear as an intensification of life processes but arises where life retreats.

It will not be difficult to agree that in our metabolism and limbs we are young. Here renewal, movement, change are in constant progress. The blood drawing its nourishment from our metabolic processes is red, passionate, in constant movement, and new cells are constantly forming throughout life, in these organs. It is here more as with young children, in constant movement and play. Activity is everywhere, building up the organism in sleep, or in outer movement and restlessness when awake.

In our middle, rhythmic system of breathing and pulse, we are, as it were, in adult life, living in relation to the present and its needs, balancing the polar functions of childhood and old age, of inflammation and sclerosis. The future streams into the child through its limbs on which it walks or runs into its future. From old age we gaze back on our lives of achievement and failure, learning to look with equanimity on the truth of it as it has been. In maturity, living more in the emotions of the present with all their battles and loves and hates, we live within the rhythmic interplay of heart and lung. Here we can achieve a little freedom in the present moment, a breathing space, as our language puts it so well. To dwell one moment longer on these issues, so important, in my opinion, in establishing a real insight into the body-soul relationship, I must recall Steiner's contribution. He connected the thinking life with the system of nerves and senses, feeling with the rhythmic system, and the will with the system of metabolism and limbs. He further pointed out that only in our thinking are we awake; in our feelings we are dreaming and in our will we are asleep. For our modern science, one-sidedly intellectual as it is and almost exclusively male in origin, it is very difficult to gain insight into these realms of feeling and will. Gifts of imagination and intuition will be needed in addition, if we are to see further into these problems. I think that the considerable part played by women in the development of homoeopathy is connected with these issues, and it is possible here for the proper gifts of woman to make their contribution in addition to the intellect which she has largely developed under male tutelage.

We may now call to our aid once more the vision of Sir Patrick Geddes. He restored the Greek Gods as ideal types of the ages of man and woman or, if you prefer, as patron saints of the epochs of our growing up and growing old. Let us plunge straight in at last. The course of life rises from Youth to Maturity and then to Decline, punctuated by four main crises, Birth, Adolescence, Senescence, Death. Within the first period we distinguish infancy and early youth; within the next, adolescence, maturity, with sex fully realized in offspring. Finally age has its earlier and later phases. These are the seven phases.

Let me quote:

> Man as lover, idealist, poet has ever created the goddesses. He worships
> each perfection of womanhood; he defers to her bright intuition, bows

before her ready spear of woman's wit, and yields his apple to her compelling charm. Each youth, in his turn a Paris, has his threefold vision; Aphrodite, Pallas, Hera are no further to seek than of old. On either side arise other goddesses, of younger and of older phase; there Artemis, the maid, still unawakened to sex, running free in Nature, and Hebe, the winning and willing child; here again Demeter, aging, saddened and grey, patient, helpful and wise.

So for her part woman creates her types of the gods; first the father in patriarchal perfection as Zeus; next Apollo, in whom manhood stands complete; then Eros, the babe of inmost longing. Between these appears Hermes, the boy messenger, swift and eager; soon giving place to Dionysos, the youth awaking towards manhood, thrilling to woman, wine and song. After Apollo, master of himself, comes Ares, armed and active in the struggle for existence; later Hephaestos, with his mastery and skill, yet limited, even lamed, thereby. Seated now in their series the Olympian Circle is complete.

But when the individual falls from the ideal what do we find? For Eros we have too often the brat, and for Hermes the gamin; Dionysos becomes hooligan or apache; Apollo falls to prig, and Ares to bully or worse. The drudge is the fallen image of Hephaestos, and the tyrant or dotard of Zeus; and similarly for the various degradations of woman.

From this briefest of sketches it is clear that our civilization lacks the ideals. We lack the differentiated ideals for the different phases of life and so the degraded forms publicized in the media have come to be accepted as the norm.

In ancient times the seasons of the year held a much greater significance for people than they do today. In our industrial age we are sheltered, insulated, and we no longer respond to the seasons and their festivals with more than a shadow of ancient feeling. So too the hours of the day were celebrated in Vedic India with different hymns for each hour. Today even night and day have lost much of their qualitative impact and the drudgery of modern occupations is merely interrupted from time to time. There is little left of the rhythmic interwovenness of our activities and moods with the greater cosmic rhythms around us. In homoeopathy we have long been familiar with the phenomena of the times of aggravation and amelioration of symptoms as they occur in patients and in pictures of our remedies. Some of our remedies are characterized by seasonal aggravation, others by the hours of the day at which symptoms occur. There is a growing body of knowledge today about what are called biorhythms. Not only are circadian rhythms investigated but others too. It was shown by Forsgren that there is a liver rhythm which runs from about 2–3 am to 2–3 pm, and König attempted to show how this cycle manifests in a range of symptoms 'at 4 o'clock in the morning'. It is a fact that most of the remedies in our materia medica with aggravations at 4 am or 4 pm or thereabouts are remedies with strong liver affinities. I have suggested that the 10 am aggravation associated with *Natrum muriaticum* is connected with the suprarenal rhythm and a maximum cortisol level at that time. It is my opinion that a most valuable field of co-operation between various schools and disciplines has opened. It is one where I believe most valuable research could be done and our remedies used as research tools. With these researches into the rhythm of life the way is opened to the rediscovery of Time as an organism with its inner structure and qualitative differentiations. I think that in this direction we can begin to gain insight into the realm of the living which is always integrated into these rhythms. As I have said, the mechanical is really indifferent to time, it is spatial through and through. The staleness and drudgery of our industrial age arise out of this, Geddes called it Palaeotechnic and looked forward to a new age of Biotechnics when we have overcome and transformed this dead vision of our present civilization. Freshness, newness, are always and everywhere associated with life coming into manifestation. The mechanical, however clever, is stale and dull and seeks only to astonish us with quantity and complexity. The living fills our hearts with wonder and rapture so that they leap with fresh hope.

Today we are faced for the first time in human history with the question of the whole. The world, our civilization, has become one world. We cannot settle a problem anywhere without the whole world being involved. The individual person is at the same time becoming aware of himself as a unique being and not only as a representative of a family, nation, profession, race or other group. The question of the individual as a whole has also become an issue. But this wholeness is a differentiated, organic, wholeness, it cannot be a mere uniformity. C. G. Jung observed four functions in the human psyche — thinking, feeling, sensation, and intuition. He described four types arising out of the dominance of one or other of these functions. Further, he showed how as one of these functions is specially developed its complementary function remains undeveloped and becomes the inferior function. Each of us in becoming a specialist in one function, becomes a victim of a corresponding inferiority, a situation which Hephaestos typified in Greece. In becoming an expert technologist he became lame. Today we are all lame. Jung saw the task of individuation, the task of becoming validly whole, as bound up with the task of redeeming the inferior function.

Now let us look at the world where the same problem faces us in the relationships between races and continents. We can take Europe and the North as specializing in Thinking whilst America has developed Sensation. Asia is characterized by Intuition, and the South, Africa, by Feeling. I am using these words in the sense Jung gave them. The task of world order and reconciliation is now seen together with the task of my own individuation process. But these twin tasks, the healing of the individual and of the world, cannot be undertaken until we learn to grasp the living interwovenness of time, its functional parts and their relatedness. To become whole, individuated, involves redeeming and integrating, revaluing one's past and orientating afresh to the future. For mankind, too, we need to begin to re-evaluate our history and evolution, and relate it to the oncoming old age of our race. At a moment like this in history when a depression and a staleness steal into all activities it becomes necessary to take stock, take a new look, a new breath, take a new forward step in a new direction. I have tried to open some such possibilities which I am convinced are all around us, awaiting our courageous efforts to realize them.

4. Holism

Everywhere today we find holism and the holistic approach put forward as panaceas. The word holism was introduced by General Smuts in his book *Holism and Evolution* and by it he drew attention to the evolutionary tendency to progressive whole-making. This tendency shows itself in the formation of ever more comprehensive wholes. Thus, a chemical compound like water is more of a whole than a mixture of hydrogen and oxygen; and a cell is more of a whole than a molecule of water; and a bird is more of a whole than a cell; higher still are minds; and highest of all is human personality. We live in a universe of whole-making. 'Holism is a process of creative synthesis; the resulting wholes are not static but dynamic, evolutionary, creative.'

When we look for instances of 'whole-making' we find at first two opposite processes. Embryological development proceeds by the original ovum dividing in two and these daughter cells again dividing and so on. A multitude of cells, differentiated in form and function, in this way comes into existence but the principle of the whole maintains itself throughout, imposing order, so that a cosmos, an organism, comes into existence. A cosmos, not a chaos, emerges. Is there perhaps in the fertilized ovum a chaos out of which the cosmos arises?

In contrast to this process we also find examples of two or more distinct organisms uniting to form a new order of organization. The lichens are a good example in which an alga and a fungus unite in symbiosis, each contributing a still distinct element to the new whole. Another example is found in the sea slugs. These humble molluscs are found to have on their backs papillae and these are loaded with sting cells, nematocysts. Now nematocysts are not normal organs of the molluscs but occur in another phylum, the coelenterates, which include for instance hydras, sea anemones and jelly-fish. The nematocyst is like a loaded pistol; a slightest touch on its trigger and it discharges. The marine biologists have discovered how the sea slugs feed on these coelenterates, rasping them with their ranula or tongue. The nematocysts do not discharge, which they normally do when touched, but are taken into the slug's stomach. From there, still fully loaded, they pass along minute ciliated tubes to the surface of the papillae and there take their place in perfectly ordered ranks, again ready to discharge at the slightest touch.

They have become integrated into the new whole of the mollusc. This 'whole' must have been active throughout the process of eating, so that the nematocyst did not react, as it normally does, by discharging at a touch, but 'recognizing' the sea slug as that to which in some higher sense it belonged, allowed itself to be directed to its predestined place. It may be added that particular nematocysts can be recognized as originating from particular coelenterates and a change of the sea slug's diet from one species of nematocyst to another results in a change, a replacement of the old nematocysts by the new ones in its papillae. This and other examples have been beautifully described by E. L. Grant Watson.

The problem of fertilization could also be looked at in this light. The unborn child acting as an entelechy directs the ovum and sperm together to initiate a new whole out of the union of two separate organisms. Schopenhauer even suggested that it was the unborn child which manifested in the love bringing mother and father together.

The principle of holism also manifests in colonies of bees and ants. The beehive with its multitude of workers, drones and the queen lives and acts as a whole. It is comparable to a single organism, and the workers pass through changing functions during their individual lives. The colony is a veritable whole. Amongst the ants one finds for example warrior ants who wage war against other ants and from the survivors of the conquered species breed slaves who have now become members of the victorious colony. The eggs have become retuned to the new whole. Innumerable other examples exist in which the whole manifests as an organizing principle to which or within which units are subdued and integrated.

The 'Portuguese man-of-war' presents a striking example of how separate organisms can unite to form a colony. These separate organisms are so specialized in function that they cannot long survive without the other functions. The interdependence of the distinctive functionally specialized organisms constitutes the Portuguese man-of-war, a new whole, but each function exists as a separate organism within the whole. A single animal of one kind forms the float; each tentacle with which the colony fishes is a separate animal, the digesting function for the whole colony is carried out by another separate lot of organisms and the reproductive function belongs to yet another animal. In addition there is a species of fish which lives happily amidst the flowing tentacles, unscathed by their stinging capacities which paralyse all other fish. Is this fish, the Nomeus, also a member of the colony? Modern ecology is on the way to finding the organic interdependence of large ranges of life, ultimately perhaps of the whole planet.

It seems obvious that this 'whole' cannot itself be simply material in nature although it may perhaps work through material entities to some extent. How are we to attempt to approach the nature of this 'whole'?

But first let us look at some other aspects of the problem. At the beginning of the century H. Bernard drew attention to colony formation as a major factor in evolution. He observed a rhythmic process in the course of which organisms of increased order of complexity came into existence, not gradually but in great rhythmic steps. Each new step arose by colony formation amongst the organisms of the earlier stage. He regarded the cell itself as already a colony of sub-cellular 'units'. On the cellular level every imaginable variation occurs and 'all variations naturally occurring are naturally selected'. The next higher stage in evolution does not arise by further variations but by a leap, by colony formation, and the characteristic form of the polyp comes into existence. Again the widest variations occur but only further colony formation raises the development to a higher stage again. Bernard suggested the annelids as the examplars of this new stage, the units entering the new colonization being already at the polyp rather than cellular stage. A further stage arises with the vertebrates and Bernard saw human society manifesting new colony formation where the bonds are purely psychic not structural in nature.

I think it can be seen that Bernard was drawing attention to a progressive rhythmic process of whole-making where each new stage incorporates the previous one as the units of the new colony or whole.

H. Jaworski understood the life processes as the rhythmic interplay of movements of interiorization and exteriorization, an idea he adopted from Dubois Reymond. Man he saw as the central trunk of the evolutionary tree from which by exteriorization the branches grow out into the great phyla branching further into orders, genera, species and so on. He saw these exteriorized organisms corresponding to the organs, tissues and cells interiorized in the human organism. For Jaworski it is only in the human that evolution proper takes place. Only in human evolution do the great steps take place. The animals fall out of the upward evolutionary progress into proliferation of forms which are only varieties of the stage reached on the central trunk of human evolution. The animal kingdom represents the analysis of which the human is the synthesis.

Jaworski, in this way, saw, for example, the snakes internalized in the alimentary canal. They were, as he put it, intestines merely served by other organs. Again, birds are lungs served only by other organs. The whole great world of animal existence finds itself again internalized, synthesized within the greater whole of the human organization. Man is the key to understanding the animals. The animals descend into fixity and specialization; only in man do we find ascent and evolution. This upward development also reveals the stages of progressive integration drawn attention to by Bernard under the term colonization.

In our approach to the riddle of the whole these stages are important. The whole is not just a conglomerate of equal cells but an ordered, differentiated cosmos and there are within it levels of integration. In spatial terms we have come to recognize the levels of the cells, the tissues and the organs. The cellular level, corresponding to the protozoa in outer space, is obvious in the white cells in our blood. It expresses a tendency to a pointwise spatial organization. The tissues, originating in the germ layers or leaves of the embryo, tend to planar spatial forms which get folded and interwoven in the complexity of the organism. They tend to two-dimensional forms. The organs arise by progressive interweaving of different tissues into three-dimensional entities. The tissues and cells are integrated into the organ which is essentially an animal expression. The tissues originating in the planar form represent more the vegetable level of organization, appearing in the form of the leaf. We can then see the cell as representing the tendency towards the pointwise structures of the physical world.

The mechanical and physical forces studied in the physical sciences are point centred.

Only the dead world and the mineral world can be grasped by mechanical models. Within a living form it is only the physical and chemical processes that can be grasped in this way. The real life of the organism manifesting as a whole cannot be so grasped. We make use of the mechanism of our skeletons to take our place and act within the physical world. But the form of our skeleton is not just mechanical. It must be grasped as an image, placed into the physical world, of a non-material, non-spatial entity, the human individuality. Images, pictures are one of the ways by which we try to grasp a whole, diagrams enable us to grasp a mechanism. S. T. Coleridge expressed it thus: 'Whatever is organized from without is a product of mechanism; whatever is mechanised from within is a product of organization.'

The suggestion just made that the human skeleton is an image of the human individuality can lead to a further insight. We meet single wholes, unique entities, in this world, in human individuals alone. Individual animals, plants and minerals are not each a real whole; they are members of a species, family, class and so on; they do not contain their unique meaning within themselves but only find their meaning within the wider groups to which they belong. Whilst human individuals belong to different ages, sexes, classes, nations and races they are also essentially individual egos and contain their centres within. Biography is the study of the uniqueness of a human individual. These individuals therefore are present to us in this world as real absolutes, wholes. The content of each of these unique and idiomatic wholes is the other absolute, the whole humanity. But this compels us to understand the idea and the reality of mankind as an organism extending over the past evolutionary development and into the future. Mankind is not only those humans who are on earth today but includes all those who have been, are, and will be on earth. Each idiomatic human is a centre of this being, which was called by Auguste Comte 'Le grand être'. V. Solovyov gave an appreciation of and a critical extension of this idea of Comte.

It is already clear that the whole is a supersensible reality conceivable as an Idea; an idea in the Goethean or Platonic sense, a reality which is formative, appears as the form and unites the differentiated functions and organs into a whole. In the inorganic world the relations between objects are grasped in the form of laws. These laws are most perfectly expressed in mathematical concepts.

They are related to the phenomena they unite only externally. In the case of living organisms the law, the idea of their being, works internally.

How does this appear? Or how does the difference between living and dead show itself? If we take a crystal, it has a structure but this structure is uniform, it is not differentiated from one place to another nor is its size in any way inherent. It may be small or large, it makes no difference to the idea, the mathematics of its structure. Further, a crystal cannot be said to have a life span, whether it lasts a second or a thousand years is a matter of indifference. In these respects we at once see the differences when we look at and consider a living organism. Size is characteristic of a living species, although it may vary within limits under changing circumstances. It is inwardly differentiated; no one part is the same as another. And it is characterized by a life span. It has origin, growth and development, maturity leading to old age and death. It is an organism in time and this time organism cannot be grasped with our physical sense organs which can only grasp the cross section of the whole organism given at any one moment. The living whole can only be grasped with the eye of imagination. The idea, the law of the organism is a higher reality than the abstract ideas with which we seek to under-stand the mineral world, and the world of the mechanical. When we employ these same mechanical ideas in investigating the living we only search out mechanisms within the living processes by means of models. We explore only the corpse present within the living. And in this way we cannot get beyond the illusion of movement and growth provided by the successive stills of the cinema. To quote S. T. Coler-idge again: 'As organisation ceases . . . mechanism commences.'

If scientific knowledge is arbitrarily restricted by definition or usage to the mechanical then holism of course becomes synonymous with metaphysics or mysti-cism, terms of abuse in science. But is there any fundamental reason to restrict the ideal component of knowledge to concepts of mechanism? Human conscious-ness and knowledge change with the centuries, a great change in consciousness underlay the origins and development of modern science, and there is no reason to think that we have reached the end of the evolution of consciousness. The laws of science never apply fully in the real world of nature, only approximately and subject to corrections. They apply fully only to the 'put togetherness' of machines, not even to the materials of which a machine is constructed. All the materials around us are on the way to death, a little life still inheres in them. The 'put togetherness' of machines is the realm of the truly dead and inorganic. It is certainly through the closest study of this realm of death that we have woken up out of a more dreamlike consciousness to our modern wide-awake consciousness which is achieved most typically in mathematical thinking. Mathematics has become therefore the criterion of science; 'there is only so much science in a subject as there is mathematics in it'.

We must now turn our attention to the phenomena of so-called metamorphosis. The word metamorphosis has been used to cover rather differing phenomena. It has been used to cover various modifications of for instance sulphur or phosphorus. Under changing external conditions the structures change in which these elements manifest. We know red and yellow phosphorus and up to six different forms of sulphur. Water and other substances also change from solid to liquid to gaseous states according to temperature and external pressure. We invent an unchanging world of atoms, behind the phenomena of our perceptions, whose varied dances are supposed to explain these phenomena in their ever-changing transformations.

A higher expression of metamorphosis comes into existence with the plants, most perfectly expressed in the flowering plants. At first appear the seedling leaves or cotyledons, then the stem grows up and there appear the spiralling expanded leaves from node to node. They may vary in form in regular progression up the stem but then a new stage is reached with a contraction into the calyx and the sepals. These are still obviously 'leaf' forms but they mark a more fundamental change than the varying form of leaf up the stem. They are metamorphosed leaves. In the expansion into petals, the losing of the green colour and the appearance of the wonderful colour of the blossoms we see a further metamorphosis. But these forms can change upwards and downwards into each other, showing that they belong together. The sepals can become coloured as in the delphiniums constituting the glory of their flowers. We can also see how the stamens are metamorphosed leaves by looking at double flowers, in which some of the stamens have regressively metamorphosed into petals. The essentially leaf form of the carpels also becomes very clear in for instance the pods of peas and beans. We can in this way watch in plants the metamorphosis up and down the stem and almost see the 'idea' which manifests in these different forms. They coexist and this makes it easy to watch the transformations.

When we turn our attention to the world of insects it is more difficult to follow the metamorphosis of, for instance, the caterpillar into the chrysalis out of which in magic transformation emerges the butterfly. We can, of course, help ourselves by the parallelism between these stages and the comparable stages in the plant: The caterpillar and the stem, the chrysalis and the calyx, finally the butterfly and blossom reveal the connection whilst such forms as 'stick' insect and 'leaf' insect manifest as final forms which in the butterfly are still 'on the way'. Here the forms do not coexist but succeed each other in time. It is undoubtedly harder to grasp these stages together in the wholeness of the butterfly than in the case of the plant. But even in the plants we can be shaken into wonder and amazement by instances like the night flowering cactus which, after long periods of dull vegetative growth, puts forth one night a marvellous blossom which has faded by the morning. Who would imagine this highly coloured and perfumed flower in the long snake-like growths of the plant? In the case of the insects one form vanishes and a new one appears. We have, as it were, to hold our breath and jump over an abyss to cross from one stage to the next.

The development of mammals and birds shows us yet more complex problems in metamorphosis. In mankind the great catastrophe of birth has always gripped the imagination and even the invasion of these sacred regions by the crudities of modern technology has not yet completely obliterated the sense of infinite wonder which can and should arise around a new-born baby. With its first breath the soul enters into the baby as with our last it departs again and all the sophisms around the concept of 'brain stem death' miss the point of the distinction between the animate and inanimate body. The body may still have some residue of life as distinct from soul in it, as the plant has life but not soul. In this world life cannot manifest without water nor can a body become animated without the interiorization of air or breath which the Romans called *anima* and the Greeks *pneuma*. We can add that during the embryonic and foetal periods, the soul and ego can be visualized as around the embryo within the membranes, the chorion, amnion and allantois.

Human life manifests metamorphoses of yet another kind. At the end of childhood, forces which up till then had been engaged in growth and formation of the body become partially free from these organic tasks. Particularly in the brain they become to a great extent free and need to be taken up through education into the new functions of memory, thinking and imagination. We think with the same forces with which we had previously grown. It seems that Hegel himself was aware of this transformation. We have now come upon the metamorphosis of forces from the sensible realms into supersensible manifestation in thinking. Are we not challenged to envisage death itself as a further metamorphosis from the sensible to the supersensible?

In discussing anatomy and the structure of the human body we sketched the metamorphosis of the body and limbs into the form of the head. Taking a deep breath and leaping over the abyss can we not begin to follow Steiner's suggestion that the body of one incarnation is metamorphosed into the head of the next incarnation? With such an idea, reincarnation which has almost become a matter of common belief in our time, begins to assume concrete reality. The phenomena of metamorphosis leaping over centuries unites together different lives in a higher concept of wholeness.

From another point of view the American psychiatrist Trigant Burrow found himself compelled to the realization that in our unconsciousness we are united with first our group and more deeply with the whole of mankind. Our individual neurosis is not explainable on a merely individual basis, the split in our nature expresses the division between that cerebral consciousness of the head and the integral consciousness of the sympathetic nervous system. In our metabolic processes, concentrated especially in the abdomen, we are in reality in empathetic unity with mankind, with the infinite interrelationships between all the individuals and groups which constitute this organic reality. In my brain consciousness I feel cut off within the fortress of my skull, gazing as a spectator at the tragi-comedy of the world. In my metabolism and sympathetic nervous system I am fully involved in this world reality but my consciousness is screened from its overwhelming majesty. Nevertheless it is the content of my individuality whose uniqueness must be looked for not in content or property but in idiom or style.

There is within the whole majestic richness of our human inheritance, the cultural achievements and traditions of our race, the concept of the divine Man, that single unique person who once carried in his consciousness the reality of the whole mankind. Other great figures have incarnated the entelechies of great nations, races and time spirits of our history, but there exists also the belief and idea that the over-soul of our whole race of Man once incarnated in a single person.

There can be no other idea of wholeness, the ideal for each one of us.

We need only add that this concept of wholeness which spans the extreme polarity between the single and the universal and which includes all the diversity of groupings, families, sexes, tribes, nations, classes, races, is expressible in the immemorial symbol of the threefold, triune. Wholeness in its full manifestation is threefold. One cannot express it otherwise, whether on the human level of experience as man, woman and child or on the level of nature with the three kingdoms; or as truth, beauty and goodness, or again as thinking, feeling and will.

In the human form and organism the greatest polarity between the upper and lower poles comes to expression. The legs have become pillars, alone amongst the encircling animals they have straight knees, given over to the forces of gravity. The head has become lifted out of gravity so that it rises balanced and poised on the summit of the vertebral column. Its spheric form is opposed to the radial form of the limbs. The middle rhythmic realm, the chest, mediates between these poles. These structural forms can be understood as the images of the corresponding functions which everywhere interpenetrate each other so that the human form can become a single whole which nevertheless includes the cosmos, from which it was created and which it reflects.

5. The nature of homoeopathy

It has been customary to define homoeopathy in terms of the so-called Similia principle, that is to say in practical terms that one should treat a disease with a remedy which can cause in a healthy person a similar disturbance. For instance, for diarrhoea one should, according to this principle, give castor oil or a similar aperient rather than an opium derivative or mixture given on the principle of treatment with opposites. One can trace both ideas back to the Hippocratic writings and indeed the treatment with similars has a much longer history, being the essential basis of much magical medicine in what we like to regard as primitive times. Sir James Fraser in the *Golden Bough* used the expression homoeopathic magic to cover a whole realm of these ancient practices. But it is not as simple as it at first sounds or as it is usually presented.

It further belongs to the commonly accepted ideas about homoeopathy that in this therapeutic system very small doses of medicine are given, the so-called potencies, and many people, both lay and professional, know only that a homoeopathic dose is one so small that it cannot harm you anyway, let alone do you any good. In addition it is often emphasized that the homoeopathic materia medica is based on naturally occurring substances from the animal, vegetable or mineral kingdoms rather than the artificially constructed and manufactured products of the pharmaceutical industry. It is probably because of this distinction and the emotive terms in which it is easy to state the difference, that homoeopathy is often grouped with natural therapies. This last distinction between homoeopathy and orthodox medicine, often referred to as allopathy, was not relevant when Samuel Hahnemann introduced his revolutionary method at the beginning of the nineteenth century. The vast majority of the remedies in the homoeopathic materia medica were and are the same as those in common use in the conventional medicine of those days, mostly traditional medical plants, many dating back to classical antiquity and beyond. Minerals and metals were also included, some also from traditional sources. Gradually additions have been made from, for instance, American-Indian folk remedies and from the poisons of serpents, spiders and so on.

It is therefore an issue which only assumes importance within the climate of present-day anxieties over the pollution of our inner and outer environment by the synthetic products of modern industry. It would be difficult, however, to find where to draw the precise line between cooking our food and sophisticatedly cooking natural substances in a modern chemical plant. Further, if what we humans contrive in our technology is unnatural, does not that imply that we are ourselves not natural, not just part of great Nature? And if so, can we confine our medicine to natural means? One remembers the trouble Prometheus got himself and us into through stealing the fire from heaven and starting mankind on its perilous path of development. Have we not today however penetrated into both a super-natural and a subnatural realm and are we not very prone to get them mixed up?

Firstly, then, let us take up the question of the similia principle, the central principle on which homoeopathy is based. In Greek times it entered into some of the Hippocratic writings in a particular form. It is indicated that some symptoms in illness are expressions of nature's healing efforts. Nature is felt to be wise, and we are contained within the womb, as it were, of nature. Our human intelligence and insight are weak and often distorted. A wise physician will therefore seek to learn from nature and imitate her. When she gives diarrhoea it is because she seeks to get rid of the poisons in the gut. Therefore a wise physician will seek to work with her and help her, giving for instance *Veratrum* which itself can produce dysentery-like symptoms.

Two thousand years later the so-called English Hippocrates, Thomas Sydenham, also stressed the healing value of the symptoms, particularly fever, and urged that the physician should avoid taking steps artificially to bring it down. Underlying all this attitude in Greece was the still present awareness of Nature as a divine goddess. Even today some children can still experience a wonder-filled adoration towards nature, and is not a nostalgia for this lost paradise world stirring within much of the present-day search for a different appreciation of nature than has been won by the methods and disciplines of our natural science?

Wordsworth's great ode gave immortal expression to such experiences:

> There was a time when meadow, grove, and stream,
> The earth, and every common sight,
>   To me did seem
>   Apparelled in celestial light,
> The glory and the freshness of a dream.
> It is not now as it hath been of yore;
>   Turn whereso'er I may,
>   By night or day,
> The things which I have seen I now can see no more.

But this was not all that Greece won of insight into nature and her child Man. In those early stirrings of the philosophic and scientific spirit that marked the beginnings of our European history, there came by stages the formulation of the world as composed of the four elements, fire, air, water and earth, and of the corresponding humours within man, yellow bile, blood, phlegm and black bile. We are far today from any appreciation of what the experience of these elements and humours must have meant to the men of those times, but we can perhaps at least grasp the idea of balance as given expression in them. Fire — the hot and dry — is polar opposite to Water — the cold and wet. Air — the warm and wet — is polar opposite to Earth — the cold and dry (Lehrs, *Man or Matter*). Health was understood as balance between the two pairs of opposites. Excess in one element, or deficiency in one, led to imbalance. When we remember how much the Greek achievement in sculpture and architecture depended on the achievement of balance, and how in Greek education the balance of body and soul was striven for, in gymnastics and study, and further how in Greek verse the balance of heart beat and breathing underlies and carries its meaning and beauty, then we can perhaps catch a glimpse of this wonderful conception of balance in Man and Nature.

But for our present purpose we can also see how when disease is grasped not just by a symptom but in the dyscrasia, the state of imbalance, in this double polarity of humours, then a plethora of one, for instance blood, will lead the physician to restore the balance by blood-letting. And we may also be more tolerant of this practice if we realize that at that time, when the fires of youth burnt high in the race and inflammatory states were the rule in the phenomena of disease, a surplus of blood in the dynamic sense was very common. Today when the balance of disease has swung to the opposite pole with the ageing of the race, blood transfusion has replaced blood letting. It is therefore understandable how out of a diagnosis in terms of the balance of the humours a treatment by opposites was adopted and plants and remedies were characterized in terms of their balance of elements as well. Pepper would be hot and dry, for instance.

Is it not only if one falls into the trap of legalistic academic definitions that one finds these two approaches really mutually exclusive? The humours are not symptoms, nor comparable with the diarrhoea of dysentery. Both methods belonged equally to the newly appearing effort to find natural causes for natural events. Before this new movement of the human spirit, disease had been understood as caused by gods, devils and ancestors. The causes of disease were supernatural. In Greece there came about this moment when the origins of natural events including disease were to be sought in natural causes.

It is however essential to grasp the emergence at the same time of temple medicine at great sanctuaries such as Epidauros. It would seem that in earlier times these two currents, the empirical craft of medicine and surgery, and the religious, magical stream of ritual healing were closely interwoven. In Greece they separated but remained in friendly co-existence as witnessed to by the friendly and professional relations existing between Galen (AD 138–201) and the priests of the Asklepieion at Pergamon.

The idea of health as balance was achieved in Greece and belongs especially to the time of Greek culture. It still runs in our day, both in ordinary commonsense feeling, in the so-called natural therapies, and even in modern scientific medicine under such concepts as homoeostasis.

Paracelsus (1493–1541) in the sixteenth century, at the very origin of modern science and medicine, grasped the Similia principle in a different way. He proposed that diseases should be classified according to their remedy. This is a most interesting idea which has to some extent been adopted by homoeopathy without always an appreciation of its origin. Paracelsus accepted the widely held view of macrocosm and microcosm. Within this concept, Man was regarded as a miniature, so to speak, of the wide universe. All processes and activities, all the organs within man corresponded with similar processes and organs in the macrocosm. When Paracelsus thus speaks of diseases classified according to their remedies, the implication is that the human disease and the natural remedy correspond to each other, almost *are* each other.

Such a formulation was made explicit at the beginning of the nineteenth century by Lorenz Oken (1779–1851), one of the great leaders of the school of *Naturphilosophie* in Germany. Oken expressed it thus in *Elements of Physio-Philosophy:* What occurs as physiology in the animal kingdom occurs as pathology in the human kingdom.

In Paracelsus also there is a strong Christian impulse and he regards illness as potentially creative for the patient. If healing really comes about, then the patient will have taken a step forward in his psychospiritual development. He will not merely have recovered his static balance, but will have experienced a dynamic metamorphosis of his whole being. His healing will be at least to some extent a new birth, not just a being rid of a discomfort and inconvenience or avoiding of death. Here the two streams which had divided in Greece, the temple medicine which was a sort of initiation experience on the one hand, and the empirical medicine of the lay physicians on the other, met again in the strange figure of the alchemist Paracelsus.

Then came the German physician Samuel Hahnemann (1755–1843) who at the turn of the eighteenth to nineteenth century began to develop homoeopathy, his system of the rational art of healing, as he called it.

It is not at all easy to enter into Hahnemann's way of seeing disease and his method of treating it. Partly this arises from the whole background of medical and scientific thought at that time, which has so radically changed since then, and partly because it was a new way which he pioneered and tried to communicate. That he is not repeating the ancient Hippocratic idea of imitating nature's healing effort is clear from the following quotation from *Organon of Medicine:*

> . . . but especially through squandering the irreplaceable blood, as is done
> by the reigning routine practice, used blindly and relentlessly, usually with
> the pretext that the physician should imitate and further the sick nature in

its efforts to help itself, without considering how irrational it is, to imitate
and further these very imperfect, mostly inappropriate efforts of the
instinctive, unintelligent vital energy, which is implanted in our organism,
so long as it is healthy, to carry on life in harmonious development; but
not to heal itself in disease. For were it possessed of such a model ability,
it would never have allowed the organism to get sick.

From this and other passages it should be clear that Hahnemann is not pursuing
the old path of imitating nature, because he is already a child of the modern age
of natural science, an adept in the chemistry of his day, the post-Lavoisier age.
But he can still hold a conviction that an immaterial vital entity animates our
organism until death when the purely chemical forces prevail and decompose it.
In this he is close to the vitalism of that time, with the German philosopher,
investigator and physician Stahl (1660–1734) and Bichat amongst its leaders. This
vital entity which he characterizes as immaterial, spirit-like, and which maintains
in health the harmonious wholeness of the organism, *is* in fact the wholeness of
it, and can be influenced by dynamic causes. How does Hahnemann attempt to
clarify this idea? He draws attention to phenomena like magnetic influences, the
moon and the tides, infective illnesses and, perhaps most importantly, the influence
of emotions and impulses of will on the organism. He draws attention to the way
in which strong emotions can cause severe illness and the imagination can bring
about cure. To quote him again:

Is it then so utterly impossible for our age, celebrated for its wealth in
clear thinkers, to think of dynamic energy as something non-corporeal,
since we see daily phenomena which cannot be explained in any other
manner? If one looks upon something nauseous and becomes inclined to
vomit, did a material emetic come into his stomach which compels him to
this anti-peristaltic movement? Was it not solely the dynamic effect of this
nauseating aspect upon his imagination? And if one raises his arm, does it
occur through a material visible instrument? A lever? Is it not solely the
conceptual dynamic energy of his will which raises it?

Now Hahnemann regards the medicinal action of substances used as remedies as
dynamic in this sense.

The medicinal property of those material substances which we call
medicines proper, relates only to their energy to call out alterations in the
well-being of animate life.

The capacity of a substance to act as medicine depends on its power to call forth
a specific alteration in the function and sensibility of the healthy organism, in fact
to produce some specific form of illness. Hahnemann next appeals to experience.
A new disease produced by a medicine can remove a pre-existing natural disease
if their manifestations are similar. It seems that Hahnemann had noted in his own
experience and collected in literature innumerable instances of an existent disease
vanishing during the course of a new intercurrent disease. He drew from this the

idea of giving a new drug-induced disease to remove in a similar manner the naturally occurring disease.

It is his idea that the totality of symptoms of a disease is the physiognomic expression of that disease and that we can know the disease in no other way than through this expression. 'Symptoms', it should be noted, cover changes both in function and sensations, it includes, in the modern sense, signs and symptoms. When these symptoms are wholly eliminated the disease, in Hahnemann's view, is cured. It is not correct to say that Hahnemann aimed only at symptomatic treatment, he grasped the disease as an entity through its deeds and appearances in the symptoms, just as in biography we seek to know a person through what he does and what happens to him. His position is that the 'idea' which unites all the symptoms into a unity is really the same idea which in a changed metamorphosis comes to expression in the remedy — the plant, for instance, as it grows in nature. Here one can call to one's aid, in the effort to understand, Plato's and Goethe's 'ideas' as the living archetypes. Whether Hahnemann was himself aware of Goethe's work in plant metamorphosis I do not know. Goethe was certainly aware of, and favourably impressed by, homoeopathy.

With this conception of Hahnemann of the new drug-given disease eliminating the similar natural disease, we approach nearer to concepts underlying modern pharmaco-therapeutics. One of the most fruitful ideas in modern therapeutics has been the use of a substance whose molecules are structurally similar to molecules in what is regarded as the disease pathways. Competition with and inhibition of the disease pathway can result. This is a very similar notion to Hahnemann's so far as the Similia idea is concerned, but it is in other respects far removed.

From about 1500, the progress of modern medicine has been dominated by predominantly structural concepts. The seat of disease was studied first by Morgagni in the gross changes in the organs of patients dying of diseases, then secondly by Bichat in the tissues examined with the microscope. After this the German pathologist Virchow (1831–1902) introduced cellular pathology and sought the seat of disease in changes in the cells. With the electron-microscope, the search has dived into the intracellular structures. The body has come to be more and more regarded as a machine to be studied with increasingly refined structural concepts even into the molecular and atomic realms. The gap between these constructed models of disease and the living, experiencing patient grows ever larger.

So it is not surprising to find that from the end of the eighteenth century throughout the nineteenth century there were repeated efforts to explore in a secular, scientific or pseudo-scientific way the psychological approach to disease, up till then almost exclusively the domain of the Church. The Viennese physician Mesmer (1734–1815) was probably the first, with his concept of animal magnetism, but the phenomena were those of what we now call hypnotism. Out of these explorations grew gradually, not suddenly, the movements of psychoanalysis and the other schools of depth psychology. Ellenberger has shown how much the ideas underlying these modern scientific disciplines are the continuation, in a changed intellectualist mode, of themes current in primitive witch-doctoring and the temple medicine of antiquity. The emphasis here is on the experience of the patient, conscious and unconscious, with no regard for the pathology.

In fact we are now faced with the results of what Barfield has aptly called the Cartesian guillotine and which Bergson at the beginning of this century described.* We have made of the body something so entirely mechanical and of the soul something so purely subjective, a mere onlooker, that real relationships between them are impossible.

How did Hahnemann, and does homoeopathy, grasp this problem? I think the clue is to be found in a most important, though largely neglected, observation by Hahnemann. He noticed that most patients present their doctors with symptoms which are partly localized to definite sites and organs and partly expressed in changed mood, behaviour and mental disturbances which cannot be so localized. These are therefore two extreme poles of the spectrum of disease. At the one pole are the diseases manifesting in a local disorder with no discernible mental symptoms, and at the other pole are diseases whose manifestations remain in the mental sphere and cannot be related to local disturbances. Between these two poles there is a spectrum of diseases with combined local and mental symptoms. Hahnemann does not state that there are no mental disturbances in apparently local diseases, or local disturbances in mental diseases, but that they are respectively too insignificant or small to be easily detected. Some years ago the Bahnsons, working psychiatrically in psychosomatic diseases, proposed a very similar spectrum of diseases from cancer at one pole to schizophrenia at the other, and with hysteria in the middle.

Further, Hahnemann steadfastly remains on the human scale of phenomena capable of observation and experience, absolutely rejecting the reductionist models pragmatically necessary for the construction of mechanistic explanations of disease. Disease for Hahnemann is a human phenomenon on the human scale. Scale is important. The emphasis therefore is on symptoms, using the word in the widest sense.

Difficulties of a very particular kind arise here which are not always honestly faced. Symptoms change in a bewildering way and very much in relation to the particular person or doctor to whom they are communicated. Physical signs and pathological quantitative findings are somewhat more static or objective, but symptoms as related are often a function of the interpersonal relationship and of the ideas and attitudes in the doctor's mind. These can determine what symptoms manifest or are confessed. In this respect symptoms approach the realm of dreams in psychotherapy where it has been noticed how the dreams of a patient relate to the school adherence of the analyst or therapist. Perhaps one reason why medicine

* Barfield, *Historical perspectives*, Vol. 1, and Bergson, *Matter and Memory*.

has been driven further and further in its pursuit of hard facts is to try and escape the kaleidoscopic changeableness of soft symptoms.

At this point one comes up hard against the issue of the personality of the doctor. As much as one must not separate the illness from the individual patient but grasp them together, so must one not separate the medicine from the physician, they too belong together. Modern medicine aims to diagnose the disease and treat it by objective measures. The two human beings, patient and physician, become increasingly onlookers. But in homoeopathy both really should be imaginatively active.

In psychotherapy as well as in ordinary life, the main method is somehow to succeed in holding the mirror up to nature. When in our neurosis, or wickedness, we have seen ourselves in a mirror held up to us by friend or doctor, or at the theatre, we may determine to change and grow and integrate ourselves a little more. We have to do it ourselves. When in the mirror of a medicine our more unconscious self sees its so-called behaviour, it too will have to decide whether to change to another way of acting. The mirror in both cases does nothing but change the state of consciousness. Here we have come up against the possibility of a medical action based on an immaterial mirror image. The point of a mirror image of course is that it is not tangible or weighable, only visible. But the look at oneself in a mirror can indeed change one's consciousness and actions. We have become accustomed to regarding real actions as being dependent on tangible properties such as weight and extension, and in fact visible qualities have been relegated to the sphere of secondary qualities or 'only in the mind'.

Now Hahnemann developed his potencies, which are produced by serial dilution, during the first decade of the nineteenth century, when the atomic theory was being developed. Hahnemann was explicit in stating that these potencies, the higher ones anyway, could not contain any molecule of the original substance. The tangible, weighable aspect of substance was reduced to vanishing point, that very quantitative aspect of substance which was being made the exclusive basis of the developing chemistry. He maintained, however, the release of the dynamic aspect of the substance. We have neglected in modern times the element of form, which we grasp in the idea and which appears to us in a mirror image. Though one cannot weigh the form, it is that which determines the morphological aspect of, for instance, plants, and enables us to classify them in orders, families and so on. It also is that which, existing as the architect's plan, determines whether a pile of bricks and mortar become built into a garage, a house, a factory, or a church.

So something very interesting has come about. A medicine, prepared from a natural substance by serial dilution until the tangible weighable vanishes, releases a dynamic aspect of form, an image, which can qualitatively change the solvent, and through this bring about change in the recipient.

The nature of the change brought about by disease or remedy, and characterized by Hahnemann as dynamic and similar to the changes brought about by emotion and will, needs further consideration. In fact this is one of the points where traditional homoeopathy is weakest. The history of homoeopathy unfolds successive attempts to understand it in terms of current physiological and pathological concepts. These were all conceived in terms of one-sided tangible properties or else equally one-sided psycho-spiritual causes. We have a very important task, to grasp the immensely complicated human morphology, a compendium or synthesis of all natural forms, so that purely dynamic influences can bring about metamorphosis of the so-called healthy, and healing as a further metamorphosis.

To grasp the different items of the symptoms and their development in a unified idea calls for an artistic creative act by the physician, as does the grasping of the details of a so-called drug picture into a whole. It is then this image-idea of the remedy which is discovered to be the unifying idea of the disease.

In antiquity medicine was largely dominated by religious ideas, in Greece there originated a period during which it has been dominated by scientific ideas. This has led to a sophisticated study of disease at the expense of any concept of healing. It seems to me that Hahnemann inaugurated a period when we can begin to discover the art of healing. It is still scarcely born.

6. The problem of potentization

The characterization of homoeopathy has to be undertaken from many different sides if we are to have any hope of grasping its true nature. Attempts to define it inevitably lead to confusion rather than clarity, as indeed do such attempts in all realms concerned with life. An example is the confusion we get into if we follow the traditional way of defining homoeopathy in terms merely of the so-called Similia principle. This is intended to convey that we should treat a patient presenting a certain complex of symptoms with that substance which produces a similar symptom complex when given as poison or in a proving to the healthy. This principle is opposed to what is usually referred to as allopathy but by Hahnemann as enantiopathy, the treatment of a symptom complex by its opposite, the substance which produces the opposite symptoms. To make clear the idea in as simple an instance as possible, we can contrast the treatments of constipation. The homoeopathic treatment would be to use a substance such as opium which produces constipation in the healthy. A choice must be made between the available constipating agents as to which most nearly matches the patient's own style of constipation and his other symptoms. The enantiopathic treatment is to give a diarrhoea-producing substance, a laxative, and opium itself would be used enantiopathically for the relief of diarrhoea. The question of dosage then arises. In enantiopathic treatment, repeated dosage of quite measurable size is, of course, called for, whereas in homoeopathic treatment it is a matter of experience that so-called potencies are most effective, often in only occasional doses. So far the traditional statement, which was good enough in Hahnemann's day but scarcely holds today.

A great deal of modern pharmaco-therapeutics is based in fact on the Similia principle. Ideas such as metabolic antagonists and competitive inhibition imply the use of molecules similar in structure to those involved in the diseased metabolic pathways. In order to clarify matters we have to look at this point into the great differences in outlook which arise from the scale of observation. In these cases, the scale is that of molecular structure; in homoeopathy, of the human being. Quite different concepts of disease are associated with these two scales of observation and the distinctive therapies are in reality poles apart, though both based on the similia principle. In the one case disease is understood entirely in structural terms, molecular or larger; that is to say eventually in mechanistic terms. In the other case, the homoeopathic, disease is understood as a dynamic disturbance arising in a human person and manifesting in the experience of symptoms. A mere structure, a mechanism, cannot experience symptoms.

At this point we have not come up against the central difficulties facing anyone trained in modern scientific medicine who seeks to approach the problems presented by homoeopathy. Hahnemann's thought, together with that of many of his contemporaries, was essentially vitalistic. He spoke of dynamic, not material, causes of disease and of the *dynamis* or vital force maintaining the organism in healthy function or, when itself becoming dynamically deranged, manifesting in morbid functions and symptoms. He spoke of the morbific influences as dynamic or spiritual or quasi-spiritual. He also spoke of the problematic potencies, based on serial dilution and succussion, as having dynamic or quasi-spiritual effects or influences.

Scientific thinking has lost all connection with such ideas which were, to be honest, too vague to be accepted into the developing scientific disciplines. And so the problem of the nature of homoeopathic potencies, for long an outstanding obstacle to a wider acceptance of the subject, comes together with problems such as the nature of life. Our present natural science cannot really get beyond the study of the corpse of the living.

Over many years a number of attempts have been made to demonstrate the action of potencies under laboratory conditions, eliminating, it is hoped, the placebo effect inseparable from clinical trials. The mere fact of being 'in a trial' influences the reaction of patients and volunteers to both placebo and drug. The late Dr W. E. Boyd conducted a number of studies, including experiments involving the mercuric chloride inhibition of diastase hydrolysis of soluble starch, the mercuric chloride being tested in rising potencies. Many experiments have been carried out using the growth of seedlings watered with potencies of different substances. Some of these trials, such as those of Pelikan, have been subject to sophisticated statistical control. Many other experimental models have been used by different workers. What remains is that orthodox scientists continue and are likely to continue to show no interest in such experiments until they can form intellectual conceptual frameworks which render the reality of potency effects understandable and until the relevance of such phenomena to their own work is evident. There is plenty of experimental evidence that potencies beyond the range of dilution which would include a single molecule of the original active substance can still produce demonstrable results. But further work in this field must be carried out with the aim of clarifying the many doubtful points.

There have also been attempts to produce theoretical models which could render comprehensible the nature of potencies. The late Dr Barnard of the National Physical Laboratory at Teddington sought to show how the structure of water, its stero-isomeric structure, would be modified by the solute and this modification could be transferred serially in successive dilutions and succussions. Currently Dr

Resch, working with Professor Viktor Gutman at Vienna University, is developing a concept of the structure of water and other media which makes it possible that a memory trace of a solute can remain impregnated on the surface of sub-microscopic holes which belong to its structure.

Both these attempts are still within traditional concepts of space, stemming fundamentally from Euclid.

An attempt of a quite different kind was initiated by the late George Adams. He drew attention to the importance of projective geometry, also called synthetic geometry. This geometry arising out of the studies on perspective initiated by Renaissance artists at the dawn of the modern age, was brought to a certain perfection by the mathematicians of the nineteenth century. Its relevance to the real world of nature has however gone almost totally neglected. Adams, working on suggestions given by Rudolf Steiner, began to discover the revolutionary possibilities in this geometry, particularly in relation to living forms and metamorphosis. Shortly before his death he contributed a paper in which he suggested the relevance of this geometry also to the problem of homoeopathic potencies.

Adams emphasized two main characteristics of this geometry which the great Cambridge mathematician Arthur Cayley had epitomized in the saying 'projective geometry is all geometry'. What were the two aspects particularly signalled by Adams? The first lies in the attention no longer being

focused on rigid forms such as the square or the circle, but on mobile *types of form*, changing into one another in the diverse aspects of perspective, or other kinds of geometrical transformation. In Euclid, for instance, we take our start from the rigid form of the circle, sharply distinguished from the ellipse, parabola and hyperbola, as are these from one another. In Projective Geometry it is the 'conic section' in general of which the pure idea arises in the mind and of which various constructions are envisaged. As in real life the circular opening of a lampshade will appear in many forms of ellipse while moving about the room, or as the opening of a bicycle lamp projects on to the road in sundry hyperbolic forms, so in pure thought we follow the transformations from one form of conic section to another. Strictly speaking, the 'conic section' of Projective Geometry is neither circle, ellipse, parabola, nor hyperbola, it is a purely ideal form, out of which all of these arise, much as in Goethe's botany the 'archetypal leaf' is not identical with any particular variety or metamorphosis of leaf (foliage leaf varying in shape from node to node, petal, carpel and so on) but underlies them all. The new geometry begets a quality of spatial thinking akin to the metamorphoses of living form.

. . . [the second aspect or insight] is perhaps even more important. Projective Geometry recognizes as the deepest law of spatial structure an underlying *polarity* which to begin with may be called, in simple and imaginative language, a polarity of expansion and contraction, the terms

being meant in a qualitative and very mobile sense . . . Think of a sphere —
not the internal volume but the pure form of the surface. One sphere can
only differ from another as to size; apart from that, the form is the same.
Now the expansion and contraction of a sphere leads to two ultimate limits.
Contracted to the uttermost, the sphere turns into a point; expanded, into
a plane. The latter transformation, though calling for more careful
reflection, is no less necessary than the former. A large spherical surface
is less intensely curved than a small one; in other words it is flatter. So
long as it can still grow flatter, a sphere has not yet expanded to the utmost
limit, which can only be the absolute flatness of a plane.

The above simple experiment in thought — the ultimate contraction and
expansion of a sphere — leads in the right direction. Point and plane
prove to be the basic entities of three-dimensional space — that is, the
space of our Universe and of our human imagination. Speaking
qualitatively, the point is the quintessence of contraction, the plane of
expansion. Here comes the fundamental difference as against both the old
geometry of Euclid and the naïve and rather earthly spatial notions which
culminate in a one-sidedly atomistic outlook. For in the light of the new
geometry, three-dimensional space can equally well be formed from the
plane inward as from the point outward. The one approach is no more basic
than the other. In the old-fashioned explanation, we start from the point
as the entity of no dimension. Moving the point, say from left to right, we
obtain the straight line as the first dimension, moving the line forward and
backward, we get the two dimensions of the plane; finally, moving the
plane upward and downward, the full three dimensions. To modern
geometry this way of thinking is still valid, but it is only half the truth —
one of two polar-opposite aspects, the interweaving harmony of which is
the real essence of spatial structure. In the other and complementary aspect
we should start from the plane and work inward. To mention only the first
step: just as the movement of a point into a second point evokes the
straight line that joins the two, so does the movement of a plane into a
second plane give rise to the straight line in which the two planes
interpenetrate. We can continue moving in the same line and obtain a
whole sheaf of planes, like the leaves of an open book or a door swinging
on its hinges. We thus obtain a 'line of planes', as in the former instance
a 'line of points'. In the space-creating polarity of point and plane, the
straight line plays an intermediate role, equally balanced in either direction.
Just as two points of space always determine the unique straight line which
joins them, so do two planes; we only need to recognize that parallel planes
too have a straight line in common, namely the infinitely distant line of
either. At last we see that all the intuitively given relationships of points,
lines, and planes have this dual or polar aspect. *Whatever is true of planes*

in relation to lines and points is equally true of points in relation to lines and planes. Three points, for example, not in line, determine a single plane (principle of the tripod), but so do three planes not in line (e.g. the ceiling and two adjoining walls of a room) determine a single point. The planes must again be extended to the infinite and thought of as a whole to see that this is true without exception.

All spatial forms are ultimately made of points, lines and planes. Even a plastic surface or a curve in space consists of an infinite and continuous sequence, not only of points, but of tangent lines and of tangent or osculating planes. The mutual balance of these aspects — pointwise and planar, with the linewise aspect intermediating — give us a deeper insight into the essence of plasticity than the old-fashioned, one-sidedly pointwise treatment.

The outcome is that whatever geometrical form or law we may conceive, there will always be a sister form, a sister law equally valid, in which the rôles of point and plane are interchanged. Or else the form we thought of — as for example a tetrahedron with its equal number of points and planes — proves to be its own sister form, arising ideally out of itself by the polar interchange of point and plane. The principle just enunciated, as it were a master-key among the truths of Projective Geometry, is known as the Principle of Duality. It would perhaps have been better had it been described as a Principle of Polarity from the outset, for in its cosmic aspect it is also one of the essential keys to the manifold polarities of Nature. The recognition of it leads to a form of scientific thinking calculated to transcend one-sided atomism and materialistic bias.*

This is how Adams himself characterized the essential features of projective or synthetic geometry. He went on to show how natural science uses the same one-sidedness of thinking in its discovery and study of the forces as well as forms of nature. The forces so far studied and with the help of mathematical thinking mastered in modern technology are pointwise forces, forces radiating from centres. He then puts forward a proposition for consideration. The forces of nature, manifesting in the world of space and time, are not only centric; there are peripheral forces also. Even as the pure form of space is in the light of modern geometry balanced between point and plane, so are the forces that prevail in nature; they are not only pointwise or centric, but also peripheral or planar. Moreover, as in the domain of centric forces the central point of the material planet on which we live, in other words the centre of gravity of the earth, is for us a centre of primary importance, so in the realm of the peripheral or planar forces, what we experience as the infinitely distant plane — in simple language the vast periphery of the blue sky — is a most important source of the peripheral forces.

* Adams, 'Potentization'.

Once this perspective has been grasped it is possible to find particularly in the realms of living forms, of growth and metamorphosis, how these more mobile thought forms illumine the problems of biology. They can indeed enliven our too rigid scientific thinking. Can they help to throw light on the homoeopathic process of potentizing medicinal substances? This process of rhythmic expansion or dilution and succussion was felt by Hahnemann to release the spirit-like essence of the substance. Adams pursued the thought further:

> If crude matter alone were concerned — if stress were laid on the domain
> of centric forces, expressed in material quantity and weight — it would
> be natural to expect that an effect, comparatively feeble in a dilute solution,
> would be enhanced with increasing concentration. We reduce the volume,
> in other words draw in towards the centre. But if the substance is the
> bearer of ethereal virtues [to use a traditional term] of which the origin
> is peripheral, experience will show — and it is equally natural to expect,
> once we get used to the idea — that the effect will be enhanced, not by
> concentration but by expansion.

We can also at this point consider how just as in Euclidean, point-wise, space we have need of the plane at infinity so in the negative Euclidean, planar space, we have need of the point at infinity. But this does not mean infinitely far away but rather a focus bearing a 'functional infinitude within'. Can we not see this in the 'emptiness' above the growing point of a plant, about which the leaves or petals form a hollow cup? This imaginary point or emptiness moves ahead of the unfolding leaves but functional as a dynamic focus or goal towards which or around which the planar forces from the periphery come into manifestation. And could we perhaps imagine that the homoeopathic potency, materially non-existent, can act as such a focus around which the planar as opposed to the atomic aspect of a substance can be intensified.

In this way, we can begin to take steps towards understanding how dilution can play its part in the enhancement of some effects. It compels us to recognize how the one-sided thought forms of Euclidean geometry acting through the centuries and allied during recent centuries with an instinctive materialism have blinded us to the observation of any but pointwise materialistic forces.

In the process of homoeopathic potentization this dilution is carried out in successive rhythmic steps. It would seem that in this way due recognition is given to the polarity playing between the pointwise and weighable stuff of the crude material on the one hand and the planar, more qualitative and imponderable side of its being on the other. This polarity must be expressed in rhythms and we can envisage the gradual descent of purely ideal, or spiritual forms through rhythmic condensation to rigid, physical structures, processes which can indeed be observed in embryology. In potentization the reverse process is undertaken and the spiritual ideal form again released from its prison house in earthly matter.

We have still to consider the nature of succussion, the shaking of the fluid in which potentization is being carried on, between each successive step of dilution. In considering this problem we are again obstructed mostly by rigid habits of thought. There seems no doubt in the minds of those who have experience in these fields that succussion does play an important part in the potentizing process and what experimental evidence exists seems to support this view. But how are we to begin to grasp the importance of this vigorous shaking?

In the first place we must rid our minds of the prejudice of the lifeless inertia of water as mere body. In nature and in organic life, water is everywhere in circulation. On the grand scale, it manifests in evaporation to the sky, and in condensation to dew, rain, snow and hail, in which it falls again to earth, to flow perhaps down river to the sea or else to rise again, directly or largely through vegetable life. On smaller scales there are innumerable minor circulations including all those within our own organisms. Water tends everywhere to drop formation, whether on the level of the whole planet with its spheric hydrosphere, or in rain-drops and so on. The tendency to form surfaces is always evident and when water is in movement innumerable surfaces come into existence throughout its body, interweaving in varied forms. Theodor Schwenk has shown the importance of these filmy surfaces which come and go continuously in all moving liquid. Into the weaving of these moving films or veils and vortices there manifest forms reminiscent of animal and vegetable forms which thus themselves can be understood as frozen or petrified moments in the coming and going of these fluid forms. Only when water becomes still does it begin to manifest the static lattice structure of ice; in motion it becomes through and through an interweaving play of surfaces, subject to the planar rather than pointwise influences we have discussed in geometrical terms.

Schwenk also shows how these surfaces are sensitive in the extreme to such influences. From the ripples thrown upon the surface of a still lake by the slightest breath to the gigantic ocean-travelling waves arising in great storms thousands of miles away, we can see how every influence is imparted to the surfaces. And if up till the present it is chiefly only wave motions which have been observed arising in response to physical forces such as wind or mechanical movements, this is only because we have scarcely begun to look for any others. If substances are the bearers not only of three-dimensional measurable and weighable content, such as we are habitually trained to observe, but also of two-dimensional planar, ethereal, spiritual, or, to use Hahnemann's term, well-nigh spiritual, essences, then it is beginning to be comprehensible that through the twin processes of dilution, or expansion, and succussion we can encourage this inner quality of the substance to be imparted to the fluid. The dilution or expansion intensifies the ethereal aspect, whilst the surface-evoking succussion, or shaking, sensitizes the fluid to these influences.

We have here touched upon the great challenge with which the problems of life and in this instance the nature of homoeopathic potencies face us. There is the habitual scientific reaction to any such problem. It is to try and reduce the problem to terms already accepted and to explain the unsolved riddle in terms of established dogma.

During the last few centuries human consciousness has contracted to an unprecedented degree. It has become very bright but very narrow. Attention is riveted on that which is measurable and weighable and all else is relegated to the fairy realm of 'only in the mind'. Our fundamental experience of measuring arises out of our limbs. We pace it out, so many feet or yards, and a horse is measured as so many hands. Weight is experienced first as the weight of our body under the earth's gravity, we weigh something in our hand. We walk from footprint to footprint and we learn our Euclidean geometry basically in this way. It is tactile in origin and the more we enquire into modern scientific theories and conceptions the more we find them developed from concepts based on touch sensation. Modern projective geometry arose from the artist's study of perspective and the sense of sight. Physiology still tries to explain the sense of sight in terms drawn from the sense of touch. The challenge is to develop our thinking, to free it from the earthbound sense of touch and to enliven our thinking, trained for so long on the study of the dead mineral world. This dead thinking must be brought into motion. We must become inwardly active, and not passive observers in the fashion of our times. This is the rub, for our inertia is very great.

In ancient times, before thinking had become entirely abstract and lifeless, it still responded more immediately to the spiritual forces present in nature which the Greeks still perceived as the goddess Natura. But this immediacy of perception did not depend on individual effort or freedom. Man was in a way moved by these forces, swayed by them.

Now we have entered into the experience of the death forces and our current thinking is an expression of these forces. If we are again to become able to study life and bring life again to the ageing, dying planet, we must enliven our own thinking so that it can observe the growth and metamorphosis of living forms. Then we may succeed in transforming our death-promoting technology into a life-restoring and renewing activity. In medicine, our current scientific medicine and therapeutics, daily more technological in character, can only promote rigidity, sclerosis and death. Can we begin to see how in the small beginning so far achieved by homoeopathic medicine, a step towards a life-promoting and real healing has been taken. To develop this we must re-educate ourselves, but we must not turn our back on the path we have come in modern science. Through the achievement of Projective Geometry it has been made possible to reopen our perception of the subtler spiritual forces of the cosmos whilst keeping the clear light of waking consciousness. In this way we can attempt to understand the problem presented by homoeopathy and its potencies without relapsing into mystical dreaminess or phrase-mongering, but rather out of the strengthened consciousness and confidence that such inner activity can bring.

7.   The nature of Man

There is today an understandable revulsion against the consequences of the technologies which arise from the natural scientific movement and threaten our outer
civilization and even the planet itself with disasters of many kinds. We have
become alarmed by the pollution of our outer and inner environments and dis-
gusted by the ruthless exploitation of Mother Nature in pursuit of commercial,
political and military supremacies. Unfortunately much of this revulsion wishes
only to go back to before this terrifying age, to a pre-scientific conception of
things. Apart from the impossibility of putting the clock back to a time which we
would certainly find morally, as well as physically and intellectually, unspeakably
cramped and unacceptable, we should also perhaps be in danger of throwing away
the baby with the bath water, were we to be able to do so. Can we hope to
discover the baby, that child of our natural science, which, to judge from the crisis
of our time, is in great need of nurture and education if it is to grow up to a
healthy and fruitful maturity? To do so we shall first have to recall the salient
features of this scientific movement and come up against the limitations of knowledge which have arisen in its path and to which Rudolf Steiner drew most particular
attention.

Man has today become overwhelmed by the avalanche of precise scientific
knowledge, based on the accurate measurements of sense phenomena mathematically developed, which accumulates in ever-increasing quantities. By comparison
with the seeming precision of this work, the world of qualities, of tones, colours,
smells and of emotions, appears as a bewildering kaleidoscope of changing dream
pictures in which no certainty is to be found. And yet it is in the midst of all these
qualities that we live and experience our life. These phenomena are not easily
shared and made verifiable; like actual dreams they are largely private and subjective, communicable perhaps only through the media of art. By contrast the world
of science appears verifiable and objective, that is to say shareable and subject to
law, but it has become empty of content and meaning, abstract and dehumanized.
Nevertheless we should recall that none other than Goethe saw and was deeply
moved exactly by the rule of law, even in Art itself.

Up until the scientific revolution, some four centuries or so ago, this stark
division between the world of human experience and the world of scientific

measurement and calculation had not been established. Nature was conceived both quantitatively and qualitatively and man was conceived as microcosm within the macrocosm. What is more, Nature was felt, and even experienced, to be peopled by elemental spirits and there were the encircling spheres of heaven with the hierarchies of spiritual beings. It was a complex, subtle conception of the world, full of meanings, purposes and mysteries, and full of wonder. In astrology and alchemy, the study of the stars and of substances in their movements and transformations was pursued out of a consciousness which still found psycho-spiritual forces, beings and qualities intimately permeating the physical bodies and substances. Everything was still living, the full impact of death had not been felt.

At the end of the Middle Ages western Man became obsessed with death and with its image the skeleton. There were dances of death, rituals of death, wrestling with the fact of death and its meaning. At the beginning of the new age of natural science the first text book of human anatomy to be based on accurate dissection of the human corpse was published by Vesalius in 1543 and marks the beginning of so-called scientific medicine. In the same year there was published Copernicus' book of the anatomy of the corpse of the solar system. The methodology for pursuing this new view of things was established scientifically by Galileo and philosophically by Descartes. A division was established between what could be measured and weighed and those other properties of colour, tone, taste, smell and so on. The first were called primary qualities and considered to be real and objective, whereas the second were relegated as secondary qualities to being subjective, and 'only in the mind'. The movement of human consciousness which from distant antiquity had progressively lost its awareness of the divine, spiritual world now curtailed yet further its scope by distinguishing that which could be known through the sense of touch from the content of all the other senses. Only what could be touched was real, that is to say in a crude way only matter. One recalls in passing how Dr Johnson refuted Berkeley's Idealism by kicking a stone. Science proceeded to turn colours and tones into vibrations and particles so as to be able to handle and measure them with its mechanical concepts, although in doing so it lost sight of and eliminated the very realities it was supposed to be studying. When Goethe opened the way to a scientific study of colour as such, the scientific establishment showed and continues to show neither understanding nor interest. Science claims to be based exclusively on sense experience, but it has not only excluded all suprasensory experience; it has also excluded all the senses themselves with the sole exception of the sense of touch, to which it has rather mistakenly attributed objectivity. To be more precise, it interprets the other senses in terms of concepts related to touch, which enables all phenomena to be treated mechanically. It should be further noted that measurements of matter and motion are then developed by mathematical techniques; and there has been a tendency to regard these as indubitably clear and self-evident, as given *a priori*, although they are in fact based on self-contradictory fictions.

Now I have had to bring forward these considerations in order to come to confrontation with the natural scientific conception of Man which is taught today to all children in our western world. Man is limited to the matter and its motions of which our bodies are composed. There is nothing special about living as distinct from dead or mineral things other than complexity; there is nothing special about animate beings as distinct from merely vegetable or living things. Feelings are the life of the nervous tissue. And Man is only another animal with a larger more complex brain which exudes thoughts. All this moreover is understood, or at any rate taught, as coming into existence under the exclusive play of blind natural forces, mechanical forces, because for our modern natural science nature herself is mechanical through and through. In so far as living things, organisms, are not graspable by mechanical models then our human intellect cannot grasp them and we must resign ourselves to helpless and hopeless ignorance. We come up against one of the limits of cognition which Steiner maintains affords us experience of the greatest significance for the future.

How then can we characterize the phenomena of living organisms which present essential problems to the human intellect? In the first place the uniformity in structure of minerals, for instance crystals, makes their characteristic form indifferent to size. A crystal of common salt has the same form whether it has the size of a microscopic grain or of a room. It is not, so to say, inwardly differentiated and organized but has only a uniform structure throughout. A living organism on the other hand carves out for itself a characteristic space, of a characteristic size neither smaller nor larger within limited variations. Elephants and mice have their characteristic sizes. Further this space is inwardly differentiated and organized into tissues and organs which, whilst distinct, are mutually interdependent and together constitute a whole. This whole lies latent in all its parts so that when we propagate, for instance, a begonia from a single leaf, it is able to develop afresh, root, stem, leaves and blossom.

There is further a relation to time which distinguishes the living from the lifeless. For the mineral, length of life is not significant. Whether a salt crystal lasts a second or thousands of years makes no difference to our understanding of it, of the laws which express its nature. But with living beings, they are characterized as much by their life span as by their size; they carve out an organism both in space and in time. The idea of the rose must comprise its whole development in time from seed and germination through unfolding of cotyledons to stems and leaves to the blossoming and fruiting. We are faced with the marvellous phenomena of metamorphosis from one form into another whilst together they are the rose. An inner realm of manifoldness comes to ordered manifestation in time.

Mechanical events, such as the collision of billiard balls and their rebound movements, can be expressed mathematically in concepts related only externally to them. These are the laws of motion, the ideal component of the whole event. In the case of living organisms the ideal component, the law of their being and growth, is inwardly active and comes to manifestation in their metamorphoses, their growth and their life processes. The ideal element in a plant, which is thus an active reality manifesting outwardly in form, is not accessible to our ordinary intellectual consciousness in the same way as the laws of motion. Here is the first serious obstacle on our path. If we are to understand living organisms we must become able to grasp this ideal element with intensified powers of cognition. To these intensified cognitional capacities Steiner gave the name Imagination. He characterized in great detail their nature and the methods by which they can be cultivated. He also pointed to Goethe as that person who had pioneered this path to the scientific study of living creatures, comparing him to Galileo in the study of mechanics. For the manifoldness, the real ideal element of living things, Steiner used the terms etheric body or body of formative forces.

It is important to realise that this Etheric body and the etheric forces do not belong to the Euclidean space in which physical bodies and forces are studied. To these belong gravity and electro-magnetic forces and characteristically they relate pointwise, between one point and another. Gravity acts from the centre and so these forces diminish with distance according to strict mathematical law. The etheric forces, on the contrary, act from the periphery and work suctionally, levitationally. Steiner indicated that the so-called synthetic or projective geometry, brought to a certain perfection in the nineteenth century, would make it possible to study these etheric forces with mathematical clearness of thought. The importance of the late George Adams' work for our present purpose is to establish that human cognition can be trained to become inwardly mobile as it has to be in projective geometry without losing that clarity of awake consciousness which is the character of mathematical thinking. The etheric forces belong to what George Adams called negative Euclidean space, which arises from the interplay or interweaving of planes as distinct from the points of normal Euclidean space. The primary polarity of space is between the infinitely contracted point and the infinitely expanded plane. Thus positive Euclidean space arises from the relationship between points, negative Euclidean space from the relationship between planes. I can of course only indicate these lines of study.

The vegetable kingdom expresses the play of these planar forces working from the periphery. That we can see them in the leaves with our physical eyes is due to the physical substances which are caught up into them as the physical body of the plant. In the plant therefore we have the etheric planar forces from the cosmic periphery in their interplay with the physical forces related to the earth centre. These etheric forces become to some extent individually organized to form what can be called the etheric body of the plant: the word 'body' is of course not entirely satisfactory.

In the plant kingdom everything is, so to say, spread out, it grows out into spatial manifestation. When we come to study the animal kingdom another gesture confronts us. A gesture of interiorization develops. Instead of growing outwards the developing organism turns in on itself and forms a cup-like form. More and more infoldings come about and gradually there arise the wonderfully internally organized bodies of the higher animals. It is not difficult to see that a quite distinct element of form here comes to expression. It pushes inwards, creating inner spaces; what in the plant was still outside now becomes interiorized into the animal. This something then manifests in movement and sensation, in desire and pleasure and pain. Something comes to expression which we must call a soul element. This in itself is not in space at all, yet it can find physiognomical expression in these formative gestures of embryogenesis. We all know how emotions such as fear and shame bring about changes in the physical body such as blanching and blushing, and how emotions and feelings of pain and pleasure find utterance in sounds issuing forth from the inner depths of animate beings. The living body can then be spoken of as becoming ensouled. A soul quality incarnates into and forms the organism as its outer expression. This quality becomes visible in the physiognomical form and observable also in its behaviour and in those sounds and tones which are its so direct utterance. For this soul element, creative of animal form and behaviour and the bearer of desires and pleasure and pain, Steiner used the term astral body or soul body. The powers of cognition needed to apprehend this element of existence must be strengthened again beyond the powers of Imagination needed for perceiving the etheric body. To such strengthened power Steiner gave the name Inspiration. Just as we can regard Imagination as a higher metamorphosis of vision, so Inspiration can be approached as a higher metamorphosis of hearing.

The mammals of the animal kingdom can now be seen as the incarnation of different soul qualities or emotions, the courage of the lion, the ferocity of the tiger, the cunning of the fox, the fearfulness of the rabbit, the bestowing benevolence of the cow. The whole world of the emotions finds its physiognomic and behavioural manifestation in the realm of the mammals. They are emotions incarnate. And the birds for their part are thoughts. The eagle soars on the majestic wings of philosophic vision. The sparrows are crowds of chattering cockneys. The lark rises and falls on lyrical outpourings, and we find the whole world of our thoughts expressed in the flight and other behaviour of birds and especially in their feathers, their plumage.

How then do they stand in relation to Man? It belongs to the commonly accepted dogmas of our time that Man is, at least in respect of his bodily organisation, just another animal, the highest and most developed mammal, the summit of the Primates. If there are certain capacities especially developed in Man these can be regarded as evolving out of the more instinctive behaviour and faculties of animals. The basic structure of the human body, its organs and systems are similar to those of the higher animals. A vertebral back bone, four limbs, a head, chest and abdominal cavities, a system of senses based on eyes, ears, nose, tongue and skin, these features compel one to acknowledge a common nature or idea which appears in varied modifications in the different species, families and orders. The question is whether the modifications of this basic vertebrate plan found in the human kingdom are derivable from the same forces and principles as underlie the animal forms. The basic building plan may be similar but the way in which it is carried out may yet reveal a quite distinct principle at work within the human organism.

In the first place we have to take note of the retention of more embryo-like features in the human development. The mature human form has not evolved further from the embryonic than the animal has, it has on the contrary remained nearer to the embryonic. If we study the development of various species through their embryonic and post-embryonic developments we find that the earlier we look the more do the various embryos resemble each other. As they mature so do they fall more and more into diverse specialization: only the human retains an omnipotentiality. The bodily organization of animals becomes specialized into instruments, the wings of birds, the fins of fishes, the claws of carnivores, the hoofs of herbivores and so on. The animals become imprisoned in these organic formations, they determine its life.

But in the case of the human, the limbs for instance do not become these specific tools. The human being on the contrary develops the ability to invent the tools and then to use them. Aeroplanes, oars of boats, boots, knives and forks and the rest of our inventions which we can freely use, these in the animals have taken hold of their bodily organization and the limb has become the specific tool not the user of it.

Further, the orientation in space of the animal and human forms points to radical differences in essential principle. The spinal organization of animals is characteristically horizontal; only in man does it become vertical, a spinal column. In animals the head is only a continuation of the vertebrae; in man it crowns the vertebral column and morphologically repeats in a synthetic mode the whole lower trunk in a new and higher form. The whole body is indeed reflected in the head. And if in the ascent to the vertical the human succeeds in giving freedom to the head, balanced, poised, almost free flying, it also gives the legs over to the earth; only the human form has a straight knee. The human, through legs, truly columns, grows down on to the earth, stands and walks upon the earth. Animals only touch the earth, mostly only with the tips of their fingers and toes. In the human form are expressed the extreme polarities, related both to heaven and earth and holding the balance between them, refusing to fall one-sidedly into any speciality. Does not this point to something active in the human being which brings about this upright stance, and also brings about walking, speaking and thinking; something which organically gives evidence of its existence in the holding back from the animal limitations. This something says no to the fall into mere animal existence, mere imprisonment in the determinism of organic form and adaptation to the special environment. This something, when it first becomes conscious of itself, manifests by saying 'No' to its mother's orders. Usually this comes about at around three years of age.

This inhibiting action also shows itself in the slow maturation of the human being, sexual maturity being achieved only at around fourteen years of age. In the human, moreover, this sexual maturity marks the beginning of the individual's mental and emotional flowering. Our organisms too go on developing into our late twenties. In animals sexual maturity marks a culmination, and gradual ageing without further unfolding of new faculties sets in. Enough has been said to indicate in which directions we must turn our attention in order to become aware of the fourth element or principle in Man which distinguishes him from the animal realm and to which Steiner points as the Ego or spiritual kernel in Man. To the yet greater cognitional power which can unite itself with the spiritual realities Steiner gave the name Intuition.

We have thus been led to distinguish four elements, constituents or principles which together form the nature of the human being. Firstly a physical body of mass and inertia, through which man is related to the dead world of the mineral kingdom. Secondly an etheric body of lightness and dynamics, through which life unfolds and which man shares with the living kingdom of the plant kingdom. Thirdly a soul or astral body, the bearer of the inner world of desire, pleasure and pain and the qualitative world of emotions. This man shares with the animal kingdom, and it finds expression also in animals' physiognomic forms, gestures and behaviour. It already marks a turning inwards, backwards on itself, of the more outwardly growing vegetative life. It expresses itself especially in the katabolic, down-breaking phase of metabolic processes, and we can see how the inner soul experience is purchased at the cost of a certain destruction of the upbuilding anabolic vegetative process. The fourth principle, the Ego principle in Man, comes to expression in the upright posture and walking, in the speaking and thinking of the human being. This principle by entering into the three bodily elements begins to transform them so that they begin a process of metamorphosis in which the meaning of the future evolution of human life can be envisaged.

We must however attempt to clarify the relationship between Man and Nature from another side, that of past evolution. The great achievements of the nineteenth century natural science compelled us all to accept an evolutionary process in which transformation of natural forms and species unfolded. In place of the omnipotent creative fiat of God, through which the distinctive forms and creatures came into existence once and for all, there was unfolded the picture of a gradual evolutionary development in which new forms came into manifestation. A real development of new, unforeseen forms came about, an epigenesis of new formations, not merely the unfolding of those already spatially present. And all this was explained by Darwin and his successors as coming about by natural forces acting blindly without aim or intention. At the summit of this process, often portrayed as a genealogical tree, appeared Man, the product of purely natural forces, the last to appear.

When however we turn our attention to actual biological events we find that a seed from a specific plant will grow only into that plant. Only an ovum from an elephant will grow into an elephant or from a lion into a lion. In the ovum no trace of the future organs and forms is visible; these unfold epigenetically. Yet a supersensible real Idea of the coming organism must be active from a supersensible or spiritual world to organize the embryogenesis so that an elephant or lion results. The modern work on genes and so on does not affect this argument, as one still has to account for the turning on or off of genetic information in different cells and regions of the developing organism. And this organizing system is supersensory, ideal in nature. Here we must call on Goethe's perception of the Idea.

Returning to the field of Evolution we are then faced with the question as to how Man appeared at the completion of the evolutionary process, which must be regarded as an embryonic process extended over vast periods of time. Must not the Idea of Man have been acting from non-spatial realms throughout the evolutionary-embryogenesis of Man? As in an artistic work, the final picture becomes clearer and clearer. We can then understand the natural kingdoms as having been cast out from the developing human form, somewhat as bits of marble are chipped away from the statue as it becomes gradually visible under the sculptor's hammer and chisel. These natural forms can then only harden and become fixed in their limitations. But the further clearing and perfecting of the human form was brought about by these lower forms sacrificing any further evolution for themselves. Only Man continued to evolve. In this sense Man was the first being in the evolutionary development, but the last to reach manifestation. The *whole* reaches expression in the human form: only partial functions are expressed in the forms of animals and vegetables. Man is synthesis, nature analysis. Steiner portrayed the evolutionary process in great rhythmic periods in which impulses from spiritual beings were active, and Dr Karl König was able to show the correspondences between these macrocosmic processes and phases and the microcosmic ones of human embryogenesis. In these evolutionary periods not only have physical forms evolved; the etheric and astral bodies have also become further developed and perfected beyond the stage of their first appearance.

We have been approaching the understanding of how the developing human form became more and more an image of the whole. We can call spirit by the name of wholeness, and so we can begin to grasp the human form as the image of the spiritual. Thus the full achievement of the evolutionary development of Man required that the Infinite, the Whole, should become fully realized and conscious of itself in a single person. The Christian revelation is witness to the truth that in Christ Jesus the Whole became incarnated in a human person: he was Infinite and he knew it. By this the Earth evolution achieved its meaning. In the periods of organic evolution, the mixed confusions of the earlier forms had first to be clarified by the elimination of the animal forms until the human became manifest. But there was still that confusion in the more spiritual nature of Man which has been known in religious terminology as Original Sin, originating in the so-called Fall of Man. Through this Man had remained unable to attain to full realization of Truth, particularly of the nature of death. Through the Christ event Man achieved his goal in one person and became the world-organ of truth-knowing. From now on the task is the gradual transformation of the old natural, unaccomplished forms in which the full human and divine are not manifest. To these belong all our social forms and institutions which like dinosaurs still stalk about, and all those old atavistic emotional aspects of our inner lives which still make us miserable with our egotistical, criminal and neurotic impulses.

But we must return from a glimpse of the future into the present and try to follow Steiner into the web of the so-called psychosomatic problem — the problem of how our immortal souls and spirits are related to our mortal and spatial bodies.

When at the beginning of our modern age Galileo and Descartes reduced objective existence to the purely corporeal, devoid of all positive properties, and consigned those properties to an attic of subjectivity, they formulated in new terms the body-soul question. They mistakenly converted what was justified as a fiction of science into an unjustified affirmation of a truth of fact. Descartes himself sought to relate the utterly immaterial soul to the utterly mechanistic and material body through the pineal gland, an effort which must leave most moderns bewildered. On the whole the dogmas of our science today seek to locate the soul exclusively in the nervous system, an equally bewildering concept; if indeed it can even be called a concept. It would seem to arise from the experience that I look out through my eyes and therefore must be behind them. But the concepts of a purely subjective soul and purely objective body are totally sundered, as the philosophers Coleridge, Bergson, Whitehead and others have understood. This association between the head and the thinking mind was first made in Greek times by the Pythagoreans in Southern Italy. But the word *phren* also enshrines the earlier Greek experience of the mind in the diaphragm or midriff. At the beginning of the nineteenth century Lavater, the creator of scientific physiognomy, related the intellectual, emotional and volitional faculties to the upper, middle and lower regions of the face respectively. It was a short step to relate these again to the head, chest and abdominal realms, a realization that led Jaworski to his biological insights and synthesis. These were attempts to find spatial homes for the soul and its faculties of thinking, feeling and willing.

Steiner took up this question afresh and sought the bodily foundations of thinking, feeling and willing in the processes of the nerve-sense system, the rhythmic system, and the metabolic-limb system respectively. Each of these functional systems is all-pervading. It is true that the nerve-sense processes predominate in the head, that rhythmic processes come to fullest expression in the rhythms of breathing and heart-beat within the chest, and that the metabolic processes are most powerfully active in the abdomen and limbs, although extending throughout the organism. Nevertheless nerve-sense processes are everywhere, even in every cell, and equally there are metabolic and rhythmic processes in every nerve cell. The three processes interpenetrate and together form the whole.

Steiner understood the soul and spirit as real entities which are effectively active, and not as mere onlookers in the manner the experimental disciplines of science have enforced on us. During the embryonic and childhood periods these soul-spirit realities are active in the building and organizing of the body as their physiognomic expression. The unconscious or superconscious thinking activity organizes the brain, and having completed this task is progressively set free from its organic responsibilities, starting from the change of teeth at about seven years of age. It can then carry on its thinking as a pure spiritual activity. That we can become conscious of this activity is due to the brain, which acts as a mirror. Without this mirror we would not become conscious of our thinking. This reflecting process wakes us up so that our consciousness in thinking is what we call waking consciousness. In this we clearly distinguish ourselves from the objects of our observation, and the logical connection of our thoughts is transparent as in mathematical thinking. It will also be evident that the mirrored thoughts of our consciousness are only images, and devoid of living reality. They can no longer rule us, we are free to move amongst them. But this killing of the living, active, thoughts into lifeless images represents also the archetypal activity of the nervous system, it is a paralysing action. The forms of our bodies are also the working of the nervous processes, which if unhindered would lead to our becoming frozen sculptured images, and to the living, moving, ever-changing processes themselves becoming paralysed. Steiner insisted that all nerves are sensory. There are no real motor nerves, only sensory nerves of movement. Almost all modern research into nervous activity has to do either with electrical, chemical or metabolic processes or else with rhythmic processes such as are revealed in electro-encephalograms. But these have to do with the metabolic or rhythmic activity in the nervous organs and not with the true nervous function. Steiner emphasized that the true nervous function would not be accessible to ordinary physiological researches, and so it has proved. We are up against another of the limits of knowledge. Only when ideation is present is there neural activity. Only during thinking is the brain a brain. What can be observed by empirical physiology is never the neural function. 'The activity of the nerves is precisely that in them which is not perceptible by the senses . . .'. To follow the nervous activity we shall have to make use of imaginative cognition.

To turn now to the emotional life, there we experience the constant interplay of sympathy and antipathy, of love and hate, and all their development into complex emotions. The bodily foundation of this feeling Steiner finds in the rhythmic processes and more especially in the breathing rhythm. Ancient languages used the same word for breath and soul, as in the Latin *anima*. Again, in the book of Genesis we read, 'And the Lord God formed man of the dust of the ground, and breathed into his nostrils the breath of life; and man became a living soul.' Throughout the entire organism there are constant and most varied rhythmic movements: not only the in and out breathing and the pulse beat, but the intestinal movements, the kidney functions, sleeping and waking, and other rhythms of all our functions and organs. One can envisage the organism as a supreme symphony with many diverse organs whose varied times are woven together into a great harmony-filled interplay of rhythms. On all this our emotional life plays in a dream consciousness. We are not in full awake consciousness in our feelings; they weave to and fro in that state of consciousness which we experience in dreams and which does not rise to the clear awakeness and conceptual sharpness of waking life. When we breathe in we awake a little, and when we breathe out we go a little more to sleep. The great rhythm of our earth life commences with our first in-breath and ends with our final expiration. To follow these processes we must rise to inspirational cognition.

The will activities are even more difficult to follow because in them the soul plunges down into the bodily processes, brings about real changes and effects, and in moving the limbs brings about objective changes in the world. Of how we do these things we are unconscious: to them the word magical can justly be applied. The consciousness of the will activities is a sleep consciousness and in them the soul and spirit continue a mode of existence characteristic of embryonic and childhood life. Only with intuitive consciousness can we penetrate consciously into these realms.

We can now characterize these three functional realms in another way and recognize that our nerve processes centred in the head are old. Death processes predominate but consciousness is most awake. Our head does very little, all our life it gets carried around and spends its time observing rather critically the goings on around. Fundamentally it is based on memory, looking back even, as Plato saw, to pre-natal existence. By contrast the life of the metabolic-limb system is for ever young. We walk into the future but look backwards in memory in our head system. In our emotional rhythmic processes we live in the present, in the immediate experiences of our pleasure and pain, our love and hate.

So do we see yet again how Man unites the spiritual, or continuum of wholeness, with the material bodily world of diversity and discreteness, and the past and future with the present. It is the nature of Man to unite two worlds, and he is that spiritual being, that Ego, whom one can meet in this spatial world, shake hands with, and come to know in his biography. For in the biography of the individual man we can find evidence of his individuality stamped on all that he does and that happens to him. It is not the events common to man as a species that constitute the biography, it is rather all that is exceptional and unique. In this uniqueness of the biography one sees the utter distinction of the human from the animal. An animal's life story is only an example of the species, the potentialities of which come to expression and vary only according to the circumstances. But in the case of Man, every biography is unique and it is the uniqueness which reveals the individuality, the spiritual kernel in the man. It is also possible to trace between the phases of a man's life the operation of a moral law of cause and effect. And we can see how the individuality wrestles with the experiences which destiny brings and builds a sort of seed kernel within the ageing, hardening husk of the body. This inner growth in man can continue right up until bodily death.

I must now approach one last aspect of our subject, the nature of man. To omit this would utterly distort Steiner's approach of the subject. But we may first agree that the basic outlines as I have presented them are in essential content the same as have been presented in Oriental religions, in Platonism and neo-Platonism, and in the thought of many mystics throughout the ages. What is most significant in Steiner's work is that he accepted as foundation the scientific revolution. As Owen Barfield has pointed out, this revolution resulted in matter being utterly freed from contamination by all psychic and even sensory qualities, and all so-called occult qualities. These were thrown into the realm of 'only in the mind'. Science proceeded to study the mineral world and its mechanisms. The mineral world is so much a dead world, excreted from and by the living, that man is related to it almost only as an observer. In his study of it and the development of the abstract thinking applied in science he was for this very reason however able to develop the germs of freedom. In this onlooker consciousness he is left uninfluenced by what he observes. This thinking now became the Trojan Horse, to use Barfield's phrase, in the citadel of science, because it was itself a supersensible element in the cognitional process. It was by strengthening and developing the potentialities in this thinking into active Imagination, Inspiration and Intuition that Steiner was able to develop the realm of spiritual science as distinct from natural science. With clear methodology he was able to develop the observation of soul and spirit as free from all traces of matter, thus complementing the natural scientific methodology which had purged matter of all soul and spirit. And this observation of the spiritual was conducted in full waking consciousness. In this relation to the scientific revolution lies the great importance of Steiner's work. It makes accessible again to modern man the fruits of man's original vision, the primal spiritual revelation to our distant ancestors, without loss of our achievement of freedom in our wide awake consciousness. This freedom we can now recognize as that offspring of the scientific revolution, which must at all costs be protected and nurtured.

The aspect which I am approaching lies in the range of the phenomena of metamorphosis. In the vegetable kingdom we can observe the metamorphosis of the leaf into sepals, petals, stamens, pistils, fruit and seed. We can see the transformation from stage to stage, and observe them lying spread out together. In the animal kingdom the metamorphoses present us with a greater cognitional challenge: one manifestation vanishes and another comes into being. The caterpillar disappears from this world, from the chrysalis emerges the butterfly. Something quite new in form appears and we are hard put to it to grasp caterpillar, chrysalis and butterfly in their unity as metamorphoses of one being. We have to hold our breath as we take a leap over the abyss.

The leap in the case of the human metamorphosis is far greater according to the observations of Steiner. Following the course of the soul and spirit after death in passing out of the spatial world and its material embodiment, he describes the spiritual metamorphoses culminating in a new embodiment. The laws of cause and effect working in these vast metamorphoses are moral in nature, traditionally known under the name of Karma. Through these studies the Ego of Man is revealed as an entity amongst others in the spiritual world accessible to the extended intuitive consciousness. But it is in this physical world and no other that we can develop the concepts with which to understand the immensely dynamic realities which are revealed to the consciousness of those who, like Steiner, have developed the faculties to observe them and to translate their observations into our customary language. This last is perhaps one of the greatest difficulties. Man is now revealed as living in vast breathing rhythms between the spiritual world — the world of wholes, of real beings and interweaving continuity — and this our present world of diversity, separateness, rigidity and death. But it is exactly to this world that we owe the possibility of freedom and understanding.

The future development of the spiritual elements or faculties of our being depends on the exercise of that free activity which we can nurture as the child of the scientific revolution. It depends entirely on ourselves whether we exercise this activity or not, but the possibility has been achieved. To the higher spiritual elements, awaiting our free activity to bring about their awakening and development, Steiner gave the names of Spirit Self, Life Spirit and Spirit Man. These are the higher metamorphoses of the astral, etheric and physical bodies respectively, and correspond to the ancient Indian terms Manas, Buddhi and Atma.

PART II

8.   Poisons and remedies

Poisons present us with a problem which has today become enormously complex and vast in range and detail. New toxic hazards resulting from technology are in themselves a highly developed field of specialized knowledge and there is an ever-increasing store of facts about plants and their poisons as well as about the venoms of animals. There is a danger of losing all perspective on the problem as a whole and getting lost in a maze of detail. The subject is one which is so coloured with emotion, drawing with it such a wealth of associative images from primordial sources, that it behoves us to attempt to grasp it as a whole. For unless we do, our emotional connection with the subject springing from unconscious depths will distort our judgments and make them dangerously unreliable. But these emotions, as we shall see, belong to the subject and can only be eliminated at the expense of throwing away the baby with the bath water.

Paracelsus maintained that it was a matter of dosage whether a particular substance acted as a remedy or a poison. However, this is obviously an over-simplified statement and we must also consider the state of the organism at the time, particularly whether it is healthy or diseased. In addition the route of entry of the poison is essential to the discussion, and we have to consider the relation of poison and remedy not only to each other but to food. Milk when taken through the alimentary tract is for most people a food, but when injected subcutaneously it can result in fever and generalized reactions. Are these reactions, mostly allergic in origin, to be classed as toxic? Again, snake venoms whilst not being foods are harmless when taken through the intact alimentary canal, but highly toxic when injected subcutaneously by the poison fangs of the snake. And although immune processes are involved in the full reaction to snake venoms, most of their action is due to proteolytic and other enzymes acting directly.

The serpent leads us to one of the primordial images connected with our subject. The story of the original poisoning of mankind, the injection of something foreign to his original nature, from which stems all the subsequent story of mankind, is known to us all from Genesis. And even if our scientists seek to escape from these traditional mythological truths, they discover the crisis of fertilization and conception when the serpent sperm penetrates the ovum and disturbs its quiescent sleep. Such is the power of the archetypal image.

The Greek word *toxin* meant an arrow. At the beginning of the *Iliad* the god Apollo, who is also the god of healing, shoots his arrows into the herds of the Greeks on the plains of Troy, causing an epidemic amongst them. Arrow poisons form another great archetypal picture and have, incidentally, led to the use of the curare-like drugs as well as of strophanthus and ouabain. The multitude of artistic portrayals of the martyrdom of St. Sebastian testify to the emotional significance of being shot by arrows and its absorbing interest to mankind.

We may link together snake bites, poison arrows and the hypodermic injection. Nor is it perhaps too wild a leap to the expressions 'to get under someone's skin', or 'to needle someone'. In all these instances there is the common motif of penetration of the defences, a breaking through a skin or barrier, a mixing of realms foreign to one another as in a hybrid. Comparable to these phenomena we may include the reactions of a group of people, a tribe or nation, to a stranger, with all the emotions of xenophobia on the one hand and on the other the shyness and fear which come over us when we find ourselves in a new and strange environment. Connected with these experiences is the range of initiation rituals marking the entry into a new society, or a new phase of life or consciousness.

We may now reach an initial insight into the distinction between food and poison. When we eat a foodstuff, it passes through a series of stages during which it is broken down, first mechanically, then chemically by means of enzymes. Only when it has allowed itself to be reduced in the digestive analysis to a state of nonentity, chaos, can it be safely absorbed and resynthesized. Analogous processes exist in the initiation rituals we have mentioned, as well as in the techniques of modern brain-washing. If it passes into the organism without this process of digestion being completed, the food acts as a poison. It must be the element of organization, not the stuff or atoms in the food, which acts in this way. It may well be that the organism needs food so that it may unfold these digestive and metabolic activities, rather than to obtain calories, and Schrödinger may be nearer the truth in suggesting that we feed on negative entropy. In that case the essential of the digestive process is the loosening and separation of the element of form, order, organization, in physics called negative entropy, from the substance to which it is bound. But as to how we deal with this loosened, liberated element of form, we do not seem to know much.

In contrast to this a poison is an entity which penetrates the organism, getting through its skin or boundaries, and unfolds within processes belonging to outer nature. A remedy or remedial substance is a bearer of this outer activity into the inside of the organism, but chosen to correspond to its own disorder. Remedy and poison we regard as basically the same but given in the one case to a sick organism to bring about health, in the other to a healthy one to bring about disease. Dosage also can be the crucial issue, as Paracelsus argued. We can, for instance, see in digitalis therapy how very critical the dosage is, and even water in excess can bring about water intoxication. The organism can be overwhelmed by quantity as well as by quality. The problem of food, poison and remedy thus brings us into the whole question of the relation of organism to environment or, as the immunologists now say, borrowing the terms from metaphysics, of the self to the non-self.

We must now inquire into the way poisons come about in nature. In plants we are concerned with what are known as 'active principles' which are responsible for the distinctive medicinal or poisonous effects of plants. The question from one side is why, or rather how, these active principles are neither rejected by the animal system and discharged nor assimilated like food substances. The other question is where and how they occur in the plants. They are not common plant products. In the life processes of the plants they are peculiar in so far as they generally represent final products and do not re-enter the energy metabolism of the plant. The plant organization, typically, unfolds in repetition from node to node, from leaf to leaf, until it is brought to a conclusion in the blossom. The blossom arises indeed as metamorphosis of the same leaf principle, contracting in sepal, expanding again in petal, contracting in pistil and stamen, and finally expanding and contracting in fruit and seed. These various manifestations can, as we know, change into each other. The glorious 'flowers' of the delphinium are mostly formed from sepals. In the exotic house plant, the poinsettia, a deadly poison, it is actual leaves which flame, the true flowers remaining inconspicuous. The fig we enjoy is blossom, not fruit, and double flowers represent the metamorphosis of stamens into petals. Further, the colouring and scent processes of the blossom can be carried down to root and stem as in beetroots and onions. But the vegetative tendency to endless repetition is brought to a conclusion in the the blossom and we can easily see how here the plant is touched by another principle of organization — the animal.

The animal organization is characterized by interiorizing gestures and processes. It arises embryologically by complex movements of invagination, infolding; from these arise the characteristic animal organs and forms. Whereas the plant gesture is exteriorizing and repetitive, the animal gesture is interiorizing and gives rise to the separation of inner and outer, with the possibility of unfolding the inner life and experience we recognize as sensation and emotion. The close connection of the flower with the higher world of the animal is seen in its relationship with the insects which hover around the blossoms, penetrating in endless ways in the complex contrivances of pollination. The very form of many flowers becomes animalized, as we can see in the orchids, and the resemblance of sweet peas to butterflies finds expression in the name Papilionacea. One could exemplify endlessly. Another phenomenon which allows us to see these connections very clearly is the occurrence of plant galls. These arise in the plant host as a reaction around the germ and developing larva of an insect. The surprising thing is the way they come to resemble the fruit and nuts of other species. The presence of the animal organization brings about a transformation and the appearance in the realm of normal vegetative life of a fruiting process resembling even that of another species. The whole development of the flowering, fruiting process in plants represents a touching, or even penetrating embrace by the higher system of force of the animal organization. Sometimes this becomes visible in the insects or birds which play this part in pollination.

It is in the fruit and seed that protein normally develops in appreciable quantities in the plant. The proper plant substance is carbohydrate, whereas the proper animal substance is protein, which incorporates the nitrogen activity from the air with all its explosive instability and inner mobility. The presence of protein in beans and peas shows the heavy penetration of the leguminous plant by the animal principle, which is already expressed in its peculiar blossom. The majority of plant poisons belong to the loose group of so-called alkaloids. These are understandable as degradations of protein by the progressive removal of hydrogen and oxygen, a process which culminates in the production of cyanide. We know that anabolic processes characterize the vegetable kingdom and predominantly katabolic processes the animal, which is dependent on vegetable anabolism for its nourishment. The origin of alkaloids and plant poisons is to be sought, then, in the too deep penetration of this animal, katabolic activity into the plant substance. The breakdown of protein is normal within the animal organization, where it is associated with the development of conscious soul life, but when it occurs within the vegetable organization it produces poisons. The principle of animal organization, instead of just touching the plant, like rosy fingered dawn, producing protein in the seed only, plunges more deeply and with its katabolic force produces degraded alkaloids, almost as excretions. In the production of alkaloids and the other groups of 'active substances' something goes on in the plant which resembles glandular processes in animals.

There are often indications, in the outer forms and gestures of poisonous plants, of this penetration by the animal process. But it is only the production of the chemically active substances which is decisive. Often only the trained botanist knows which particular species is poisonous and which is not. This is especially the case with mushrooms, which in any case represent a very animalized form of plant existence — without chlorophyll, living katabolically on decaying organic matter. In other plant families we can trace the disturbance in differing gestures. In the hemlock (*Conium*) purple patches develop on the stem and leaves, revealing the displacement of the flowering process, and in the water hemlock (*Cicuta*) air cavities develop in the root where the virulent poison is gathered. In the Belladonna plant the dark tubular flowers are displaced down and through the plant, and in the allied thorn apple (*Stramonium*) one can observe how quickly the strongly-growing stem is cramped and the plant development frustrated. In *Colchicum autumnale* the flower is brought prematurely to birth six months before the vegetative leaves appear and the seed develops within the dark earth.

If one recognizes the different systems of organizing force, one can begin to observe their action in form and gesture and in the production of distinctive chemical substances.

We must now consider how poisons come about in the animal kingdom. They are produced by glands. Can we form any idea of what really happens in a gland, what glandular processes are? Normally we only consider the chemical composition of the secretion and calculate the energy involved in separating it and the biochemical pathways by which its components are formed. But if we consider it from another point of view we are faced with a separation of substance from the living unity of the organism, from the systems of force which enlivened it and ensouled it. What happens to these forces? Let us take the example of weeping, as a simple instance. The person is overwhelmed by an experience and the whole organism weighed down. Then a clarification occurs, grief separates into conscious emotional experience and the tears are excreted; with this the organism regains vigour. The poisoning of the whole organism which had come about through too deep a penetration of the experience into the organic has been healed. The experience is now lifted up into the realm of the soul, the emotions can be digested and absorbed, enabling the personality to grow and develop. The organic or physiological realm has been detoxicated, purged. In glandular secretions we have always to inquire not only into the chemistry of the excretion but into the psychic, emotional activities which are involved. And if we can come to understand that these psychic, emotional activities belong to the same system of organization as the animalizing forces we have previously considered, then many important connctions begin to appear.

To return to the excretion itself, which in the case of the animal venoms has been produced by the so called poison glands. There are many chemical connections and near identities between some of the vegetable and animal poisons. As examples we may mention the quinones in *Coccus cacti* which closely resemble those in *Rumex crispus*, *Sticta pulmonaria*, and *Drosera rotundifolia*; the formic acid in ants which also occurs in bacteria and mainly in the seeds of higher plants; and the bufagins of the toad which closely resemble the scillaridin of Scilla. As far as one can see, the plant poisons do not serve any useful purpose in the plant life, they do not aid its survival and are the expression simply of the exaggerated penetration of the vegetable by the animal type of organization. In a sense they are in plants what disease is in animals and man. In animals on the other hand the production of poison is intimately bound up with their behaviour and life adaptation. We have only to think of the snake or spider using its venom in catching and killing its prey, or again of the bees almost instantaneously killing any rival insect intruder into the hive. Similarly the ink of the cuttlefish is released in the elaborate escape behaviour of the creature. Whereas the penetration of the plant by the animalizing forces results in the production of poison, these forces would in the animal result in disease, were it not that the glandular processes bring about a detoxication and healing. Poison in the vegetable and disease in the animal are therefore really equivalent, and this close connection of the animal venoms and secretions with many plant poisons and active principles is understandable; they are both produced by the same system of forces.

The really distinctive reactions typical of the animal substances are, however, the allergic and immune reactions. These arise in relation to protein. They have to be distinguished from the toxic reactions in that they arise as a result of sensitization. Whilst they are very specific in this sensitivity, the reactions are fairly stereotyped according to the site of the reaction, for instance hayfever and asthma. Where the sensitivity arises to vegetable substance it is most frequently to the pollens which, as we have seen, are strongly animalized, or to fungi and moulds which show similar features. The bacteria are certainly in their metabolism also animalized, which accounts for the prevalence of immune type reactions in relation to them and their products.

So it begins to appear that the penetration of the human organism by vegetable substance which escapes digestion leads to what we call toxic processes. These are most likely to occur with what we call plant poisons. The toxic symptoms are specific to the particular poison which is often common to a family of related plants. On the other hand the penetration of the human organism by animal substance leads to the complex processes of immunity and allergy. The toxic symptoms are not specific to the particular foreign proteins, they are simply typical of an immune reaction occurring in certain tissues and cells and this differentiation is related to accidents of sensitization. What is very specific is the sensitization itself, not the particular site of action which determines the clinical picture. Hayfever, asthma, urticaria and the other manifestations are not specific to particular foreign protein but only typical of allergic reactions in general occurring in these sites.

Research is now discovering that the lymphocytes are the main active agents in sensing and reacting to foreign proteins by producing antibodies. The lymphocytes reveal themselves through form and life history as mainly vegetative. They live for long periods just circulating around blood vessels, lymphatic vessels and nodes, rather as a plant just goes on living and producing repetitively node upon node. Then one day they are touched by a foreign protein and transformations are set going. They become metamorphosed into plasma cells and start producing antibodies. It is not difficult to see that here we have a process similar to the one which transforms the plant into a blossom. The foreign protein or antigen essentially belonging to the animal level of organization acts into and arouses changes in a vegetative type of cell.

On the other hand the vegetable poisons seem to act more into the animal, psychic level of the human organism. The substances which produce the great changes in human consciousness are of vegetable, not animal, origin, such as opium, belladonna, LSD, mescaline. The specific drug pictures are expressions of the differentiating forces in man. In plants this differentiating principle shows itself mostly in the blossom, which is why the flower is of such importance in plant classification. In the human it manifests in the system of psychic or emotional forces. The immunologists, to account for the immense diversity of pre-existent antibody producers in the cell, invented a few years ago a new principle which they call the Generator of Diversity, G.O.D. for short, which does not get very far. But it is more valuable to discern that the principle which manifests in the vegetable kingdom, differentiating its essential unity into diversity, is the actual animal system of organization and that this is also active in us in our psychology.

If one accepts that all phenomena are on the same level of existence and that mechanical models are equally applicable in all spheres, then chaos arises. But if one begins to distinguish the levels of organization and the distinctive principles of organization in the different kingdoms of nature, a surprising order begins to appear. The human interiorizes the lower organisms in its organs and functions. The animal kingdom displays these functions separated in space in a sort of divine vivisection. In the human they exist in synthesis, in the animal they are displayed in analysis. In disease, when the synthesizing force is too weak, there develops the tendency of an organ or tissue to become autonomous, to become 'non-self'. Auto-immune reactions develop. In healthy digestion we exercise a synthesizing action which transforms outside nature, non-self, into self. The activation of antibodies is like the activation of complexes in the unconscious and the laws of immunology are decipherable in psychological and not mechanical terms.

I have sought in this chapter to pursue a thread through the labyrinth. We found the thread in the picture of the penetration of the outside as poison into the organism and we followed it in the strange interaction of animal and vegetable organization in the plants. In the animals and humans we came upon the fascinating realm of immunology and were forced into new views concerning the psychosomatic relationship.

A curious suspicion now arises that disease, poison, differentiation and diversity, the G.O.D. of the immunologists, are all manifestations of the same principle which in us is known as the Psyche. In its unconscious action this psychic world penetrates the organic and becomes the organic. In its conscious action we experience its endless play of emotions and become identified with it. This world of psyche is the principle of poison which has compelled the world into manifestation. We can now see that disease and poison are essential for human life and progress. Through them manifestation and consciousness come about and grow, through falling ill and overcoming illness personality develops. And if we can agree that personality and consciousness are the values and meaning of human life we should be grateful and appreciate the essential value of disease and poison.

9. Sulphur

It is often helpful to discover and study the polarities within various processes and entities. Light and dark, past and future, sleeping and waking, we always have to find our way between opposites and discover the middle realm whether colour, the present, or dreaming which arises between them. We have come upon the polarity between the metabolic system and the nerve system in man from many sides and have noted the relationship of willing to the metabolic processes and of thinking to the nerve processes whilst our feeling life plays in the rhythmic processes. Now it is not difficult to see that sulphur is related especially to the metabolic processes centred in the abdomen, whilst Phosphorus, burning with a cold flame, is equally related to the nervous system. Sulphur is connected with warmth; it burns with a hot flame and mediaeval imaginations portrayed Hell with burning brimstone. Pictures of the Last Judgment portray the archetypal configuration of Man with heaven in the brain and hell down below in a belly world. In the middle realm some souls go up and others down and Christ or Michael is usually portrayed in what we can grasp as the heart. Down below the fires of hell burn. This is the realm of sulphur and we can easily see it also macrotellurically as the realm of volcanic phenomena.

Along the north coast of the bay of Naples one comes to the Phlegraean fields. This is a strange area of pot holes and subterranean volcanism. There is Lake Avernus and Cumae where the Sibyl's sanctuary was, which Aeneas visited and which was excavated in the 1930s. The Sibyl guided him to the underworld to meet again his dead father Anchises. An underground sanctuary was discovered after the Second World War at Baia with an underground river Styx. Such may well have been the Chthonic initiation site where Aeneas carrying a branch of the golden bough and accompanied by the Sybil hazarded the fearful journey through the realms of the dead. Virgil himself came to live there and then Dante invoked Virgil as guide through hell and purgatory on the way to heaven. There is in this area, where the whole land moves up and down over the centuries exposing and submerging in turn the Roman ruins, the Solfatara. This is a volcano but not on a mountain. It is, to look at, a flat disc, some hundreds of yards across, surrounded by a low rim of hill. It is like an ulcer. In places the crust, on which one can walk, is holed and a black treacly fluid, the fango, boils away. Around the rim are occasional little vent holes and if a lighted wand of smouldering paper is waved over one of these then immediately it starts to belch forth clouds of steam and simultaneously all round the rim all the other vents, quiescent till then, also start to belch. The result seems completely out of proportion to the stimulus. One can only really understand this bewildering phenomenon by putting it together with the rising and falling of the whole land there. The land appears to be in an equipoise between levity sucking up and gravity pulling down. Only a slight stimulus is needed to move the balance see-saw.

In the phenomenon of the volcano, matter from subterranean depths is hurled upwards. Lehrs has placed this in polar relationship to the phenomenon of the avalanche. Again a slight stimulus, even a shout, can result in thousands of tons of snow tumbling down. From the upper reaches of the atmosphere snow crystals fall and gathering into flakes cover the ground in stillness with their white covering. The crystalline stillness, each crystal unique in its distinct variation of the hexagonal pattern, this infinitely differentiated white covering of the earth stands in opposition to the turbulent molten, sulphurously stenching world of the volcanos. Here we always find sulphur.

Sulphur shows itself as a substance in which the imponderable warmth is intimately interwoven with the elemental sulphur. Sulphur lies quiescent on the table in the reduced state. Only at high temperature does it combine with oxygen. But phosphorus bursts into flame on exposure to the air and has to be kept under water. The imponderable light is always trying to get free from the substance.

There are no references in Shakespeare to phosphorus, which had not yet been discovered. It was accidentally discovered in urine in 1669 by Brandt. But Shakespeare uses sulphur and sulphurous in the accepted traditional sense.

Roast me in Sulphur! Wash me in steep-down gulfs of liquid fire!
(*Othello*, V, 2)

My hour is almost come, When I to sulphurous and tormenting flames
Must render up myself. (*Hamlet* I, 5)

You sulphurous and thought-executing fires . . . (*Lear* III, 2)

Of course Shakespeare was writing out of a cultural background in which the old doctrines of the four elements and the alchemical three principles of salt, mercury and sulphur were still accepted. Robert Boyle (1627–91) is the best-known figure in the attack on these traditional ways of seeing and understanding things which led gradually to the establishment of scientific chemistry. There can be no reasonable doubt that the new age and consciousness which were coming into existence at that time called for this scientific revolution. But consciousness is again changing and in crisis in our time, and what was right three centuries ago may not be right for all time or for our present. The presentation and working out of these problems by Ernst Lehrs in *Man or Matter* seems to me to merit most careful consideration. The ancient principles Salt, Mercury and Sulphur were not substances in the modern sense. Lehrs has shown how real elemental sulphur, real elemental oxygen and so on are not experienced by our senses. They begin to appear rather as Ideas in the Goethean sense. We do not come upon elemental oxygen, O, but only O_2 or O_3. Sulphur is known to us in nature in six different metamorphic forms, the real elementary, unchanging; sulphur is not a matter of experience; it is the Idea manifesting in these different forms. In the human kingdom this ideal sulphur, which we could also call functional sulphur, manifests through all the metabolic processes. In these it warms and cooks, mixes and pervades it all with a spirit of togetherness or gregariousness. Gregariousness breaks down barriers and distinctions of class and rank. It brings about equality but in the loss of distinctiveness, consciousness is also lost, submerged in the ocean of unconsciousness or sleep consciousness. In our metabolic processes real processes go on, our will is here action but we are not conscious of it, unconsciousness prevails. It is at the nerve pole where the cold phosphoric light of consciousness burns that distinction and consciousness light up. From this pole originate hierarchy, ranks, and all the discrete differences without which dull stupor prevails. The soul submerges itself in the activities of the metabolism but separates from and reflects itself in the brain and nerve processes. In the old sense of the polarity dry and wet we can see that sulphur is wet, phosphorus dry.

We can now begin to penetrate the homoeopathic drug picture of sulphur. Warmth and sensations of burning run through the whole picture, which is not surprising. Sulphur patients are usually warm and like the colder weather and open windows. They complain of burning pains whether of gastric ulcers, of eczemas and skin diseases, of redness at the muco-cutaneous junctions of mouth, eyes, anus, vagina, urethra. The volcanic warmth process may erupt in boils or acne as examples. Further, the instability we noticed in the land in the neighbourhood of the Solfatara, appears in a corresponding instability in the circulation. Flushes particularly menopausal hot flushes but also headaches with warm feelings which may be frankly migrainous. Feelings of congestion anywhere become a key to the picture. The liver, the centre of the metabolic world is sluggish and congested and this may so to speak pile up backwards as Caspar Blond elucidated. Then arise haemorrhoids and varicosities and a multitude of disturbances within the portal circulation draining into the liver. One can also understand some eczemas as originating in the liver. If this organ does not metabolize the nutritional stream, if it is sluggish and lazy, then the skin or other organ may have to undertake these functions. The skin has to perform liver functions.

All the digestive functions belong to this sphere of activities. We can relate purgatory, purify, purges, the root *pur* being connected with fire. Sulphur therefore had a traditional use as a laxative, to purify the system, in the form of brimstone and treacle. But it also has, in potentized form, a use in early morning diarrhoeas which may even awaken the patient and drive him from bed. König showed how uch phenomena were related to the liver.

The sulphur patients are proverbially untidy and even dirty and smelly. They are so dominated by the digestive, metabolic, functions that they put these all around them. One has only to contrast them with the arsenicum patient or the phosphorus, who need to have everything tidy or elegant. These put the nervous system around them.

Sulphur mixes and combines chemically very freely. Again the typical sulphur patient is gregarious and social and even the love of argument belongs in the same direction. The argument is to irritate and get under the skin of the opponent so as to break down the barriers and establish relationship and community.

The anxiety of sulphur is the liver anxiety, anxiety depression. The sluggish liver, the sluggish metabolism are part and parcel of a torpidity of will. Therefore the demands of life which disturb the sluggishness cause anxiety. This sleepiness spreads over the nerve pole as well, causing drowsiness particularly after eating. In order to preserve the torpidity and avoid disturbance from a full waking life of thought, the sulphur patient craves alcohol. This inhibits the thinking, wakeful activity, and encourages the gregarious propensities. But the sulphur patient may awake at 3–4 am, the critical hour of the liver and be unable to sleep again till morning. Then out of the whole characterology he falls asleep, unable to face the daytime tasks.

Apart from these particular indications of symptoms and conditions calling for sulphur as a remedy, there is a much wider sphere of action. When there is with a patient a failure to respond to treatment, a continuing ill-health, or chronic conditions such as arthrosis and other rheumatic conditions, then a sulphur treatment may enliven the metabolism, and loosen and dissolve deposits. Sulphur waters at spas have an age-long tradition of effectiveness and the Fango mud is greatly valued in treating rheumatism. In homoeopathy Hahnemann introduced sulphur as his main remedy in combating the chronic miasm of Psora. It seems to me that much confusion has arisen through attempts to understand these miasms in similar terms to the modern ideas of diseases. We have seen how functional sulphur or ideal sulphur is not the same as the material forms of sulphur which we can handle. In a similar way Hahnemann's miasms should not be confused with what we nowadays call a disease. They are ideas, but ideas which manifest in various metamorphoses, are causative in a form-creating sense.

Sulphur then is a purifier, enlivener of the metabolism or anti-psoric according to the school of medicine from whose stand-point one is speaking. It brings about healing from within outwards.

10. Phosphorus

Solidity, massiveness, weight, ponderability are some of the words we use to indicate one pole of our experience of things; they indeed weigh heavily upon us and reduce us to inertia and sleep. The other pole is known to us as light through which we awaken to the created world around us, which indeed emerges from the empty chaos of darkness only when light strikes in. Light is opposed to heavy, to dark; it arouses us out of the unconsciousness of sleep to the alertness of waking conscious life. What is this light, which we cannot weigh, which has a velocity which cannot be outpaced and which we also meet as the light of understanding and as enlightenment?

Today light is grasped with concepts which belong properly to the sense of touch. Either it is handled as little particles, photons or quanta, or else it is conceived as wave-motion, vibrations, a portion only of the whole electro-magnetic spectrum. Neither approach, as far as we can understand, is more than a mathematical way of describing certain phenomena in the realm of optics as if they were material. Some of these phenomena need the concept of discrete particles and others of continuous waves for their description. Understanding the real nature of light is not attempted but it is interesting, though hardly surprising, that even in this ultra-abstract mathematical treatment, the inherent paradoxes of our understanding come to light. In our own bodily organisms we find the system of nerves and the system of the blood. The nervous system is composed of separate nerve cells, discrete entities, whilst the blood is a continuum in perpetual movement and circulation. Our concrete experience arises in the interplay of these utterly polar processes. These problems were focused in Greek times in the paradoxes of Zeno, and Leibniz's invention of the differential calculus was necessary to bring into existence the whole of modern technology. This calculus takes it that two things infinitely little different can be treated as identical. To a Greek this would have been unthinkable and to the Greek in each one of us it remains so. Through it we can handle the rational absurdity of motion.

Michael Faraday, whose genius pioneered our electrical technology, finished one of his lectures in these words:

> Assuming heat and similar subjects to be matter, we shall then have a very
> marked division of all the varieties of substance into two classes: one of

these will contain ponderable and the other imponderable matter. The great source of imponderable matter, and that which supplies all the varieties, is the sun, whose office it appears to be to shed these subtle principles over our system . . . The properties of known bodies would then be supposed to arise from the varied arrangements of their ultimate atoms, and to belong to substances only as long as their compound nature existed; and thus variety of matter and variety of properties would be found co-essential.

The importance of the imponderable element in things is asserted in these words of Faraday.

Now can we take a step into the consideration of actual examples of how the ponderable and imponderable are bound up together? We may note in passing that modern chemistry was born exactly through paying attention exclusively to the ponderable. The balance was the tool by means of which Lavoisier and his successors established chemistry, the atomic theory, the conservation of matter. The imponderable accepted by the ancients, the principle of levity, had been banished. But let us take Sulphur and Phosphorus as representing a certain polarity, a suggestion we owe to Ernst Lehrs. In sulphur the material is bound up with the imponderable element of warmth whilst in phosphorus it is united with light. Sulphur only burns at high temperature with a hot flame but phosphorus burns at room temperature with a cold flame. An immediate association is well-nigh inescapable. Sulphur is related to our metabolic processes centred in the abdomen polar to phosphorus and the cold light of consciousness in the head and brain. Phosphorus is an essential component of nerves, of the myelin sheath of nerves in particular. R. Treichler has brought forward reasons for regarding the myelin sheath as the essential nervous substance. The nerve cell and central nerve fibre are concerned with the metabolic and rhythmic processes within the nervous system, not with the true nervous processes. It is in fact doubtful whether these are accessible to empirical research. Is the brain really a brain except when we are thinking? And is the direct experience of thinking accessible to empirical research? Attendant changes, chemical and electrical, can be measured but these can only be reflections, shadows thrown into these realms by real activities in that region where we are the measurers and not only measurable objects.

The phenomena of the cold flame are familiar to us in phosphorescence. Phosphorus itself burns with a cold flame in which one can hold one's hand. It depends on ozone as distinct from oxygen, and other phenomena of phosphorescence such as the light of glow worms, fire-flies, etc. are also bound up with ozone. Today alarms are sounding because there is evidence of damage to the ozone layer in the upper atmosphere. This layer shields us from too strong exposure to the so-called ultraviolet and other radiations. But is it not also the realm where the visible light of our daytime atmosphere originates? Beyond it the cosmos appears dark.

Lucifer — Phosphorus, the Greek Prometheus, stole the light of heaven to bestow it on earthly man. He brought it to earth and was chained to the rocks of the Caucasus. Apart from the phenomena of phosphorescence, light on earth is mainly a manifestation of combustion and heat; it is bound to the material processes involved in combustion. These processes are dependent on oxygen, the more earthly form, as contrasted with the ozone, the more heavenly metamorphosis.

Phosphorus exists in three forms, yellow, red and dark red. The red form only phosphoresces in the presence of ozone. The yellow creates ozone, whilst the dark red form, the most earthly, scarcely phosphoresces at all.

Now turning to phosphorus as a remedy and the so-called homoeopathic drug picture, what do we find? We find excessive sensitivity of all the sense organs. The eyes, ears, nose in particular are hypersensitive, and there is sensitivity to cold. Phosphorus patients love to be massaged in order to soothe the excessive irritability of the sense of touch. The sense of balance is easily disturbed, giving rise to various symptoms of vertigo. In the realm of the higher senses we find sensitive responsiveness to other people and either a quickness or slowness in response to questions, the spoken word. They are, for short, over-awake in the realm of the senses, and the destructive effects of this awakeness may appear in actual destruction of the organ as for instance in retinitis and other eye diseases.

Out of this extreme sensitivity it is easy to see arising the phobias which are characteristic of the phosphorus patient. Fear is attached to particular situations or things, to the dark, to thunder and lightning. Fear of disease and death, of drowning and water, of evil, ghosts and imaginary things and many other specific fears are recorded. In all these, fear as a general experience tends to be fixed on specific situations. One could also say that anxiety arises from more general unrest into the awake pole of the nerves and senses and assumes more the nature of specific phobias. The aggravation of all these fears when one is alone emphasizes the element of fear proper as distinct from shame, both of these being components in what should be called anxiety. Shame avoids company, fear seeks it.

Another feature arising out of the overall hypersensitivity and awakeness is the need for sleep and the improvement these patients experience after even short intervals of sleep. I incline to understand their 'desire to be magnetized', mentioned in old books, in the same way. Hypnotic states and relaxation relieve the over-awakeness of the nerves and senses. Prolonged, drug-induced sleep has of course been used for breakdowns brought on by sustained and repeated fear and over-awakeness, such as was experienced by bomber crews in the late war. Bjerre, the eminent Swedish psychiatrist recorded how at the end of the last century Wetterstrand in Stockholm ran a most remarkable and therapeutically successful clinic in which fifty or more patients at a time were lying at rest in hypnotic sleep for very long periods of time.

Besides its relationship to nervous function, phosphorus has a relationship to bone both as a constituent and through enzymes, phosphatases, etc., to its forma-tion and dissolution. The skeleton has its focus of concentration in the head just as the nervous system does and these two systems may be said to manifest the element of form to its greatest extent. One can even feel how from the head pole and the nervous system flow the sculpturing, formative forces, which guide the embryogenetic development. Light is a formative force and phosphorus containing enzymes enable this 'ideal' entity to act formatively into the organism. The phenomena of rickets illustrate these connections between light, Vitamin D and proper formation of the skeleton, in which phosphorus is closely involved. In the days when industrial phosphorus poisoning was common, through the inhalation of phosphorus fumes in the manufacture of matches, 'phossy jaw' was not uncom-mon. The jaws, maxillae and mandibles, could be attacked and destroyed in a most painful and hideous condition.

Severe phosphorus poisoning can also result in acute fatty degeneration of many organs, particularly of the liver, kidney, heart and muscles. The destruction of the liver is said to resemble closely 'acute yellow atrophy' of the liver. In the days when chloroform was commonly used as an anaesthetic, a small number of patients used to suffer from jaundice due to hepatic poisoning, and in some death followed the destruction of the liver. Phosphorus in homoeopathic dosage earned a repu-tation in preventing this condition when given prophylactically. Chloroform and many other anaesthetics are taken up by the fatty substances in the brain, the constituents of the myelin sheaths of the nerves. They act polarically to the phosphorus, resulting in unconsciousness as opposed to the awakeness of function-ally acting phosphorus. That heavy material doses of phosphorus also destroy the liver is understandable. The Promethean myth is obviously related to these phenomena. Lucifer-Phosphor-Prometheus acting in the brain as the Eagle who soars aloft, the symbol of highest philosophic thought, plunges as vulture to peck at and destroy the liver. Our conscious waking life is purchased at the expense of destruction to the life-organs of which the liver, as its name implies, is the centre. That the phosphorus poisoning brings fatty degeneration to the liver could perhaps be seen as its tendency to metamorphose the liver into brain, to awaken to consciousness an organ which should remain unconscious.

When tuberculosis was common phosphorus was a frequently used remedy. It was also one of the most frequently used remedies when acute lobar pneumonia was commoner than it is today. It seems to have had a tendency to be more related to the right lower lobe of the lung, lying just above the liver. In pneumonia the lung becomes more like the liver, as the term hepatization indicates, it loses the capacity to take air into itself. Instead of air and light penetrating into the lung it becomes filled up with fluid-solid material.

The rest of the drug picture fits into these general lines of thought. The phenom-ena of tuberculosis point us to some further considerations. Patients with tubercu-losis of the lung were known to be very sensitive to the effects of sunlight. Carefully graded exposure could be helpful but too intense or prolonged amounts could bring about a severe deterioration. In bone tuberculosis the effects of sunshine were more predictably beneficial. Such relationships can lead one to envisage an inner light-metabolism. Light entering the organism must be metamorphosed into inner light else it can act as poison, in a manner comparable to other foreign entities. Outer warmth also must become metamorphosed into one's own inner warmth if it is to be wholesome. The well-known phenomena of after-images points in a similar direction. If one fixes one's gaze on a light or a coloured figure for a minute or so and then looks away at a neutral surface, then the visual form arises in complementary colour. Even if the eye is shut the forms arise and their colours can be watched going through rhythmic changes for some minutes. These phenomena point to an inner light which always confronts the outer phenomena of observation. One can observe that in many or most patients with multiple sclerosis there is a severe incapacity to produce these after-images. It is as if the outer light entering the eye and not being met by the inner light, acts destructively on the nervous system.

We can now attempt to grasp these problems more completely in relation to the universal problem of light and darkness. These themes were given incomparable expression in the essays of the Russian philosopher Solovyov on Beauty. Starting from the contrast between a lump of coal and a diamond and between a cat's caterwauling and the singing of a nightingale he shows how beauty arises in the 'transfiguration of matter through the incarnation in it of another, a super-material principle'. This super-material principle he goes on to show is an 'idea'. 'Beauty or the embodied idea is the best portion of our real world, namely that portion of it which not merely exists but deserves to exist'. In the diamond the black carbon is transfigured by light and in the nightingale's song the crude sex instinct is transfigured by love.

He goes on to determine the criterion of worthy or ideal being in general as the 'greatest possible independence of parts combined with the greatest possible unity of the whole'. The aesthetic worth is determined by the degree of complete and many-sided embodiment of this idea in the given material. From this it follows that a small degree of 'idea being' may be perfectly embodied whilst a lofty idea may be poorly embodied. He instances a tape-worm and a diamond. The ideal content of the tape-worm as an animal is indeed higher than that of even a diamond as mineral but the aesthetic value of the diamond is higher than that of the tape-worm. This latter is 'an extremely imperfect embodiment of a comparatively high idea but is aesthetically incomparably lower than a diamond which is a complete and perfect expression of the poorer idea of a luminous stone'. The stone is only illumined from outside, the animal is inwardly enlivened.

> Matter is inert and impenetrable being — the direct opposite of the Idea
> as positive all-penetrability or all-unity. Only in light is matter liberated
> from its inertia and impenetrability.

. . . The cosmic artist knows that the basis of the animal body is ugly and tries in every way to cover it up and adorn it. His purpose is not to destroy or thrust aside the ugliness, but to make it, first, clothe itself in beauty, and finally, transform itself into beauty. Therefore by means of secret suggestions which we call instinct he incites the creatures to make out of their own flesh and blood all kinds of beautiful coverings; he causes the snail to get into a fancifully coloured shell of its own making, which for the purposes of utility (if it had any) did not in the least need to be ornamental; it impels the caterpillar to put on multicoloured wings which it had itself grown, and induces fishes, birds and beasts to cover themselves completely with sparkling scales, bright feathers, smooth and fluffy fur.

. . . the cosmic mind, in obvious opposition to the primeval chaos and in secret agreement with the world-soul or nature — rent by that chaos and more and more amenable to the mental suggestions of the architectonic principle — creates in it and through it the complex and magnificent body of our universe. This creation is a process having two closely interconnected purposes, the general and the particular. The general purpose is the embodiment of the real Idea, i.e. of light and life, in different forms of natural beauty; the particular purpose is the creation of man, i.e. of the form which together with the greatest bodily beauty presents the highest inner concentration of light and life, called self-consciousness. Even in the animal world the general cosmic purpose is attained with the help and co-operation of the creatures themselves, through exciting in them certain inner feelings and strivings. Nature does not build up or adorn animals as some external material, but makes them build up and adorn themselves. Finally, man not merely participates in the activity of cosmic principles, but is capable of knowing the purpose of that activity and consequently of striving to achieve it freely and consciously.

I have quoted these brief selections from Solovyov, which of course call for full study, to help us enter into the story of the fall and redemption of light. Prometheus-Phosphorus stole the light from heaven and was bound to the rocks of the Caucasus. But his gift became the source of all the arts and crafts of man. The pure light of heaven became materialized into the warmth-light gradually permeating and transfiguring the chaos of original inert and formless matter. In human self-consciousness this light principle begins to shine again and in the attainment of the free spiritual deeds of men realizing the aims and intentions of Providence, the realm of what should be as contrasted with the necessity of what must be, we can see the redemption of Prometheus, *Prometheus Unbound*. The lost tragedy of Aeschylus was so titled and became the theme of Shelley's great poem. The immensely detailed knowledge of material processes within the human organism calls for its completion in an understanding of man which transcends the material and sets man free. Kerenyi undertook the interpretation of the Prometheus figure as the archetypal image of human existence and our studies help us to see that the inmost nature of Phosphorus becomes revealed in the Phosphorus process in Man.

11. Salt (*natrum muriaticum*)

We live in an age of continuing crisis. It is of course true that all ages of history are times of crisis, but some are more overwhelming in scope than others, just as in the life of the individual puberty and adolescence and again menopause are moments of transformation on the grand scale. Birth and death, or perhaps rather conception and death, mark the greatest of the turning points but the crisis of the noon-tide is the greatest between birth and death. Gutkind wrote of the crisis of the noon-tide:

> The terror of noon-tide is more frightful than any terror of night. It is the extreme of tension, when the height has been reached, the day can rise no more; there must be a decline.
>
> Today there is this tension; we are experiencing the suffering of limitation, of finiteness, of being able to grow no more — the suffering of death. Yet this time is no time of decadence — it is the mightiest of all world crises. The world is passing its noon-tide height; it will change, and a new thing, unheard of before, will come to pass.

From this critique of modern man we can gain a deeper insight into our troubled times. There is an immense tide of energy, a spiritual momentum gathering in the so-called unconscious. Yet this gathering pressure of libido can fundamentally find no outlet within the established forms and order of our present intellectual establishments and their embodiments, the modern nation-states. All current forms are too narrow, too limited for the vast currents of our time, and crack under the great pressure. In the midst of it all, feelings of despair and exhaustion arise and even characterize our time as one of overwhelming depression and impotence. Yet it is only the despair of the old modes of thinking unable to cope with the unheard-of new life seeking birth. The terrible crises of our days are birth-pangs. The grim and shattering experiences of the two world wars lie heavy still, unrepented, on our human conscience; in the life-time of my generation uncountable millions, probably hundreds of millions, have met their deaths in the wars and revolutions through which we have lived. Yet we must try and see these catastrophes, spasms, convulsions, more in the light of birth-pangs than of decadence. It is only the fact that the new cannot be grasped with our cold intellects that accounts for our despair and sense of impotence. 'Life has not weakened upon the earth. More vehement than ever before seems the thundering of secretly yoked suns and worlds soaring through ages', affirmed Brezina, the poet of Czechoslovakia.

The gathering hurricane of spiritual life breaks again and again against the rigid concepts of tradition, habits of thought, dead rituals of bygone times. The faces of our time betray our plight. Even a century ago the faces of our forebears were strong and full of content, whilst today the term 'faceless' has been coined to characterize a whole civilization. The old spirituality is gone and now into the faces of emptiness must come the new spirituality, born truly in the hearts and souls of the mere individuals, men, women and children. It must be a spirituality which is the expression of the free individuality, not possessed by tribal oversoul or instinctive unconscious forces. To those still seeking to be possessed, driven, moved by vast collective forces, it will therefore appear as weak and insignificant.

Against this background of our time we must seek the expression of the universal crisis in the experiences and diseases of the individual. There is no doubt that the forms of disease have greatly changed in this century and very particularly since the last war. Epidemic febrile diseases have declined in severity. Deaths from tuberculosis of the lungs have been replaced by deaths from carcinoma of the bronchus. Deaths from rheumatic carditis have given way to deaths from coronary thrombosis, myocardial infarction. Accidents are now the commonest causes of death under twenty years of age. Nervousness and sleeplessness have become well-nigh universal, so that universal sedation by day and night seems necessary for the full enjoyment of the benefits of the welfare state.

The concept of stress was introduced by Selye to cover the non-specific syndrome which occurred in response to all sorts of specific injuries at the same time as the specific responses also developed.

The post-war years have seen the accumulation of enormous new factual knowledge about the functions of the suprarenal glands and their hormones. Much of this has been in relation to the stress adaptation syndrome. There is little doubt that many disorders regarded today as stress disorders have increased in occurrence during recent decades, and the growth of the researches into these hormones seems to correspond to the growth in their importance.

At the same time, during and after the second world war, the late Dr John Paterson was noticing, in the course of his work on bowel bacteria, that an increasing number of patients showed the organism Proteus in their stool cultures. (It should be noted that the nomenclature and method of typing these organisms is according to the technique described by Dr Paterson, and based on Bach's original description.) Before the war Morgan had been the commonest organism, but Proteus became more and more common. Now in his work on the bowel organisms and nosodes, Paterson was gradually able to associate the various non-lactose fermenting organisms in the stool with specific groups of homoeopathic remedies. The main remedy associated with Proteus was *natrum muriaticum*, and

Paterson associated the greater frequency of indication for these remedies with the long stress of the war crisis. The use of the word stress by Selye is of course not quite the same, but their relation is obvious. Paterson therefore noticed that the type of reaction in the organism resulting in different organisms in the stools had considerably changed from the twenties and thirties of the century, at the same time as clinical observation showed such changes in the forms of disease, and at the same time as the interest in the suprarenal glands had exploded in the medical world.

Now John Paterson considered the keynote of the Proteus nosode and its associated group of remedies to be 'brain storms'. An obvious example of what he means is migraine. Leaving alone all the detailed maze of physiological mechanisms in the migraine attack, the term brain storm fairly characterizes the phenomena from the patient's point of view. There is often a prodromal period of tension, followed by the lightning flashes of visual spectra and the thunderclaps of headache, culminating in vomiting and followed by peace.

Now in these symptoms we can follow a certain conflict between the cool awareness of our head, very much become in our day an onlooker consciousness, and the irrational forces buried in our unconscious depths. These dynamic, ultra-dynamic forces are frustrated of expression, the onlooker's world becomes more and more shadowy and unreal and yet is unable to accept the life-giving impulses from the blood in other than recurrent convulsions, storms, crises. In English literature the figure of D. H. Lawrence gave expression to this conflict and the sexual reaction against cerebralism. Today all this has become symptomatic of the age. Youth is in rebellion against the unreal, shadowy mirage of our culture and civilization, and seeks in sex, drugs and orientalism to reach reality, experience. The question is whether what is reached is not yet still more illusory.

The characteristics of *natrum muriaticum* patients can be interpreted in these lights. Often very nice, very sympathetic persons, in ordinary life mild, they find the proximities of family life and the challenge of strong emotional relationships unbearable. As Paterson observed, they make bad wives. Under the stronger emotional challenges they become irritable, even impossible, and I think this accounts for the oft repeated phrase that they object to sympathy. It is not sympathy discreetly, tactfully, offered that they object to, but they fear to become involved, overwhelmed in an emotional situation beyond their control. They excel in a gentle sympathy which keeps uninvolved and hence many go to them with their troubles. But the deeper currents erupt in migraines and the emotional outburst which we recognize.

When we turn to associated remedies, we find *Ignatia, Cuprum, Chamomilla, Secale*. The same idea runs through them. In *Ignatia* it manifests in nervous instability and contradictoriness, in *Cuprum* in sudden cramps and angers, the cramps appearing in varied organs; in *Chamomilla* mainly in fevers and tempers. *Secale* offers a most important contribution to our task. *Secale* itself, extract of the Claviceps purpura growing on rye, gives rise mainly to cramps of digital arteries, though history suggests that the epidemics of St. Anthony's fire also gave rise to acute insanity. From the crude extract, chemical sophistication has produced many substances: ergometrine acting primarily on the uterus, ergotamine with its selective use in migraine, and lysergic acid with its characteristic psychic phenomena. Could we not call an LSD trip a psychic migraine?

John Paterson related the Morgan nosode and associated remedies particularly with the liver. The Dysentery Co. nosode he related to the heart and epigastric regions. It seems to me reasonable to relate his Gaertner to the lungs and I wish to suggest that Proteus and its remedies, including *natrum muriaticum*, find the basis of their action in the kidney and suprarenal system. I think the empirical findings of modern research justify taking kidney and suprarenal as parts of a common function. Their closely interrelated actions in the renin-angiotensin mechanisms of hypertension, the peculiar kidney phenomena in the adaptation syndrome, the role of the kidney in maintaining electrolyte balance and homœostasis, and the suprarenal influence on sodium and potassium do, I think, give a basis for thinking of these organs together. It is not by accident that the suprarenals sit like hats on the kidneys. Rudolf Steiner and his school have pointed to a higher function of the kidney, other than urinary excretion. This they have called the kidney radiation. If urine is excreted, there must be a counter thrust into the organism, the kidney radiation. Some of the phenomena of this are mediated through the suprarenals.

The kidney mostly performs an eliminatory and katabolic activity, the suprarenals more an 'inliminating', or 'incretory', and anabolic action. The pictures of Cushing's and Addison's diseases can serve quite usefully to focus our attention on an extreme form of hyperadrenal and hypoadrenal syndromes, complex and varied though these are. The hypertensive, florid, overactive pyknic Cushing contrasts with the hypotensive, pale and pigmented, fatigued, depressed, asthenic Addison.

Embryologically, both the kidney and the suprarenal gland are formed by a combination of polar forces and systems. The kidney originates in the pronephros at the cephalic pole which, as it were, calls forth the metanephros from the sacral pole. The adrenal gland also combines a nervous medullary with a metabolic cortical portion. From this inner tension of origin and function arise the rhythmic phenomena of the kidney and suprarenal function. I would draw attention particularly to the rhythmic changes in cortisol level. This level rises during the morning and there is a corresponding fall in the number of eosinophils in the peripheral blood. By 10 to 11 am these have reached a minimum, the cortisol a maximum, and this is maintained over noon-tide. In the afternoon reversal begins, and by 10 pm eosinophils are nearing a maximum, cortisol a minimum. Now *Natrum mur.* is characterized homoeopathically by a 10 am aggravation and *Chamomilla* by 10 pm aggravation. I suggest that the depressed, often hypotensive, fatigued, wasting picture of *Natrum mur.* lies in the direction of hypoadrenalism, as has often been suggested before, but also I suggest that the strong, angry, flushed, screaming *Chamomilla* who by contrast wants to be held, points rather to the hyperadrenal side of the balance.

That *Natrum mur.* quite often proves of value in rheumatoid arthritis is now understandable, and its great value after times of emotional stress, bereavement, unhappy love, when depression, fatigue, emaciation supervene, is justified. Migraine has found its place, and the peculiar combination of gentleness and irritability. *Natrum mur.* patients often have a tendency to watery secretions. They weep easily, or have watery nasal secretions, suggesting allergic rhinitis; they may have pale, watery polyuria. The water drops and drips from them, they cannot hold it and stress incontinence also arises. The whole picture is a drooping and a dripping, and this is one aspect of the condition we are studying, it represents the exhaustion of the up-building, invigorating adrenal forces. Near to it is the hypoadrenalism of *Sepia*. We can also relate the water-retaining tendency of sodium chloride.

Finally, I should like to mention the occurrence of aphthous ulceration in the mouth. I know no other remedy so likely to relieve the severe recurrent cases of this painful condition. Is it related to the equally common recurrent herpes simplex on and around the lips? The virologists say no. Are the herpes psychogenic, from the reluctance to kiss or be kissed? Do they point to a state of actual nervous exhaustion? But they come in crops, explosively, probably from the nervous system, and bring us back to Dr Paterson's brilliant characterization of this group of remedies and disorders associated with his Proteus nosode — 'brain storms'.

We have attempted to see how far one can understand this remedy, *Natrum mur.*, as the mirror of our age. The terror of the noon-tide is the terror of our time, and we have seen how this is corroborated even into detail of empirical research. Empirical research, traditional homoeopathic drug pictures, the researches of Dr John Paterson come together and even help to throw light on and build a bridge of understanding towards the remarkably illuminating ideas of Steiner and his school.

12. Lead (*plumbum*)

To explore the ramifications of the *Plumbum* drug picture let us start from common usage and experience, from myth and legend, and from the poet's imagination. Shakespeare can always, with sure eye and pen, point to the salient issues. His world vision is impregnated with the correspondences of earth and man and heaven. The response of the poet's imagination must be added to the crude responses of 'the too solid flesh' in a proving or poisoning, if we are to catch the true inwardness of the archetypal process represented by the metal lead;

> Is not lead a metal heavy, dull and slow?
> I say lead is slow, — you are too swift, sir, to say so:
> Is that lead slow which is fired from a gun? (*Love's Labour's Lost*)

> But old folks, many feign as they were dead:
> Unwieldy, slow, heavy and pale as lead. (*Romeo and Juliet*)

> Leaden age, quickened with youthful spleen and warlike rage.
> (*1. King Henry VI*)

Already the dull heaviness of old age and lead are highlighted and suddenly the contrast with the spleen bursts forth. Ancient insight always linked lead with the spleen and also with the skeleton, distinguishing the planet from its planetary sphere and the organ from its corresponding system. In this case the planet was Saturn, the outermost planet in the old models of the solar system. The polar opposition between the planet and its sphere is caught by the poet in the contrast between leaden age and youthful spleen. Today we know of the birth of cells in the bone marrow and of their graveyard in the spleen. Shakespeare seems to have known something of these processes out of his deeper understanding of correspondences:

> Thy bones are marrowless, thy blood is cold. (*Macbeth*)

The spleen seems to correspond both to anger and merriment:

> Brief as the lightning in the collied night,
> That in a spleen unfolds both heaven and earth.
> (*Midsummer Night's Dream*)

12. LEAD (*PLUMBUM*)

> If you desire the spleen and will laugh yourselves into stitches,
> follow me. (*Twelfth Night*)

Both anger and laughter can become enthused out of measure from the forces of
the spleen and everything be dulled down in the heaviness of bone and lead and
old age. As we find that silver is concerned with youth and reproduction, lead is
concerned with old age, death and perhaps resurrection.

Saturn, or Kronos as he was called in Greece, is known to us as Old Father
Time with his scythe or sickle, the figure of death and the skeleton. And yet in
Greek mythology, which may well in this case originate with the Hittites of
Anatolia or even earlier, Kronos was, before his dethronement by Zeus, ruler of
the Golden Age. He had come to power by rebellion against his father Ouranos.
Ouranos, the sky, used to come every night to mate with Gaia, the earth. She
bore him many children, amongst them six male and six female Titans. These he
hated and used to bury deep in folds of the earth. Gaia conspired with the
youngest, Kronos, and when Ouranos came at night Kronos crept out of his hiding
place and, with the sickle which Gaia had given him, castrated his Father. The
father's manhood he threw into the sea and from the foaming was born Aphrodite.
In parenthesis we might comment that the Oedipus legend seems to have even
older mythological backgrounds.

Kronos was married by his sister Rhea who bore him children. These he
promptly swallowed as soon as they were born, on account of a prophesy that he
in his turn would be dethroned by his son. There are indications that this age of
Kronos, The Golden Age, was a period of matriarchy and after Zeus, the youngest
son, had been saved by Rhea in conspiracy with Gaia and even Ouranos himself,
and had grown up and defeated his father, he is said to have established Kronos
at the outermost edge of the world where he still reigns over the Golden Age,
husband of Rhea, the goddess enthroned above all.

That Time consumes its own children is known to us all and the age of Kronos
was succeeded by the age of Zeus, the age of Space. The mystery of birth and
death for each of us is deeply connected with the coming from the realm of Time
into the realm of Space and our return again to the realm of Time.

We can now begin to see how our life experience here is bounded by the sphere
of Saturn, itself in the traditional picture, the outer limit of our solar system. The
limits of our life and space are set by Saturn — it is also true that the formal limits
of the movements of our bodies are set by the bony skeleton.

Now we can approach lead more directly. Its common uses have made it familiar
to most of us. Lead pipes have been used from Roman times and only recently
have the dangers of lead poisoning led to its replacement by other materials.
Plumbers, as their name indicates, were originally workers with lead. Lead also
has been greatly used in buildings for roofs and for sealing corners. It is used to
cover and protect cables. As lead paint it has been used for protection against the

weather and it has played a great part in the glazes on china and pottery. In these uses it has set limits and protected against outside penetration. In electrical accumulators it stores and locks up the elusive electricity and again it offers the greatest protection against the penetration of radiations such as X-rays.

It is used in manufacture of pigments of striking colour and these pigments show little translucency, reflecting the light from their outermost surface and allowing no penetration. It is lead, too, which added to glass conveys added brilliance approaching that of diamonds. Here indeed we approach the paradox of lead again, the brilliance and colours concealed within its dull grey exterior, the renewal within death.

Lead has played a very great part in the history of the written word. Lead was used to write on paper before graphite became the core of lead pencils and lead type became a central material in the printing processes. The living word became imprisoned on the paper, paralysed.

Lead occurs mostly in the Western hemisphere; even in antiquity it was found in Western Europe, in Spain. At Broken Hill in Australia zinc deposits are found under the lead, and this reversal is commonly found, with the heavier lead lying nearer the surface whilst the lighter zinc is more deeply concealed. The commonest form of lead ore is galena, lead sulphide, heavy grey metallic-looking crystals in which the sulphur nature is entirely locked up and paralysed in the lead. Mostly it is found in rocks of calcium carbonate and associated with silver. This association of lead and silver together is very striking, a conjunction of polar opposites. Lead is also found as cerussite, lead carbonate, consisting of lattice structures of interlacing crystals resembling the structures found in the heads of our long bones. As green lead ore, pyromorphite, chlorophosphate of lead, it reveals similarity of structure to apatite, a natural phosphate of lime. Lead, then, shows strong connections in nature with limestone, calcium carbonate and with calcium phosphate, and in man 90% of lead gets stored in the bone.

Chemically lead combines easily with acids, alkalis and other elements, but these are mainly insoluble, and so reactions are quickly sclerosed and paralysed. It is notably averse to water. Its crystalline compounds have no water of crystallization. Its ores are completely moistureless. Water is essential for all chemical reactions, and for life itself to manifest. It is not surprising therefore to find that lead is a powerful poison, really antipathetic to all life processes. In its bivalent compounds it is closely related to calcium and in its tetravalent to silica.

It is soft yet brittle, and has very low conductivity of heat and electricity, but it expands and contracts strongly in response to heating and cooling. It has a dull grey appearance, lacks resonance, even absorbing and deadening vibration, yet to the touch feels rather soft and warm and oily.

Whilst its chief ore galena is gloomy like lead itself, many of its more uncommon ores are of very bright colour, mostly yellows, oranges and red, full of inner fire, as in croconite and wulfinite. In this we again glimpse the inner paradox of lead, heavy deadness opposed to inner fire. We can contrast its relationship to light with that of silver. Silver salts are broken down by light and the silver set free can assume the whole range of colours according to the colours of the light to which it is exposed. Lead and its salts are not changed by light, but the light itself is taken hold of and united strongly with the darkness of their own substance, giving rise to the stable, strong, impenetrable colours. Or else, as in the refraction of the light in lead glass, very brilliant spectra are produced. Silver points to the substantial changes characteristic of the metabolic processes, lead to the sensory phenomena of the nerve processes.

However, we must also take note of the bivalent and tetravalent forms of lead. Bivalent lead is related to calcium and barium and other metals of the same group. Through calcium lead is related to the bones, and barium and lead are important in the treatment of arteriosclerosis and related conditions. Tetravalent lead is more related to silica which is a polar opposite to calcium and related more to the nerve and sense systems. Hence it is understandable that the lead additives in petrol, such as tetraethyl lead, work their destructive actions mostly in the nervous system. But even before the introduction of these compounds older forms of lead poisoning had been known to produce their neurological syndromes. In his helpful review of modern work on lead toxicity P. Fisher draws attention to progressive muscular atrophy, or motor neurone disease. It has been 'recently' recognized that a condition indistinguishable from this disease can be caused by lead poisoning. Dr Richard Hughes in his *Manual of Pharmacodynamics* draws attention to the striking similarity between progressive muscular atrophy and effects of lead poisoning, mentioning that Trousseau admitted the differential diagnosis to be difficult. Hughes had drawn attention to their similarity in 1869 and advocated the homoeopathic use of *Plumbum* in this disease as well as in paralysis of extremities, particularly of the extensor muscles as in the famous 'wrist drop'.

Fisher also draws attention to a synergy in the actions of lead and alcohol in porphyria and in their effects on the nervous system. This is important. He does not give an explanation of the classic symptom of chronic lead poisoning, the colic, with painful spasms and indrawn abdominal muscles and severe constipation, although he compares it with the similar symptoms in porphyria.

When we try to draw these observations together for clinical use we have to admit to much uncertainty, largely due to inadequate use of this remedy in serious diseases or in trials.

Its usefulness in arteriosclerotic conditions has led to a fairly wide use. Experience has shown that it is most effective when given for some one or two months at a time in 10th potency. It seems particularly helpful when combined with honey in the preparation *Plumbum melitensis* (Scleron A). When the sclerotic phenomena are mainly cerebral, higher potencies, 20x or 30x, are more helpful. It would also seem sensible, and much experience has confirmed it, that prophylactic courses of such treatment should be instituted in persons with hereditary or constitutional tendencies to sclerosis. It would be important to compare *Plumbum* with the *Baryta carb.* and *Baryta mur.* often used in homoeopathy. They are of course closely related.

It has been used in the treatment of chronic, obstinate, painful constipation with hard and lumpy stools; when associated with colic and when firm pressure relieves the pain, the indication for *Plumbum* is even stronger. The spasms have been described as present also in the rectum and make one think of this remedy for those prone to proctalgia fulgax. These abdominal symptoms play a large part in the classical drug pictures, but I have the feeling they are not so much used by modern homoeopathic physicians.

Anthroposophical physicians have used *Minium* (red lead oxide) in the treatment of chronic alcoholics. It has been used in 3x and 6x doses (obviously for limited periods of time) and the similarity of its action to alcohol enables it to offer a mirror effect whilst the personality is helped to regain strength for the battle.

Cerussite (lead carbonate) has proved very helpful in controlling the pain from bone metastases in malignant disease. Here sub-cutaneous injections of the 8x potency have been most useful. It might also be helpful in the not very common disease myelosclerosis.

The use of lead in neurological conditions has probably been neglected. Apart from the interesting suggestions both from Richard Hughes and modern workers as to its relevance in amyotrophic lateral sclerosis, it is probable that very little work has been done with it. Lead in potency could probably increase the elimination of lead from the body and therefore might be useful in conditions where decalcification of bone leads to freeing of lead into the circulation. It might therefore be, at least, protective in these circumstances. It seems that the action of lead on the nervous system is complex, partly involving the myelin sheath of the nerves and partly interfering in synaptic transmission. Traditionally, in classical homoeopathic literature, its use was recommended in epilepsy and motor paralyses of the 'wrist drop' type.

The toxic effects on the kidney were certainly made use of by earlier generations of homoeopaths. The gout mentioned in the literature was probably brought about by the failure of the kidney to eliminate urates and the hypertension was probably also secondary to kidney damage.

Lead poisoning is particularly associated with abortion and there seems to have been a widely held opinion that even the wives of men who worked with lead were especially prone to abort. In this respect lead is polar to silver which promotes fertility.

In children in whom bone formation is disturbed, as in rickets, lead has proved helpful and in children of a too dreamy disposition potencies of lead have been shown to alert them. This of course relates with the observations of the hyperkinetic children suffering from lead poisoning.

It is interesting that whilst nearly all lead poisoning results from inhalation of dust or vapour, the lung is one of the few organs little affected by the poison.

Slowly a picture emerges. Lead is indeed a death-dealing poison. It destroys the life processes everywhere, it puts limits to our existence in space and time. But without these death processes in us we should never wake up, we should only dream.

The death processes in us come in especial expression in the bony skeleton and nerve-sense system, both of which grow from their centre in the head. The action of the nerve system is really an inhibitory function, a paralysing force, and lead acts in a similar way. Lead wants to bring everything to rest, to death. The victim of chronic saturnism becomes cachectic, pale, lethargic, melancholic, just skin and bones.

Yet, to return to Shakespeare, we come in the *Merchant of Venice*, to the scene when Bassanio opens the leaden casket and finds the portrait of Portia within. Not within the golden, nor the silver caskets, but within the dull leaden one lies the image of this ideal woman. Full of wisdom she is, but a wisdom transformed by the quality of mercy. Full of love, but bubbling with mischievous fun and wit.

What was written on the leaden casket?

> Who chooseth me must give and hazard all he hath.

And how did Bassanio address the lead?

> But thou, thou meagre lead,
> Which rather threatenest than does promise aught,
> Thy paleness moves me more than eloquence;
> And here choose I: joy be the consequence!

The appeal of the silver and gold caskets has been emotional, that of lead certainly not. Bassanio's 'And here choose I' makes clear, the choice is a challenge to the very ego, and the decision a free decision of the individuality, opening the door to a new destiny and not merely the satisfaction of old desires.

Lead therefore, according to Shakespeare, is related to the ego, the spiritual kernel of Man. It is this which gives the human form to the skeleton, with its uprightness and head balanced supreme over all. It also finds external expression in the outer form, where the senses are concentrated. Lead poisoning destroys this form, but lead in the right amount is necessary for its development. The ego also works destructively within the human organism, our wide-awake consciousness being purchased at the cost of death. At this moment in the development of Man, when self-consciousness and the possibility of freedom are achieved, the choice lies open. Bassanio avoided the temptation to lower desires and attained to the vision of reality of Portia representing the path to higher spiritual wisdom. A wisdom, however, which also sought to enter into and transform the worldly Venice, not merely to live in blissful contemplation on the heights of Belmont.

At such moments we need the enthusiasm for the spiritual and it is perhaps this that the spleen offers. Where the blood dies, forces are set free which the ego can transform into enthusiasm for spiritual ideals, which is to say, in other words, ideals for the whole, the whole world, the whole mankind, eschewing the partial and sectarian interests that seduce us. Lead then is not only a danger of our time but a challenge to our highest endeavours.

13.   Tin (*stannum*)

Let us take it in a provisional, heuristic way, that the ancients' intuition or their clairvoyant sense of the correspondences between the cosmic, telluric and human realms may have been in some way true. It may be that if we accept them in a provisional sense we can come upon relationships between various phenomena that would otherwise escape us. Let us then consider the age-old correlation between the planet Jupiter, the metal Tin and the Liver. The planet Jupiter was also related in some way to the god Jupiter, the Roman Zeus. That the root *Ju* is related to Zeus is evident and so the Romans in giving the name Jupiter to Zeus emphasized the fatherly side of the supreme god at the expense of his child aspect which constituted a major element in the Greek myths. There is also the Latin Jove from which comes jovial:

> Our jovial star reigned at his birth. (*Cymbeline* V.4)

Is there no etymological relationship to joy, and through the French *je* to I and even Yahweh, 'I am the I am'? At any rate, after the overthrow of Kronos, Zeus-Jupiter became supreme god of Olympus. The world government was distributed between him and his two brothers Poseidon and Hades. Zeus received the realm of air, Poseidon the oceans and Hades the subterranean kingdom of the dead. However, as Seltman emphasized, the earliest Hellenic tribes to come down into Greece, the Minyans, had as their supreme god Poseidon and it was only a later tribe, the Achaeons, who named the supreme god Zeus. It is even possible, as he points out, that Zeus and Poseidon were not only brothers but one and the same supreme god. In any case, historically Poseidon was the senior and in the hilarious story in the *Odyssey* of the adultery of Ares with Aphrodite, it was Poseidon, not Zeus, who was not amused and as the senior god amongst the Olympians restored seemly decorum. There may be then some justification for associating Zeus-Poseidon with the watery realm.

Zeus is also most intimately related to Prometheus; both are sons of the Titans. In the great war which Zeus waged against the Titans, Prometheus sided with him. To a great extent Zeus's victory was thanks to Prometheus. As the story further relates, Prometheus had compassion on the race of mortal men, whom Zeus was leaving to their fate, and stealing the fire from heaven bestowed it on men and undertook to teach them the arts and crafts needed for survival and bettering their lot. Zeus was enraged and, also because Prometheus possessed a secret essential for Zeus to know, he had him chained upon the rocks of the Caucasus. There, as we know, an eagle came from Zeus every day to gorge upon the liver of Prometheus which grew again every night. Eventually, after the eagle is shot by Herakles and the centaur Cheiron has offered himself as sacrificial substitute for Prometheus, Zeus and Prometheus are reconciled. It would seem as if Prometheus comes to represent the chthonic, underworld, side of Zeus which in Zeus' ascent to an exclusively Olympian respectability has been, as the psychologists would say, repressed. We could also describe the events as Zeus' battle with and ultimate integration of the shadow. What is more, the reconciliation is brought about through the action and mediation of the sun hero Herakles.

We have now Zeus reigning on Olympus over the world-encompassing and ruling thoughts, Prometheus active and willing in the metabolic realm of the liver, which in all of us is subjected by day to katabolic destructive processes and at night is restored through anabolic reconstructive processes. Between them Herakles, who as a sun hero is related to the heart, mediates.

Liver, Brain and Heart, These sovereign thrones. (*Twelfth Night* I.1)
and:

Which I will add to you, the liver, heart and brain of Britain.

(*Cymbeline* V.5)

Related to the liver is the whole muscular system, as we can see for instance in the complementary glycogen metabolisms. The will comes to expression in motion and action largely through the liver and muscle system. We saw in our discussion of lead a similar relationship between the spleen and skeletal system. In the ancient view, the planets and organs correspond, whilst the planetary spheres and systems are correlated.

These considerations lead us to grasp the Zeus-Jupiter function in the world-ordering creative imaginations, the thunder and lightning, from Olympus. Also we can pursue the same function when Prometheus leads man into action and mastery of the earthly realm through the arts, crafts and technologies of civilization. We have also glimpsed an opening into the watery realms through the close connection between Zeus and Poseidon. In the Athens museum is a superb statue of Zeus or Poseidon prepared to cast thunderbolt or trident. It is uncertain whether the statue is of Zeus or Poseidon.

We must now turn to the metal tin and see what are its main characteristics and what purposes it has mostly served.

Tin enters upon the human scene at a very early date, probably 4000 or even 5000 BC. It became of major importance in the manufacture of bronze, an alloy of copper and tin. Copper by itself is too soft for the manufacture of weapons and tools. Tin confers on it a capacity of firmness and strength of form, so that the bronze swords carried all before them until the later arrival on the scene of iron. It is not certainly known where the first sources of tin were found. It was probably very early, 2000 BC perhaps, that the tin of Cornwall was discovered in the streams and became a major item in the commercial trading in the Mediterranean dominated by the Phoenicians. Incidentally, Britain had had a large export trade before this, of flint arrow heads from Grimes Graves on the Norfolk-Suffolk borders. Flint knappers continued to work at Brandon until after the Second World War.

Tin occurs in Cornwall in the form of cassiterite, tin oxide. Today the world's main sources of tin are found in South East Asia and in Bolivia. Cassiterite, when pure, occurs as clear brilliant crystals, tetragonal in form. Usually, however, it is brown or black, from traces of iron. It may occur in fibrous woody form. It is found mainly in granite which it modifies by its presence. In the Bolivian fields, the main tin ore is tin pyrites, a copper-iron-sulpho-stannate.

Tin as a metal is shiny, silvery, soft. It can be bent and then emits the 'tin cry'. This arises from the crystalline structure of the metal. So we find it, at the same time, almost fluid and yet crystalline and rigid. It has peculiar relation to warmth. It has a low melting point, at 232°C, but a rather high boiling point, 2300°C. It maintains a fluid state over an exceptionally broad temperature range. Further, we find that if tin is kept for any length of time in the cold it is reduced to a powder. It develops 'tin sickness', and this is even to some extent infectious. If tin below the temperature of 18°C is scratched and some of this powdery tin rubbed in, the transition from the soft ductile tin to the powdery form is greatly speeded up. On the other hand when tin is heated to above 160°C, instead of becoming softer it suddenly becomes harder and brittle. These three modifications of tin correspond to three different crystal systems, cuboid, tetragonal and rhomboid.

One can perhaps see in these relations of tin to warmth a certain rejection of the usual responses. It refuses to soften with heat, and instead of hardening with cold, it powders. Further, having melted, it retains the fluid state for a long time before it consents to vaporize. Tin seems in its reactions to heat to show a peculiar relation to form. In the solid state it can change its crystalline structure easily with changing temperature, but in the liquid state it shows a prolonged resistance to further change. Is this perhaps an echo, within the purely mineral realm, of Zeus' characteristic proneness to change shape, particularly in pursuit of his erotic intentions?

In its many alloys somewhat similar tendencies manifest. In bronze, tin confers form and resilience on copper, and in pewter it does the same for lead. In other alloys such as the babbitt metals, alloys with antimony and copper, it confers a softness and pliability which have been used in bearings. A further closely related realm is the solders used to unite other metals. Here easily fusible alloys of tin are used to join other less fusible metals. It forms a solid joint between two other harder metals, whereas in the case of bearings the join is freely mobile. Again tin seems to play in a realm between form and formlessness.

Tin has played an important role in dyeing, as a mordant. Here again it confers a permanence in fixing the dye to the fabric and it also in some instances brings out the colour in the colourless vegetable extract. Colour arises in the interplay of light and darkness, as Goethe demonstrated. When a light source is viewed through a dark translucent medium it appears reddened. And when a dark, black, surface is viewed through a lightened translucent medium it appears blue. These phenomena can be seen in the sunset and in the blue sky. Does tin act, in producing colour from colourless extracts, by acting as a joint between the lightness and darkness in the fluid? Without it the dynamic relationship between light and dark necessary for the appearance of colour is lacking.

Can we at this stage perceive something of the tin nature, of its peculiar character? Firstly we have noted its unusual relation to form, manifesting pliability yet crying when bent, fluid and crystalline at the same time. Then secondly we have noted its relation to joints, both solid soldered ones and freely running bearings. Thirdly we have recalled its use in alloys such as bronze and pewter, and in type metal, to confer firmness of form, a character echoed in its use as a mordant. Finally we may mention its use in tin plate where the tin surfaces preserve the form and integrity of the steel and of the food contained in tin cans.

For a metal associated with the supreme God of Olympus, tin does seem rather unimportant, lacking in the sort of industrial or artistic uses we might have expected. It is after all mostly as an alloy that it has been used. But Zeus's own sphere of action was the airy realm and so we should perhaps not expect to find the character of tin strongly active on the solid physical plane. Zeus would seem to represent the ruling thoughts, the living forms, those ideas that as Types and Species actually create and bring about the determination of living beings. To grasp the reality of this realm we must overcome the Nominalism of our time and attain to a new experience of Realism. These ruling thoughts should be sought in the sculpturing forces of the organisms. In the embryo the head forms first and from it gradually grow down the trunk and limbs. It is reasonable therefore to look for the seat of these sculpturing, formative forces in the head. These are the Zeus-Jupiter forces. But since the victory of Nominalism, thoughts have become mere names, powerless to effect anything, no longer Types but typed. The living word, the Logos, has fragmented into bits and pieces, as tin itself becomes powder under the influence of cold. But in the same way as this powdered tin is restored to its 'metallic' form under the influence of heat, so can our dead and abstract thoughts be enthused with new life and become the means of perceiving the realm of the ruling ideas. These normally we experience only as images reflected in the silver mirror of the brain.

So now we are led over into the realm of the Will, that mysterious region which escapes our conscious attention, but which makes real and gives life to all our shadowy existence of dreams and images. Out of primordial unity, mankind had to experience the gradual separation of will and idea which in Greek mythology became the separation of the upper Gods from the lower Gods. The upper gods of Olympus are ruling still in the realm of our nerves and senses, producing the whole phantasmagoria of our vision of the world. In the inner world of our metabolic organs and processes are to be sought the mysteries of the Unconscious which were the realm of chthonic gods of the ancients.

As we have already noticed, Zeus had originally a chthonic depth to his being. Only with Homer did his Olympian shining aspect become clarified and the separation of the domains of Zeus, Poseidon, and Hades established.

The chief or central organ of the metabolism is the liver and this was associated by the ancients and by Paracelsus and the alchemists with the planet Jupiter and the metal tin. So we find Zeus-Jupiter not only in those ruling thoughts emanating from our head pole, but in the great metabolic centre of real material processes in the liver. This raises the question of the relation between the lower organs of our trunk and our head. Shakespeare, who still lived at a time when the correspondences of macrocosm and microcosm were part and parcel of cultural inheritance, pointed clearly to liver, heart and brain for the realms of will, feeling and thought. Let us take it that the liver is psychosomatically speaking the central organ of our will, together with its metabolic counterpole in the muscular system. This then must represent the chthonic side of Zeus which is closely related to Prometheus. The name Prometheus signifies foresight, which is certainly an attribute of our unconscious and our will, whilst his brother Epimetheus possessed only hindsight, the knowledge of our reflective, mirror, head consciousness. In the myth it was Epimetheus who was seduced by the fake beauty of Pandora and in opening her box let loose all ills on mankind, Hope only remaining. It seems that here is portrayed that basic split in human nature to which Socrates referred in his utterance that all men were mad, only some knew it and others did not, Socrates being one who knew it. The great American psychologist Trigant Burrow substantiated this in his fundamental and constructive critique of Freudian psychoanalysis, laying incidentally the basis of group analysis and synthesis. The split, in terms of our modern jargon, is between the consciousness of the brain and the consciousness or rather unconsciousness of the sympathetic nervous system and the belly world. In Greece, at Delphi, the two gods Apollo and Dionysos, both sons of Zeus, had their sanctuaries. Apollo was representative of the upper and Dionysos of the lower gods. They divided summer and winter between them. Nietzsche focused our attention on the Apollonic and Dionysiac, contrasting impulses in Art which were reconciled in Greek tragedy. We should be able to see in this whole Greek world a preparation, as much as in the Hebrew world, for Christianity and its saving utterance 'I and my Father are one'.

It is of course true that all the organs of the trunk appear again in the head which is indeed the synthesis, polar to the body as analysis. For example the molluscs are at the same time female genital organs and heads. The birds are at the same time lungs and the thoughts on which we fly. And so with the rest of our inner organs. Gradually we must establish the dialogue between the two modes of head and trunk, between synthesis and analysis, noting that the head is indeed structurally the synthesis, but the seat of our analytical thinking, whilst the trunk is analysis into distinct organs, but the seat of our synthetic consciousness or will.

We must now turn to the drug picture of *Stannum* as developed in homoeopathy together with extensions of its use in practice.

The outstanding feature in all accounts is of great fatigue and weakness both of body and mind. There is no will or ability to do anything. A few steps exhaust, and on going to sit down the knees and legs give way, so that the patient drops into the chair. With this weakness there is aching and fatigue in any and every portion of the body. A characteristic mentioned in the accounts is that the weakness in knees and legs is greater when going downstairs than upstairs. Further, there is a particular weakness of the voice, both in speaking and singing. Any speech exhausts and the voice itself may be hoarse. There is no will to contemplate or carry through any task. There is depression, in the sense that depression is not an emotion, like sadness, but a paralysis or weakness of the will. There is also a headache, as if overworked, and a difficulty in raising the head. With the depression there is irritability, dislike of others speaking and a restless anxiety which quickly exhausts. The descriptions easily fit the picture of Anxiety-Depression. That this often arises from the sphere of the liver is made manifest in hepatitis in its subjective aspects. A symptom in the *Stannum* picture also points in this direction: nausea or vomiting from the smell of cooking. The weakness extends also very much to the female genital system, manifesting in symptoms of prolapse and leucorrhoea, similar to those of *Sepia*. Richard Hughes seems to have found it a major remedy for such conditions and *Sepia* also has depression and irritability and other symptoms pointing to liver affinities. The peculiar symptom 'weakness more marked on descending than ascending stairs' fancifully relates to the probability that Zeus was weaker descending to lower realms than in his own true home on Olympus.

The next important sphere of action in the homoeopathic drug picture is that of chest diseases, bronchitis and perhaps tuberculosis characterized by profuse sputum and exhausting coughs. The sputum is described as yellow or green and sweet-tasting and there is also described a hollow empty sensation in the chest, a sensation again relating *Stannum* with *Sepia*. The profuse expectoration, taken together with the profuse leucorrhoea and another symptom, swollen ankles, helps to build a bridge to a valuable new field of action opened up by the anthroposophical school of medicine — that of oedemas and disturbances of the fluid organization. But before considering this, we may follow the ascent of *Stannum* from liver to lung, to speech weakness, to the headaches. These are often migrainous and, arising slowly in the morning, reach a climax in the middle of the day, and gradually decline towards evening. We are reminded of *Sanguinaria*, a close relative botanically and pharmacologically of *Chelidonium*, which also shows this ascent or metamorphosis from liver to bronchitis or pneumonia, to tracheitis sinusitis and migraine. *Sepia* also, of course, rises from uterus to liver to head, and we recall how Zeus once had a severe migraine which turned out to be labour pains culminating in the Caesarean delivery of Pallas Athene from his skull. The tracing of a theme through the different organic functions can be of great help in interpreting the drug pictures, of gradually revealing the essential unity that underlies the confusion of symptoms.

One of the themes in *Stannum* has to do with the fluid organization. Are we here in the realm of Poseidon-Zeus? The liver is a watery organ, its very name indicates its relationship to life whose very own element is water. The life-liver process can be grasped physiologically, not anatomically, as pervading the whole organism. The liver itself can suffer from congestive, dissolving liquifactions on the one hand and from sclerotic hardening, drying processes on the other, culminating in acute yellow atrophy at one extreme and cirrhosis at the other. We can look for comparable processes elsewhere in trying to discover something more of the *Stannum* range of action.

Stannum brings inner organization, formation, into the fluidity of the organism. This watery realm should be a living whole. When some of the fluid-watery element falls out of the organic wholeness it tends to form oedemata, ascites, pleural effusions, effusion into joints, and in children hydrocephalus. In all these conditions *Stannum* has been found useful. The joint effusion leads on to the *Stannum* action in arthritis. *Plumbum* acts right into the bony skeleton, but *Stannum* works only as far as the gelatinous cartilage. It has been found of use in revitalizing cartilage in arthrosis, a drying condition, as well as in fluid exudations. The Zeus-Jupiter forces work to give inner form, the ruling thoughts, to the substantial processes, into the fluid and as far as the cartilaginous processes. This play of softening and hardening, of loosening and tightening is well seen in the whole muscular system. How much of the sculpture of the body, outwardly seen, is due to the play of muscles. There is a commonly used expression 'to loosen his tongue' which leads us further. The tongue plays a great part in giving form to our words, further it tastes our food, a process entirely within the fluid element, discerning the inner form of substances. Does not the liver continue this chemical tasting right into the unconscious depths of the metabolic processes? Now it has been found that the content of tin in the tongue is as much as ten times its average distribution in other organs. Only in the skin does the tin concentration approach that in the tongue. Here in the tongue we find the acme of the plastic activity of muscle, enabling us to achieve the plastic modelling of words and speech. Here, in the tongue, we find the most conscious achievement in the whole range of the chemical, metabolic, mostly unconscious processes. Taste has become extended to cover aesthetic appreciation and judgment. We speak of good and bad taste in matters of art, though we may not all agree on what is good taste. Here the most subtle discernment of the inner and outer forms and of their harmonious unity comes into play.

Finally let us look once again at the soul manifestation of the *Stannum* process. We have noted particularly the depressional pole with inertia of the will, but the liver can be the source not only of depression but of manic overactivity:

I will inflame thy noble liver, And make thee rage (2 *Henry IV*. V.5)
as against:

Reason and respect make livers pale and lustihood deject

(*Troilus and Cressida* II.2)
So Treichler out of a large psychiatric experience draws attention to the value of *Stannum* in manic-depressive disorders. It has its use in awaking the inert will in depression and in helping to establish balance between the manic and depressive poles.

In less serious conditions such as premenstrual tension and fluid retention I have found it of great value together with *Sepia*. Most often I have used *Sepia* 30 weekly and *Stannum* 6 twice daily.

With the extended study of tin, as here attempted, the impression grows that we are only at the beginning of the therapeutic uses of this metal. It will certainly need concerted efforts to determine which preparations of *Stannum* and which potencies should be used in differing conditions and circumstances. Thus we may find a powerful remedy for overcoming our discouragements and the agnostic atomism of our thinking and, with Zeus and Prometheus reconciled, find again the way for our tongues to speak truth.

14. Iron (*ferrum*)

It would be difficult to overstate the importance of the metal iron in the three kingdoms of nature any more than in the human organism itself or in the civilization in which we live. This civilization is a definite phase of the Iron Age and we can look back to earlier civilizations before the use of this metal was mastered. There are in myth and legend many pointers to the origins of the iron age. The figure of the smith arises mighty in the great Finnish epic the *Kalevala* and we all know the verses of 'Under the spreading chestnut tree'. My own childhood memories are full of the magic of the village blacksmith with his forge and bellows and the hammering of the burning red horseshoes. The hammer beats of the pulse here met the breathing rhythms of the bellows and we stood spellbound before the open mysteries. Across our country are many memories of Wayland the Smith and we can trace his ancestry to the great source of human freedom in the figure of Prometheus and to the Olympian Hephaestos. Today when the figure of the blacksmith is lost to our village life we can nevertheless in the iron foundries and mighty steelworks experience on a gigantic scale these same basic themes.

Iron is the fourth commonest element in the earth crust known to us, coming in order after oxygen, silica and aluminium. It is essential to vegetable and animal life and of course to human life on earth as well. In haemoglobin it enters as a quantitatively important constituent into the blood organ, contrasting with those metals whose more qualitative presence is required in only trace amounts. It is strange therefore that its use as a remedy in medicine is relatively limited, in academic medicine to supplement the natural sources in food in cases of iron deficiency anaemia and in homoeopathic medicine to the rather thin indications for *Ferrum met.* and *Ferrum phos.*

I believe that there should be a greatly extended therapeutic use for this metal and I hope to point to some of the fields in which it can be a healing agent. Indeed it does seem to me that as we approach the parts that this metal plays in various natural realms we begin to see it as a healing force, a real undoer of poisoning over a wide range of phenomena.

The principal iron ores are distributed in the northern temperate zone where they lie close to large coal deposits. Iron in the metallic state occurs on the island of

119

Disko off Greenland, in meteors and finely distributed in various basalt rocks. The main ores are the sulphides, oxides, carbonates and hydrates. The main sulphur ore is pyrites which is almost metallic in appearance; here the iron overcomes the sulphur. There are various forms of these iron sulphides. When exposed to air and water the ores are changed to rust and salts, they are stable only if imprisoned and protected in deeper layers of rocks. With oxygen, iron forms ferrous and ferric oxides and the ferrous salt of ferric acid occurs as magnetite, notably at Kirunavara in Sweden. As ferric oxide it occurs as haematite which gives a reddish colour to the rocks, whereas ferrous oxide conveys a greenish colour to olivine for instance. With carbon dioxide it forms carbonates, such as siderite which bears striking resemblances to calcite. This siderite can dissolve in carbonic water to form bicarbonate of iron. In this form it appears in the chalybeate springs. The changing seasons bring about varying concentrations of carbon dioxide and iron in the water. With water, iron forms various hydrates important in the German deposits. Arsenic occurs in combination with sulphur and iron in the form of arsenical pyrites and here we can see that iron can subdue both sulphur and arsenic, rendering the latter non-toxic. Iron also combines with arsenic acid to form insoluble scorodite.

Hauschka has pointed to the appearance of two main dynamic tendencies in the crystallization or rather the pattern of crystallization of iron compounds. Firstly there is a radial formation most clearly seen in marcasite, a centripetal radial pattern of crystals being especially characteristic. Secondly a tangential arrangement is typically found in haematite and limonite. These two tendencies are further combined in spiral arrangements as in many examples of siderite:

> The spiral tendency always arises when time enters space and develops towards a centre. The fact that this dynamic shows up so clearly in iron ores points to the fundamental role played by the iron process, for it transforms spherical forces quite unrelated to the laws of the earth into radial forces working towards a centre. Or we can say that the function of iron is to help cosmic, weightless elements to enter the sphere of gravity.

This is a characteristic of iron to be found at every level of its functioning.* We have noted the capacity of iron to unite with arsenic, rendering it non-toxic, and have seen that in pyrites the metallic nature of iron masters and overcomes the sulphurous tendencies. It further has the capacity to combine with cyanide to form the prussian blues and ferrocyanides and render the cyanide harmless. In the chalybeate springs, the changing seasons dissolve or precipitate the iron compounds, showing how iron responds to these rhythmic processes of the earth. We also find that in its compounds with oxygen, the ferrous and ferric oxides, it shows a wonderful responsiveness to light. These two forms easily change into each other, the iron taking up and giving up oxygen with equanimity and showing no

* Hauschka, *Nature of Substance*, p. 176.

preference for the bi- or tri-valent forms. Light is a powerful agent for converting ferric to ferrous oxide. These phenomena led Pelikan to characterize iron as the 'breather among the metals'. A further example of the detoxicating function of iron is found in the rivers and seas. Lead, copper, arsenic, mercury and other metals are constantly being washed down to the seas where they would make life impossible were it not for the hydroxide of iron washed down with them which combines with them and precipitates them to the floor as mud.

Not only is iron responsive to light and the warmth of the seasons, it is also responsive to magnetic fields and takes up magnetism. Pure iron is soft and malleable and will scarcely maintain its form. But it has a remarkable quality of absorbing carbon which confers upon it the rigidity of the earthly state in cast iron. Together with various metals such as chromium and tungsten, carbon gives qualities to iron which then as steel fit it for the enormously varied needs of technology. Not only can it be made rigid, elastic and so on, but it will retain magnetism — which pure iron almost immediately loses when removed from the magnetic field. So that we see that iron can also respond to the qualities in carbon and these metals, absorbing and retaining their forces. It is responsive both to the influence of light and to the gravitational and magnetic forces of the earth.

We can now turn to the functions of iron in the vegetable and animal kingdoms. Our attention is at once gripped by the green chlorophyll of plants and the red haemoglobin of animal blood. These two substances are basically very similar, only chlorophyll contains magnesium whilst haemoglobin contains iron. Chlorophyll cannot be formed in the absence of iron, but it cannot take it up into itself. In haemoglobin and chlorophyll, the porphyrins are so to speak the break-down product. Introduced into the animal organism, these open it to the poisonous effects of light. The porphyrins are constructed out of four pyrrole rings and pyrrolidine enters into many plant poisons such as the alkaloids of tobacco, belladonna and coca. In these phenomena we can see the metals iron and magnesium antidoting or overcoming the poison and even converting it into life-building substance. Are the porphyrines themselves the destructive agents or do they act as media through which the destructive action of, say, light penetrates into the organism?

When the animal organism and particularly the human is exposed to light, the pigment melanin is formed. This happens in the eye, or again in the skin as a response to sunlight. Melanin pigments do not contain iron but, like chlorophyll, they can be formed only in its presence. The ink of the cuttlefish is also related to its extraordinary and wide open eye.

Pelikan has shown how in the plant kingdom the appearance of alkaloid poisons comes about, as forces akin to the specifically animal forces penetrate too deeply into the vegetable sphere. These forces, often referred to as astral, normally contact the plant in its blossom. There they paralyse vitality and growth and eliminate the green colour. If they penetrate more deeply then poisonous substances are found. In the human, the nervous system is the specific organ for these forces which here penetrate into the organism as paralysing, katabolic destructive processes. But it is on the basis of these destructive processes that consciousness can arise, the price being a constant sickening from the nerve pole of our organisms. Against this sickening the iron in the blood provides a constant healing activity comparable to its healing of the poisonous porphyrins. We have already seen that iron can subdue the sulphur processes which, arising from the metabolic pole, strive to overcome consciousness in a polar form of disease. Iron acting as a rhythmic breathing element works to balance and heal both tendencies to illness which we forever carry within us. This rhythmic balancing function also makes it possible for iron to become the bearer of our ego freedom and presence of mind.

If we look at the homoeopathic drug picture of *Ferrum met.* we find headaches with a distinctly migrainous character conspicuous. They are full bounding headaches revealing a bursting through of the sulphurous metabolic processes into the realm of consciousness. Iron can help to subdue these too turbulent, exuberant forces. The *Ferrum* patient is chilly, and deficient in warmth. Iron enables the imponderable element of heat to enter into the organism. The blushing and blanching reveal the sensitive responsiveness of iron which we have noted and this responsiveness is further revealed in sensitivity, particularly to noise. Gentle, slow movements are said to help these patients and we can guess that such movements act into the general rhythmic system in contrast to the vigorous ameliorating exertions of *Sepia* which relieve rather the liver and portal congestions.

Ferrum phos. helps in inflammatory conditions, particularly of the respiratory tract, and in a less acute phase *Pyrites* is of help in tracheitis and bronchitis.

We have seen how iron is in a sense a real remedy for the inherent illness of the nervous system. Treichler has suggested the use of Catoptrite and Berthierite in multiple sclerosis. Catoptrite is an iron antimony compound and in Berthierite sulphur is added. In the earlier time when acute poliomyelitis was epidemic, zur Linden reported on the very useful action of Scorodite (iron arsenate) in this disease. In multiple sclerosis the earliest lesion is probably in the optic nerve and visual tract. Not only is retrobulbar neuritis often the earliest presenting symptom, but recent studies have shown that in practically all cases of multiple sclerosis there is a demonstrable delay in conduction from eye to visual cortex. I have personally noticed a great deficiency in the capacity to produce 'after-images' in these patients. Can we perhaps interpret these phenomena as indicating that light itself is here again acting as a toxic agent? Can we not take it that normal light is digested in the eye and does not pass into the nervous system as a foreign element? It is met by the blood in the retina and the sclerosing, destructive effects of light are met by the metabolic dissolving inflammatory forces of the blood. Anyone who will spend a little while observing the phenomena of after-images can soon observe the rhythmic play of colours continuing for some minutes. In these rhythmic phenomena, can we perhaps see the iron again playing its 'breathing' role and how it helps in a healing manner to mediate between the sclerotic and inflammatory tendencies we have mentioned? We can, following Treichler, envisage the morbid process in multiple sclerosis as consisting in the process normal on the retina being displaced further and further, so to speak, into the brain and spinal cord. The first phase of the attack, demyelination, is an extension of the normal dying, sclerosing 'life' of the nervous system which then arouses an inflammatory, explosive, counter movement from the blood. This inflammatory reaction is often more destructive than the original demyelination. The plaques can in this way be understood as displaced eyes, attempts to form eyes within the nervous organ itself. We can hope that iron may help to antidote the toxic effects of light, that it may help to bring this imponderable constructively within the earthly realm, and may restrain a too violent inflammatory reaction. By exerting its rhythmic tendency it can mediate between the two poles. Something of all this can be seen in the psychic phenomena of these patients. On the one hand their thoughts and mental life become very scatterbrained even for our scatterbrained generation; they find it difficult to bring the synthesizing force of the will into their thoughts to enliven what have become excessively dead and abstract items of mental existence. On the other hand they cannot infuse their life of will with ideals and conscious goals. The life of will becomes blind impulsiveness, they cannot inform the will with purpose. In the course of working with these patients I have found that these remedies do seem to help this divided state of soul even when the organic state does not respond. I have the impression that one can often act therapeutically in this way and can have an idea of what one's therapeutic goal can be.

Another of the great epidemic diseases of today may also call for iron. I refer to depression, that state of paralysis of the will which is so common. *Aurum*, gold, is the most famous homoeopathic remedy for severe depression, but we should also consider *Stannum*, tin, and *Ferrum*, iron. The relation of depression to the liver is obvious in the experience of hepatitis and tin and iron have a special relation or affinity for the parenchymatous and bile functions. Whilst tin may be said to arouse and unlock the torpid and paralysed will, iron serves more to fan it with enthusiasm and gives it individual force to take its place in the world, to fight for its place. Gold is concerned more with the despair of existence and those depressions whose solutions point to a transformation of life's goals and meanings. It has to do with the transformation of material into spiritual goals. There are of course many other remedies needed in depression, but these three give a certain orientation in penetrating the dark enigmas of this state. There are many preparations of these metals to choose from. I must draw attention particularly to the vegetabilized metals, the metals potentized by the passage through corresponding plants. Particularly of use in depression are *Taraxacum Stanno cultum*,

Chelidonium Ferro cultum and *Hypericum Auro cultum*. They also can be given by injection.

Finally there is the possibility of using iron in various potencies and forms in the treatment of rheumatoid arthritis. This suggestion from Selawry still lies perhaps for the future to take up and work out.

This is a very compressed sketch as an introduction to the study of iron and its extended therapeutic field. It is far from comprehensive and needs working out and expanding in all directions. I am indebted for the basic contributions on which I have drawn to the anthroposophical school and in particular to Pelikan's book *The Secret of Metals* and the relevant section in Hauschka's *The Nature of Substance*, also to Treichler's work on multiple sclerosis and his contribution on depression.

15. Golden Apollo and the heart

There was an early Greek mythology dealing with the Titans which affords a glimpse into the abyss of pain, suffering and cruelty which lies at the bottom of things. After the Titanomachia, the victorious Olympians arose in happy, laughing blessedness, a dazzling vision of immortal beauty and joy. Amongst these immortals of Olympus, Apollo was the sun god, successor to, or identical with, Helios. At his first appearance, with tight strung bow, in the banqueting chamber, the other gods trembled. Was not Apollo the true centre of the Olympians, their sun? But Apollo was moving towards the earth and so Zeus continued to rule supreme. Could one say as regent?

At his birth on the island of Delos, Apollo was surrounded by gold, as was his twin sister Artemis by silver. They were both expert marksmen and those whom they slew with their arrows died peacefully as if falling asleep with a smile on their lips. Apollo also carried his lyre and became the inspirer of music and the arts, the leader of the nine Muses. According to one story he received this lyre from the new-born Hermes as a peace offering, in token compensation for the stolen cattle which Hermes had rustled from him. Hermes had taken a tortoise shell and strung it with sheepgut, creating the first seven-stringed musical instrument, and this he gave to Apollo. The two instruments, the lyre and the bow, became the very insignia of Apollo.

Apollo held aloof. With his arrows he slew from a distance. In his statue at Olympia he brings order by his gaze alone. He is the bestower of order, law, balance and harmony. Inspiring Orpheus, he brought healing and peace to nature and man through his music. He is the chief of the healing gods, Asklepios is his son. He incorporated Paeion, the physician of the gods, the Paeans were sung at his festivals. When before Troy he was challenged by Poseidon to a duel, he disdainfully refused to be embroiled on behalf of mere men. He turned away.

From his sanctuary at Delphi he ordered through his oracle the life of all Hellas, maintaining the balance between the three tribes, the custodians of the thinking, feeling and willing life. He arrived at Delphi, according to some accounts, riding on a dolphin from Crete. On arrival he had to overcome a female dragon, the Python. He achieved this victory with his bow and arrows, but had then to undergo rites of purification on account of the shed blood. He became the purifier, the protector of the rites of purification.

In his study of the Olympian gods, Walter Otto characterizes Apollo as the mightiest after Zeus. His greatness is ennobled by loftiness of spirit. Of the statue at Olympia he comments that

> the artist has perpetuated a moment of overwhelming magnificence. In the midst of the wildest tumult the god has suddenly appeared, and his outstretched arm enjoins calm. Loftiness shines out of his countenance; its wide eyes command merely by the superiority of his look; but about the strong and noble mouth there is a delicate, almost melancholy suggestion of superior knowledge. The manifestation of the divine amidst the desolation and confusion of this world cannot possibly be represented with greater forcefulness.

During part of the year, Apollo regularly departed from Delphi to the remote and mysterious and blessed country of the Hyperboreans, a land perpetuating the primordial undisturbed state of harmony before discord entered. In his absence, Dionysos enjoyed sole rule at Delphi.

Radiance, beauty, measure, moderation, balance characterize Apollo. 'In his music resounds the spirit of all living forms. It is hearkened to with delight by friends of the lucid and well-ordered world, which is governed by the lofty thoughts of Zeus; but to all immoderate and monstrous beings it is strange and disagreeable.'

His conquest of the Python seems, as do so many other similar myths, to commemorate some ancient event through which order and balance were restored to a disturbed and endangered development of man. Apollo had to intervene and in doing so became involved in a deeper way in human destiny, even needing purification himself for his deed.

What possible relevance can such stories and characterization have for an understanding of the heart and of gold? For this is our problem; can the ancient correlation of Sun, Heart and Gold, with Apollo as spirit of the sun or at least as image of that spirit, help us today in our efforts to understand the heart?

Let us start with gold which has always been the noblest of the metals. Radiant with its yellow lustre it yet maintains itself in serene aloofness and does not allow itself to fade away to the circumference after the manner of ordinary yellowness. The most precious of metals, by which we mean that it resists earthiness most powerfully, it yet is immensely heavy, showing a relationship of great intensity to earth gravity. What do we mean by saying that it resists earthiness? It enters only with the greatest difficulty into combination with acids and alkalis. It dissolves only in *Aqua Regia*, a combination of nitric and hydrochloric acids. It is not subject to rust, tarnish and corrosion after the manner of other metals. In this it shows how it remains true to its cosmic origin, it rejects earthiness. Yet it is the heaviest of metals. So it holds the balance between earth and cosmos. In colour it has the radiance of yellow, but in moderation; it holds itself together and does not lose itself in dissipation. Its radiance is a royal radiance which magnanimously gives without becoming empty. It holds a middle place in the order of the traditional planetary metals. This can be confirmed in the order of conductivity for heat and electricity. Pelikan has elaborated this theme of the middle or central position of gold amongst the seven metals. It holds the balance between the outer planets and the inner, between Saturn, Jupiter and Mars on the one hand and Venus, Mercury and the Moon on the other. In colloidal solutions it shows enormous colourfulness; it can be greenish-blue, violet, reddish, violet-blue, or pure rose. In these colours it avoids only the yellow and orange which the metal itself manifests. When beaten into gold leaf it becomes translucent and then the transmitted light is a lovely green.

In all its properties it shows a balance between earth heaviness and sun lightness and these polarities are balanced with a fluidity which manifests in its extreme malleability and ductility. It can be reduced by beating to sheets of gold-leaf $\frac{1}{10,000}$ of a millimetre thick and can be drawn into wire of invisible fineness without breaking.

Again with our modern education and prejudices we find ourselves perplexed. What has any of this to do with the heart? After all, are we not taught that the heart is a mere pump, necessary to keep the blood moving round the circulation, which the great William Harvey discovered? And yet that same William Harvey, one of the heroes of the scientific revolution, wrote that it was not his view that the heart moved the blood but rather that the blood moved the heart. And he also affirmed that no one would get very far in the study of embryology without the help of astrology.

Movement and circulation of fluids in living organisms is not dependent on a heart. In the unicellular Paramecium the flow in the protoplasmic content can be seen to follow a lemniscate or figure-of-eight course, in Hydra and the Coelenterates fluid circulates in and out and through the tubes which make up their structures. In the Echinoderms the circulation becomes more interiorized, still without a heart, and only in the Amphibia do we begin to find anything approaching a heart organ. Movement of fluid and circulation precede the heart in embryological development, the movement of blood in vessels is visible before the heart becomes incorporated into the circulation. The eminent Polish cardiac surgeon, Professor Manteuffel-Szoege has brought forward cogent reasons from his experience and experiments to question the doctrine of the heart as a mere pump.

Taking a physiognomic look at man, where the heart rises to its highest perfection, becoming even the organ for love and conscience, we find the heart occupying a central position. It comes to its central position between the upper and lower poles of man from a position in the throat region. It holds a balance between upper cephalic and lower metabolic abdominal poles. It also holds a balance between left and right, or between arterial and venous blood. To hold this balance it comes slightly to the left of the mid-line. The axis of the heart is from above; behind, on the right, to below, forwards, to the left. It also holds the balance between behind and forwards. Do we not walk forwards into the future remembering the past which is behind us? Do we not need to balance the one-sidedness of our past actions with our future deeds? If we did not believe in this possibility, should we not be condemned to despair?

The polarity of left and right is also the polarity of female and male. The right is right, the left is left out or behind, it is sinister whereas the right is dexterous. The left side is the defensive side of the shield, the right the active side of the sword. And the woman walks on the left arm of the man. Where can we find the reconciliation of man and woman? The child is the reconciliation and synthesis. When we are able to listen to the voice of the heart we experience always again the freshness of the newborn child, the breath of the eternal in the present. Is it surprising that, in our age, when our hearts are so overburdened and when our reason and hardhearted reality-sense have become so rigid, even the physical heart organ suffers so much?

The upper and lower polarity is also mediated by the heart. From above descend the world-forming thoughts of Zeus. From the brain proceed those sculpturing, shaping forces which inwardly and outwardly sculpt the forms of our organs and body. When we are overcome by fear, and become over-awake in our senses, we become frozen to the spot, we become a veritable white block of marble until our blood releases us again into movement. From below come the dissolving, moving dynamic metabolic processes, which would make everything gregariously equal in a formless togetherness. The blood carries these processes. When shame overwhelms us we become covered with a blush, our thoughts become muddled and confused, our knees give way, we wish to lose our self-presence and vanish from the sight of all.

In the rhythm of systole and diastole the heart holds the balance, continuously restores the balance between these upper and lower forces. In systolic contraction the heart responds to the form-giving impulses of the head, whilst in diastolic expansion it gives way to the flooding blood forces. We can even see how in the leptosome asthenic person the heart assumes a more vertical and contracted appearance, corresponding with the predominantly nervous make-up. In contrast, in the pyknic, the heart becomes fuller, rounded and more horizontal in appearance, showing us the predominance of metabolic processes in this constitutional type.

Could we dare to say that, when we are in harmony with ourselves and our environment, we breathe freely and our heart feels at ease, responding to every nuance of feeling? Is it not true that at such moments we have no sense of the heart working, but rather that in the perfect balance of its rhythmic dance it can hold its place by the slightest variations in its beat? Only when things are thrown out of balance by disease or unaccustomed exertion does the heart labour.

There may be yet a further higher function of the heart to be unveiled. The heart has an immense richness of nerve endings. Should we not suspect that the heart is also a sense organ, besides being an organ of balance? Was Steiner right in pointing to the heart as a sense organ by which the upper conscious pole of man could perceive the processes within the lower unconscious pole? And if so, how are we to understand these processes which proceed within the metabolism and the metabolic organs proper?

At Delphi, the spiritual heart of ancient Hellas, two gods had their sanctuaries, Apollo and Dionysos. How intense is the polarity expressed in these two divinities. The measured, balanced, aloof Apollo in contrast to the frenzied, drunken, mad Dionysos. Nietzsche who introduced these two gods into the language of art criticism characterized the Apollonic inspiration of art as akin to dream vision and the Dionysiac as erupting out of the drunken orgiastic experience. He interpreted Greek tragedy as the synthesis of these two streams. In Delphi they met, in Delphi was the heart of Hellas. The word Delphi or Delphos signifies a womb, and Apollo came to Delphi on a dolphin also signifying a womb. At Delphi was the Omphallos, the navel of the world, and the stone called by this name is preserved in the museum. The heart and the womb have many connections, outwardly apparent in their hollow muscular form. Dionysos, the mad, raving, raging, drunken divinity, had a mortal mother. He was brought up by women, dressed as a woman and was attended by women. He was not, however, particularly promiscuous sexually and his closest woman companion was Ariadne whose thread of intuition guided Theseus out of the labyrinth of the brain and its thinking. Divinity bursts the bonds of mere sanity and reason, the ecstatic also belongs to the human experience of the divine. To lose oneself is also to find oneself. In Greece the Dionysiac orgiastic frenzy was not characterized as in the corresponding Asiatic cults by excesses of sadistic horror. But it was the women who were caught up into the rituals on Mount Parnassus which called for outstanding physical endurance.

It was moreover Dionysos who was the key divinity in the mystery religion of Greece. Apollo had spoken through his oracles voiced by the sibyls at Delphi and elsewhere. The way to Dionysos was through the mysteries, and at the height of the Eleusinian drama came the revelation of the god Iacchos in the mother's arms. Iacchos was Dionysos. But Heracleitos uttered the saying that Hades and Dionysos were one, and at Delphi Apollo and Dionysos are revealed as two aspects of one divine essence. Dionysos also was, above all, the masked god. The players on the stage of the Dionysiac theatre were masked, and huge and varied masks of the god were central to his cult. The Greek word for a mask was *persona*. Through the *persona*, the god became manifest in mortality and through our personalities our own immortal selves become active in history. Dionysos, the mad god who dies and is reborn, confronts us with an immediacy of experience both in the dramatic art of tragedy and in the intoxicated dances on the mountains. Death and birth become one in Dionysos whose essence is paradox and the union of two worlds. Plato who was regarded as the reborn Dionysos taught by means of the paradoxes of dialectics and for him the highest wisdom was dependent on the soul's mania.

Apollo with his lyre rules in the nervous system. His lyre is the nerves radiating from the spinal cord. But Dionysos with his flute rules in the blood. Death and resurrection are the immediacy of the blood process but the nerves radiate their influence into the body from their aloof citadel in skull and spine, detached and observant. Looking at the movement of descent and interiorization of the heart during embryological development, could one say that the heart sought out and united with the blood system as Apollo sought out and united with Dionysos in the heart-womb of Delphi? In the museum at Delphi is to be seen the charioteer who in perfect poise and balance holds the reins of the charging steeds.

Is not the heart both sense organ and organ of the blood pulsation?

We can also approach these riddles with the help of psychology. The important American psychiatrist Trigant Burrow was concerned to expose the morphological split in human nature which has arisen between the 'I'-centred consciousness of our head and brain as against the integral or collective unconscious-consciousness mediated by the autonomic nervous system. In our waking consciousness we experience ourselves looking out on the world from behind our eyes. This consciousness is bound up with all our inherited ideas and value judgments as well as those acquired in the course of life. We accept or reject aspects of reality according to accepted canons of true and false or good and bad. These standards are based on partiality, of sex, age, class and so on. Our 'I' consciousness has been purchased at the cost of partiality and being cut off, alienated, from the whole, integral reality. This integral response does however operate in what has become for us our unconscious. Our organic processes are related integrally, not partially, to our environment, our social environment in particular. These organs and processes are related to the autonomic nervous system. Trigant Burrow understood the chaos and crisis in our human affairs as arising out of our mistaken attempts to understand the integral responses of our organic unconsciousness with the modes of interpretation developed and appropriate for the phenomena of our partial awake, 'I' consciousness which is mainly based on our visual and auditory and laryngeal experience.

It seems to me that we are here approaching the same riddle of human nature as we have approached through the mythological figures of Apollo and Dionysos. Our human nature is the union of two worlds. Dionysos as the cosmic representative of the ego is the mad god. On the one hand he is the revelation of finding one's true self through losing it in intoxicated immediacy and on the other he is the masked god hiding behind the *persona*.

Into the abyss between Trigant Burrows' divided worlds there has descended the heart which listens to the intimations from the 'other' world of the unconscious.

Our real conscience, not our moral conventions, would speak though our heart. Between the awake but partial consciousness of our heads and the asleep but universal awareness of our metabolism and organic processes arises the conscience of our hearts still largely in a dream consciousness, the consciousness also of our emotions.

The language of our souls is poetry and art, whilst the language of our bodies is prose. The totally inartistic language of modern scientific literature and in particular of medical papers effectively screens out any trace of the soul's experiences and activities. We must envisage that fruitful studies in psychosomatic medicine will in the future show the problem of the relation between soul and body to be kindred to that between poetry and prose.

Can these considerations help us to take up the medicinal uses of Gold-Aurum and find the underlying unity in the diverse phenomena of the homoeopathic drug picture and clinical experience? Amongst the latter must be included over fifty years' work with gold salts in the treatment of rheumatoid arthritis.

The main spheres of action of *Aurum* in the homoeopathic drug pictures seem to be on the heart and circulation, on the genital organs, uterus, ovaries and testes, on the sense organs, particularly eyes and ears, and on the bones. Above all depression and suicide are emphasized. In an earlier time it was a main remedy amongst homoeopaths for dealing with advanced syphilis and the ravages of intense mercurialism arising in its treatment. Bone pains and nodes and gummata seem to have been particular indications, but these problems have vanished from the clinical scene.

From our considerations, the actions on the heart and circulation are really central. Congestion and hyperaemia are described in many organs. Orgasms of blood as in menopausal hot flushes are common and these circulatory imbalances culminate in the heart itself. In the older homoeopathic literature, irregular heart action, extrasystoles, etc., figure together with sensations of fullness and actual dilation and hypertrophy of the heart. Angina pectoris, rheumatic and syphilitic heart disease come in. Kent remarks on wandering arthralgias and rheumatic pains culminating in the heart. Together with these functional and organic symptoms Kent connects the affective disorders rising to suicidal depression. There is extreme sensitivity to insults and disagreements, with suppressed indignation, and to grief and bereavement. But it is above all sadness and depression, often associated with irritability, that characterize the mental picture. The depression is combined with fear of death, or its opposite, longing for death, and may lead to suicide. But *Aurum* is also characterized by industriousness rising to hypomanic and manic intensity. Kent, out of his Swedenborgianism, relates all these 'mental' symptoms to affective disorder and the heart, in contrast to the intellectual disorder of *Argentum* related to the lung and brain.

We have here, in the fear of death and the longing for death, in the depression and mania, two poles which should be balanced in the heart, in the heart's courage.

Both the wild enthusiasm and the fearful depression belong to Dionysos; does not Apollo bring the balance and healing in calm courageous self-presence. Courage is not the opposite of cowardice but the solution of the polarity of cowardice and foolhardiness. There is a distinction between the fear of the heart and the fear of the liver. In the case of the sudden heart attack there is fear of imminent death, that the next moment will not be, whereas in the depression and fear of hepatitis there is rather dread and fear that the day will come and that one cannot face it; it is a fear of life.

In the drug picture of *Aurum* we come next to the senses which are oversensitive; so the *Aurum* patient may find light and noise unbearable. In the mental sphere this may find expression in phobias, fears of the other world, in which the lung dynamic also comes into play. It is contrasted with the inner organic restlessness and anxiety arising out of the sphere of the kidney, and this polarity of inner and outer must also be balanced in the heart. We find that *Aurum* had a valuable role in homoeopathic practice in inflammation of the eye, iritis, choroiditis, on to corneal opacities, and in otitis media and chronic ear discharges with mastoid involvement. Here it seems we have the polar opposite to the hyper-acuity of the senses, blindness and deafness.

The polarity of the two major senses, the eye and the ear, is related to the polarity of exteriorization and interiorization. The eye develops by an exteriorizing gesture of the brain, the most withdrawn and still of the organs. The brain sends out the so-called optic nerve to form the most mobile, outward looking eye. The eye becomes a limb with whose glance we finger, as it were, the objects we look at. To see we must keep our glance moving over the objects, we must not stare. But the ear develops by interiorizing gesture. The three elements of a limb — thigh, leg and foot — become interiorized in the ossicles. The inner ear bores deep into the petrous bone. To listen we must become inwardly still and silent.

This polarity of the eye and ear, of seeing and hearing, which dominates our sense experience is repeated in a major polarity in the reproductive sphere in the male-female distinction. The female reproductive organs are interiorized, pregnancy develops inwardly almost as a tumour, whereas the male organs are anatomically exteriorized and functionally also inflammatory and exteriorizing. We find that the *Aurum* sphere of action extends to both male and female organs. Inflammations and tumours of ovaries and uterus, presumably fibroids, are found in the drug picture, as well as pain and swelling and atrophy of the testes. The old descriptions are admittedly not clear in terms of modern diagnostic criteria. A nice point is recorded: *Aurum* acts preferentially on the left ovary and the right testis.

We must now turn to the rheumatic and bone pains in the drug picture. The bone pains were related by older authors to syphilis and mercurialism. These have almost completely disappeared from clinical practice. Would gold be of use in bony metastases or in the pain in Paget's disease? The old experience of the

132

relationship of gold to bones, including periostitis and 'nodes', may be related to the great heaviness of the metal, heavier than lead and the other planetary metals, lighter only than Platinum.

For over fifty years now gold in the form of various salts has been used in the treatment of rheumatoid arthritis. Its use is complicated by toxic effects particularly on the skin and on the kidneys. Nevertheless a beneficial effect on the course of the disease has been demonstrated beyond doubt. New orally administered preparations are being tried at present, probably less toxic than the previous drugs given by injection. Can these actions, assuming they are related to the gold rather than the sulphur in the salts, be brought into the picture? Kent probably referred to the cardiac complications in rheumatic fever and this only helps us in so far as some relationship between arthritis and carditis is indicated. The other phenomena we have been considering, centred in the heart, all had to do with the meeting of polarities in that organ or of the other polarities expressed in the male and female duality in the genital and sensory organs. A functional relationship, reminding one of the rheumatic fever heart connection, but in a way opposite to it, meets us in the frequent remissions in rheumatoid arthritis during the course of pregnancy. It is as if the uterine pregnancy replaced pregnancy processes in the joints.

Here we can call on the genius of language and the poet's imaginative insights to help us. Homer sang of the future lying in the knees of the gods. The usual English saying 'in the lap of the gods' is close to this. Shakespeare used the expression 'in the pregnant hinges of the knees'. Here the emphasis falls on the gn, kn, ng root and, as Groddeck showed, this root leads us into knowing, gnosis, gynae, generation, join and joints, especially the knee joint, the genu, genius and many other words. In the Bible the same word to 'know' is used for sexual relationship, a use persisting in our current use of the expression 'carnal knowledge'. We can go a little further and find in the word heart and in carditis the rt, rd root. In fact the word root itself has the same rt as do ratio, radius, and arthron, the Greek for joint, which gives us arthritis.

All these words have the common meaning in them of joining together, the union of opposites or polarities.

In the old conception of the planetary metals the outer planets and metals were in polarity to the inner.

Saturn-Lead	was polar to	Moon-Silver
Jupiter-Tin	was polar to	Mercury-Mercury
Mars-Iron	was polar to	Venus-Copper

But the Sun-Gold was central and contained all the polarities within itself; it was the very heart of the system.

The tragedy of gold has been in its descent from the sphere of divine kingship, its use restricted to priestly and royal cult purposes. From Egypt the Persian Cambyses removed the gold and it became coin of the realm. In turn the Great Alexander acquired this wealth and replaced divine images with his own on the coins. He was himself proclaimed divine. In time the gold passed into the vaults of the bankers and into Fort Knox but continued to rule the destinies of mankind, not perhaps entirely for their good. From the sacerdotal realm through the imperial realms to the economic and financial regions gold has passed and drawn mankind from spiritual heights and intuitions into the confined hells of our modern materialism.

Can medicine find the way so to use gold that we may be aided to find our way upwards again from our one-sided obsession with material and economic values to an all embracing and balanced existence? An existence where universal spiritual values and earthly instrumentalities find their healthy harmony. In the despair of modern existence when all material values and possessions turn sour, medicinal gold can help to lead over into a consciousness of wider, universal values. The mad enthusiasm for mere material gain and possession can be metamorphosed into the inner enthusiasm for wisdom, greed into compassion and understanding.

16.   Copper (*cuprum*)

The ancients took it that Aphrodite-Venus was in some sense the inner quality and being of the metal copper. The old story told of the birth of Aphrodite from the sea-foam. Ouranos or heaven lay every night on Gaia or mother earth. All her children he concealed in folds of her body when they were born. At last she managed to contrive with the youngest, Chronos or Saturn, that when Ouranos came at night Chronos would come out of hiding and with a sickle cut off his father's genitals. This he did and threw the members into the sea. From the foaming gradually appeared the form of a most beautiful girl.

According to some stories she frolicked for ages in the sea with a beautiful boy companion, but eventually, sailing upon a cockle shell, came to land first on the island of Cythera and then to Cyprus at the bay of Paphos. There she was quickly decked out with clothes and jewels by the Hours and led to the assembled Gods of Olympus who promptly fell in love with the ravishing beauty. She is thus a goddess of very ancient origin who assumed her customary image of an overwhelmingly lovely and irresistible girl on her adoption into the family of the Olympians. On her stepping ashore at Cyprus, nature blossomed into spring time, and this gives us a first key to her nature; she manifests in all the blossoming of nature. Further, in other stories such as her seduction of Anchises, the father of Aeneas, we hear how at her coming all the wild animals paired off two by two and lay down in shady places. Her portion of honour amongst men and gods is 'girlish babble and deceit and sweet rapture, embraces and caresses'.

Art has expressed these stories in incomparable images; Botticelli's *Birth of Venus*, and the relief in the Terme Museum in Rome showing the goddess rising from the sea are just two of the most lovely. She is the spirit of enchantment of blooming nature. 'Thou, goddess, thou dost turn to flight the winds and clouds of heaven, thou at thy coming; for thee earth, the quaint artificer, put forth her sweet-scented flowers; for thee the levels of ocean smile, and the sky, its anger past, gleams with spreading light.' She was patroness of safe voyages, and sailors on return to port have always been wont to celebrate her festivals. The Homeric hymn begins: 'Muse, tell me the deeds of golden Aphrodite, the Cyprian, who stirs up sweet passion in the gods and subdues the tribes of mortal men and birds that fly in the air and all the many creatures that the dry land rears, and all that the sea: all these love the deeds of rich-crowned Cythera'. Alone amongst the immortals three goddesses could withstand her power — Artemis, the young pre-adolescent maiden, Athena, goddess of wisdom and Hestia, the maiden-aunt of Olympus.

The miracles of grace and charm, sheer beauty, are the manifestations of Aphrodite; they inspire, excite, enchant, filling with desire. It is the charm which attracts and then yields rather than the wild pursuit itself in which Eros comes to expression. Mostly her impact on men is kindly and brings good luck, but on women she can bring disaster, as the stories of Medea and Phaedra told. It is dangerous to reject her influences, for then she can indeed exact terrible punishments for being scorned. Her true worship, openness and gratitude for beauty, brings blessing; the scorn of beauty, as in our modern civilization, brings the curse of violence and crime as punishment.

How do these imaginative responses of the psyche to the Aphrodite-Venus archetype relate to the metal copper and to the corresponding organ in the human organization, the kidney? For to the ancients these were all expressions of one and the same reality and it is our heuristic endeavour to enquire what value is to be found today in such a view-point.

It is commonly held that copper acquired its name from the island of Cyprus. Copper mines were worked there from at least 2600 BC and it was a main source of the metal throughout the bronze age for Egypt and the Eastern Mediterranean. But from what did the island of Cyprus derive its name? Some have connected it with the Greek name for the henna plant which grew extensively there. At Paphos, in the south west of the island, was one of the main sanctuaries and cult centres of the goddess. There she had come ashore.

Copper itself is a warm reddish golden metal. In nature it combines with all acids, and assumes wonderful greens and blues as well as yellows and reds. In fact no metal appears in such wonderfully coloured ores as does copper. Copper pyrite shines golden yellow, azurite is blue, malachite green and bornite delights the eye with all colours of the rainbow. The metal is an excellent conductor of heat and electricity, second only to silver, and when melted it greedily sucks in gases such as hydrogen, carbon monoxide and sulpher dioxide, only to expel them again in spattering little explosions as it hardens, a phenomenon reminding us of the behaviour of silver with oxygen. The wonderful colours in which copper salts and ores shine forth proclaim that here heavenly beauty is brought to earthly form, truly a deed of Aphrodite.

Chemically we find copper salts crystallizing with much water. Indeed without this water of crystallization the colour vanishes and the crystals disintegrate into powder, which however quickly reabsorbs water and regains its colour. To the realm of water, the realm of life, copper brings colour. It is a painter. Soul qualities are brought to expression in the otherwise merely living, vegetative realms. It is a lively, chemically active element. It forms multitudes of different salts and complex organic compounds. It, so to speak, ensouls the fluid and living realms with lively movement and transforms the vegetative and merely growing nature into blossoming and colour. Desire, love and yearning are added to growth and form, inward experience is added to outward growth. Copper is happy to enfold, to form vessels or to cover domed roofs, it is easily hammered into such forms imitating the invaginating forms which characterize animal development.

Alloyed with tin it gives rise to bronze. Now in Homer we find another story of the birth of Aphrodite from the marriage of Zeus and Dione. However, it appears that this is a cover-up for the actual marriage of Zeus and Aphrodite herself. Can we see here in picture form the origin of the bronze age which was that age of which Homer sang. And Homer was the creator of Olympian gods almost wholly purged of those earlier stories of strange births such as the more primitive stories of the birth of Aphrodite.

Traces of copper are essential for healthy growth of the higher plants; it is an essential trace element. But unicellular plants, low types of mushroom, algae are killed by minute traces of copper. These are all plants which cannot attain to flowering.

In animals we find first of all that copper forms the basis of the blood pigment haemocyanin which in certain invertebrates enables the oxygen breathing process to be mediated. Many molluscs and arthropods depend on this copper compound, whereas the vertebrates make use of the iron-containing haemoglobin. Gastropods and cephalopods in particular depend on haemocyanin, though a few gastropods living in very poorly aerated media have developed haemoglobin. The sedentary lamellibranchs mostly do without breathing pigments. Very small amounts of copper are necessary for haemoglobin synthesis but additional supply of the metal is not required in practice. In a similar way small amounts of iron are of course also required for the synthesis of chlorophyll, a pigment which contains magnesium instead of iron. There is therefore a close functional relationship between iron and copper in physiology; both can form pigments mediating respiratory function. Through breathing, oxygen is taken up and carbonic acid eliminated, the reverse of the process in plants. We can see here, yet again, the importance of copper in the transformation from vegetable to animal life, the animating, ensouling transformation.

Aphrodite-Venus and Ares-Mars were always falling in love, every nice girl loves a soldier. Ares was related to iron and the iron age replaced the bronze age as did haemoglobin haemocyanin. Can we discern any significance from the evolutionary-psychological standpoint in this movement from copper to iron in the blood-stream, a movement approximately parallel to the movement from invertebrate to vertebrate? Does it not represent a further stage in the ensouling process when iron strength of will, the courage to fight and wage war, is added to the more feminine soul qualities of yearning, love, charm and beauty? And Aphrodite's husband was Hephaestos, the lame artist craftsman who according to some accounts was a dwarf but of supreme ability to forge the very weapons used by the votaries of his wife's lover. Hephaestos is the shadow of Ares.

How are we now to relate the function we are beginning to discern in the archetype Aphrodite-Venus to the function of the kidney? This is an organ whose function is usually confined to the elaboration and excretion of urine, together with its role in maintaining the balance in the electrolytes, acid-base balance and so on in the blood. What does it have to do with ensouling the organism?

We can make a start with certain, as it were, gestures associated with the kidney and its functions. Firstly we may mention the descent of the kidney from the pronephros to mesonephros and further to the definitive metanephros. This meta-nephros also is seen to rise up from the region of the bladder and gential organs. Does this find its mythological expression in the story of the origin of Aphrodite from Ouranos, the heavens descending to earth and further in his genitals to the sea? From there she rose again to earth which blossomed at her coming. But with this descent of the kidneys must be associated the ascent of the lungs and, as König has shown, these two, lungs and kidneys, come to mirror each other. This too may find expression in the old story of Hermaphroditos.

Secondly the kidney is related intimately to nitrogen metabolism and to the excretion of urea and uric acid, end-products of that metabolism. We get a hint of the role of nitrogen in the contrast between carbohydrates, the characteristic stuff of plants, and protein, the characteristic stuff of animals. That element in animal nature which brings about sense perception, desire and movement, the essential characteristics of animals, brings about also the incorporation of the nitrogen, its interiorization. Where proteins do occur in plants, it is often obvious that this same element, sometimes called the astral, has touched the plant. For instance in the Leguminosae with their rich protein-bearing seeds we can also see their butterfly-like flowers. Nevertheless, we can perceive that these vegetable proteins are distinct from the animal; the astrality has touched from outside only, not worked from inside to incorporate the nitrogen as in the animal.

Thirdly, the kidney plays a miraculous role in maintaining the balance of body fluids. It senses the fluids, it tastes the constituents and responds by reabsorbing from the tubules fluid and constituents exactly in amounts to maintain the fluid, electrolyte, acid-base balances. One can follow König's suggestion that the glomerulus, like an eye, sees into the fluids, the tubula like a tongue tastes them.

Fourthly, we must understand that the kidney irradiates the organism, lifting it up from mere vegetative life, to blossoming, sensing, motion, as did Aphrodite when she came ashore at Paphos. Some aspect of this irradiation acts through the renin and other products released by the kidney into the blood stream. But even more important may be the two suprarenal glands which sit so significantly on top of the kidneys to catch the radiation and transform it into the adrenal hormones. We can also grasp the active agents in the action of these hormones as immaterial radiations which only require the hormone substances as slippers with which to

138

gain entrance to the different organic realms. We can indeed say that these active principles are astral forces which do not themselves belong to the space of Euclid but with the help of the hormone substances as catalysts can work into the physical spatial organism.

These kidney radiations, to which Steiner drew attention, can be regarded as the backthrust into the organism corresponding to the effort expended in separating and excreting the urine from out of the living whole of the body fluids.

We can in another way approach the nature of these phenomena through the contrast between a patient with Addison's disease and one with Cushing's syndrome. Addison's disease may arise through destruction of the suprarenal glands. In the absence of the hormones, the kidney radiation then cannot find a foothold with which to work into the organism. What do we see? A patient reduced to an almost vegetative state. Too fatigued to move or stand erect, pale and pigmented, a dangerously low blood pressure and a reduced level of sodium in the blood as against the potassium. Potassium belongs to the world of plants, whereas sodium belongs to the animal organism. As against this picture we have the patient with Cushing's syndrome which may come about through over-activity of the suprarenal glands due to a tumour. This patient will be red, florid, over-active, a bit obese and with a high blood pressure, restless and excited, full of inner anxiety.

To the action of the kidney radiations, mediated by hormonal substances, in many physiological processes, we must add an important role in the nutritional processes and the upbuilding of protein. Again we are indebted to Steiner for most fruitful suggestions as to the synergistic action of four principal organs in these processes. We must look for these actions in a generalized dynamic sphere rather than in localized structures. These four organ systems are the heart, kidney, liver and lung. The nutritional stream has to be enlivened by the liver, aroused, ensouled by the kidney, raised to be a fit ground for the ego-individuality by the heart and related to the earth through the lung. Of the essential chemical elements in protein we can then relate oxygen to the liver, nitrogen to the kidney, hydrogen to the heart and carbon to the lung. Again, it should be clear that we refer here to the dynamic processes rather than to merely inorganically conceived atoms.

In these ways, very briefly sketched, we can see an indication of the ways in which the kidney organ plays an ensouling function, arousing the organism from vegetative sleep to animal dream. When the kidney system is overactive, then great restless anxiety comes about which may go so far as visual hallucinations and schizoid states. When it is inactive, apathy, sleep and inertia come about. The polarity in the action of coffee and barbiturates, which are both closely related in their molecular structure to urea, confirms these indications; coffee arouses, awakens; barbiturates sedate and put to sleep.

We must now approach the drug picture of copper in the homoeopathic materia medica and then enquire into further extensions of the therapeutic use of copper.

When we search through the items recorded in the materia medica we find a theme running throughout. It can be characterized as cramps, or spasms, or convulsions. These terms must be understood as gestures. We find the cramps may appear mostly in the limbs or even in the peripheral arteries. But they also may occur in the uterus as dysmenorrhoea or in severe cramping colic. In the severe colicky pains of cholera, copper is a most valuable remedy. In the stomach the pain may be associated with gastric ulceration. Continuing our ascending study through the organism we find that copper can prove valuable in angina pectoris, cramping pain in the heart, and in asthma where the cramp is in the airways. It has been found to be one of the important remedies for the spasms of coughing in whooping cough and in laryngismus. Then there are various convulsions, jerkings, chorea and in the mental and behavioural field, impulsive actions, piercing shrieks, delirium or melancholic sullen withdrawal. These extreme mental disturbances are also recorded: mania with biting, beating, tearing, foolish gestures of imitation and mimicry, full of insane spiteful tricks, illusions of imagination, does not recognize his own family. There is a further symptom recorded: tongue darts in and out rapidly like a snake.

Of other features noted one stands out as significant. Deeper disturbances develop when a rash or fever is suppressed or fails to develop, or when emotions are suppressed.

All in all it is a picture of some violence and suddenness, ranging through cramps, including tetany, severe colicky pains and violent diarrhoeas, asthma and whooping cough, to spasmodic coughs which may culminate in unconsciousness. The mental spectrum seems to range from temper tantrums to full blown insanity whilst also, at the polar extreme, appearing as apathy, perhaps boredom, rather than real depression. Restless excitability stands against lethargy and lassitude.

We record here in briefest statement the symptoms attributable to *Cuprum* in homoeopathic provings and in clinical experience. Can we relate this picture to the image of charm and beauty that we found in the stories of Aphrodite? In these we meet the charm of early womanhood arousing sweet desire, and inducing springtime loveliness, gentleness, harmony and calm of season and the elements. Surely this grace-bestowing being is what comes to mind when we think of the sanguine temperament. The temperaments belong properly not exactly to the realm of psychology, but rather to the living world of physiology. They impress themselves both in the soul world of behaviour and into the more structural world of the physical body and even skeleton. The sanguine temperament is essentially the airy temperament. It represents therefore within the fluid living realm of physiology, sometimes called the etheric, the impress of the soul which finds its home in the airy element. It can therefore colour, as a painter, the living realm and bring all the colours of the rainbow to play in the personality. The beauty and charm which a sanguine woman spreads around her is the working of Aphrodite and finds its organic basis in the kidney system. When slighted, Aphrodite becomes a demon of destruction driving to madness and disaster. She speaks the prologue to Euripides' *Hippolytus* and exposes this extremity of her nature, charm turned to revenge and jealousy. Is this the meaning of the peculiar symptom, the tongue flickering in and out like a snake's? This strange symptom is found again in the drug picture of *Lachesis*, a snake-venom.

It has been found clinically by Treichler amongst others that copper and its salts are important remedies in the treatment of schizoid and even fully schizophrenic conditions.

The restless, excitable conditions arising out of overactive kidney radiations can also pass into the hyperthyroid processes of Graves' disease. In these conditions also copper, as *Cuprite* 3x, has been found of great use.

Of recent years attention has been repeatedly drawn to the phenomena of hyperventilation. Some patients are very prone under stress to overbreathe, and washing out too much carbon dioxide from the blood, upsetting the acid-base balance and chemistry of the blood. We have indicated the close relationship between the lung and kidney systems which König has depicted in more detail, showing the importance of the kidney and bladder for the dynamics of respiration. The over-breathing of these patients would, from this viewpoint, seem to have its origin in the kidney system, and such patients can usually be found to be of sanguine temperament. A causative treatment should then be aimed at this system, in addition to symptomatic re-training of the breathing. The symptoms recorded as provoked by hyperventilation cover almost the whole field of 'psychosomatic' and 'psychoneurotic' phenomena.

Returning to the homoeopathic experience, we find that *Cuprum* is associated by Paterson with a group of remedies around the bowel nosode 'Proteus', of which he gives as keynote 'brain-storms'. The other remedies included in this group besides *Cuprum* are *Natrum muriaticum* and the other chlorides, *Ignatia*, *Secale* (*Claviceps purpurea* from which ergot derivatives are obtained), *Apis*, *Borax*, *Conium*, and to these *Belladonna* and *Chamomilla* should probably be added on clinical grounds. The linkage of these remedies with the kidney is established by *Natrum muriaticum* (sodium chloride). Not only is the kidney concerned with maintaining the proper concentration of salt in the blood but the sodium ion is intimately involved in the level of the blood pressure. Further the homoeopathic indications for the use of *Natrum mur.* as a remedy include periods of severe strain, stress and grief. In this way the connection with the suprarenal glands and the stress adaptation syndrome of Selye is also established. *Apis*, the venom of the bee, is related to the kidney and produces diuresis. Actually all the insect remedies used in homoeopathy have a relation to the kidney. The ergot derivatives have a spectrum of application or action very similar to that of *Cuprum* itself. It ranges from spasm of peripheral arteries, through contractions and cramps of the uterus and smooth muscles of the alimentary canal to those peculiar cramp-like phenomena in the circulation, associated with migraine, to the full schizophrenia-like trip of LSD.

Paterson saw the main action of this group of remedies, in which he found the organism Proteus appearing in the bowel as a marker or indicator, to be sudden disturbances in the brain and central nervous system. This is an interesting observation and raises one more question. How is the central nervous system dynamically related to the kidney system? This question leads us again to consider that system of forces which are sometimes called astral. It is this system of forces which gives rise to the animal form by repeated gestures of invagination or interiorization. Hence arises the central nervous system as a main organ of these astral forces which from and through it act formatively, sculpturally on the organism. Their action from the nervous pole is primarily paralysing and katabolic. It is these same forces which are switched by the kidneys into constructive anabolic forces playing their part in the upbuilding of protein. In these two modes of action we see the play of polarity which always characterizes these forces and which we experience also in their expression in the feelings. The emotional life plays between sympathy and antipathy, love and hate, pleasure and pain, all of which originate out of these astral forces in their development.

One further feature of the kidney corroborates these connections with the nervous system. It is the lack of regenerative capacity and the very high oxygen consumption they both share. These astral forces are opposed to the regenerative, merely living, forces, and only their very high oxygen consumption keeps these organs alive. They are quickly damaged beyond repair by quite short periods of oxygen lack.

So we see the brain and central nervous system, with which the voluntary muscles are connected, even if not in the way still commonly believed, stand opposed to the kidneys and the involuntary muscles and inner movement. The role of the central nervous system is rather to paralyse and sculpt purposeful movements from out of the vast ocean of potential movement. From the kidney system in its full sense arise the inner impulse and stimulus to movement, happily in gracious and charming gesture, unhappily in restless excitement and violent irrationality. Something of all this was present in the old use of the word for the kidney, the reins:

My reins instruct me in the night season. (*Psalms* 15:17)

My reins shall rejoice, when thy lips speak right things. (*Proverbs* 23:16.)

and in Shakespeare we find

Look thou be true; do not give dalliance
Too much the rein. (*Tempest* IV, 1.52)

Cold as if I had swallowed snowballs for pills to cool the reins.
(*Merry Wives of Windsor* III, 5.24)

I have begun, And now I give my sensual race the rein.
(*Measure for Measure* II, 4.160)

142

When she will take the rein I let her run; But she'll not stumble.

(Winter's Tale II, 3.51)

Some of these quotations seem to refer to the reins with which we guide and control a horse and some more to the kidney. And now giving rein to our imagination, are not these two meanings related? Do not the reins draw down the nervous excitableness from the horse's head and bring it under control, as the kidneys were drawn down from the head region to the abdomen? Are the horse's reins and the ureters related?

Leaving aside these speculations, we can however see that the confusion which arose biologically long long ago when the kidney system fell downwards and assumed excretory functions and became connected with the genital system, still persists to trouble us. It is more difficult on anatomical grounds for men than women to distinguish the excretory from the reproductive function, the profane from the sacred. Today the sacred is profaned and Aphrodite is dragged through the mire and mud. She takes her revenge, drives us into restlessness, nervousness and cravings for sensations and drugs — even into mad destructive violence. Art and beauty alone can help us restore her to her true function as the bestower of grace, charm and the freshness, loveliness of a new springtime, perhaps to flower now in a new spiritual culture in the souls of individual men and women and children.

17. Quicksilver (*mercurius*)

The figure of Mercury-Hermes stands as a particularly enchanting and likeable image amongst the gods of Olympus. Full of mischief, with an amorality more happily innocent than that of some of his relatives, he idealizes in some respects the pre-adolescent boy, playful and essentially healthy. The story surrounding his birth epitomizes much of his character, his archetypal psychic functions. On the very day of his birth he stole forth from his cradle, journeyed long, until he came to the herds of cattle belonging to the gods and to his brother Apollo. Detaching fifty of these he drove them off, cleverly reversing their hoof marks and himself walking backwards. Having secreted them safely, he returned to his cradle through the key-hole and snuggled down, prepared to lie like a trooper when his brother furiously turned up. But he had also found a tortoise and of its shell together with sheep gut constructed a lyre, the first seven-stringed instrument ever. In due course, when he had admitted the theft, he gave his brother Apollo this lyre and peace and friendship between the brothers was sealed, Apollo giving Hermes the caduceus.

The hymn from 600 BC in which this is recorded is so full of light humour and fun that Hermes cannot but be loved. For Apollo trying to catch him fast in accusation and truth he was indeed a drop of mercury, breaking into innumerable droplets, coming together again somewhere else.

He is a herdsman, a traveller, a thief, a liar and so we find him as protector of cattle and guide to travellers; herms were originally heaps of stones set up to mark the way for those on journeys. Later herms were bearded heads set on square bases with prominent phalli at gates of cities and doors of houses. As thief he became patron of merchants and pickpockets whose task it is to redistribute wealth and keep up the circulation of goods. Night and darkness are congenial to him. As liar he became the symbol of herald and ambassador and politician and now of journalists. As guide to travellers he became also guide and messenger between gods, men and the underworld. He was the psychopomp, the guide of the souls after death. He is not a threatening god, always lightness and humour, quick-wittedness are his happy weapons.

He is guide to herds, leading them, to travellers and to souls. He guides to the place and time where good luck befalls. His blessings come as unexpected windfalls. How much good luck is needed for successful business or successful theft. Always under Hermes' guidance things move and thoughts fly. He had winged feet and wings upon his helmet, he carries the caduceus.

And Mercury, lose all the serpentine craft of thy caduceus.

(*Troilus & Cressida* II, 3.13)

He is master of hidden ways, sleight of hand and magic conjuring tricks. It is easy for him to become Hermes Trismegistos, patron of occult wisdom. His caduceus, the herald's wand of office, has two gold serpents twisting up the staff. Asklepios was always portrayed with one serpent coiling up his, on which he is often portrayed leaning.

We know that in Christian times Hermes-Mercury became the Archangel Raphael, patron of healing, whilst in the north he had become Odin-Wotan the chief of the northern gods. His name survives in our Wednesday, the French *mercredi*. As Raphael he has been the inspirer of the ideals of healing within the Christian world and belongs with St Rocco and his dog and St Sebastian with his arrows to the iconography of healing saints and gods.

Should we as physicians be offended at being lumped together with thieves and merchants and perjurors under the banner or caduceus of Mercury? Is there not something, some theme connecting these diverse activities? Does not healing often imply a re-ordering, a redistribution of functions, so that a content repressed into the unconscious may be restored to the realm of light and consciousness? Disease can be understood as a right thing in a wrong place and to rectify these states of affairs merchants, Robin Hoods and physicians labour, and all need much good luck.

Now if these are some of the images produced in the human mind by the Mercury archetype can we follow them through into the realms of physiology, pathology and the drug picture, as well as finding support in the properties of the metal mercury?

It belonged to the ancient view of things, which sought the micro-macro-cosmic correspondences, to correlate the planet and sphere of Mercury with the metal of the same name and with the lung as organ and with the glandular system. The lung corresponded with the planet and the glandular system with the sphere of mercury. The god Hermes or Mercury was so to speak the planetary genius. Accepting this again in a heuristic or 'as if' way, we hope it may help to bring to light the wholeness which lies fragmented in the materia medica. We can also regard the mythology of Hermes as the response of the collective psyche to Mercury, planet and metal, and therefore as a sort of mental proving.

Mercury the metal is familiar to us today as the sensitive content of thermometers. Its property of expanding and contracting readily to changes of temperature together with its fluid state at ordinary temperatures makes it ideal for this purpose. In barometers and sphygmomanometers, its heaviness allows these instruments to be of convenient size. Up till recent times it found a place in toys for children. A drop of mercury under glass in a box had to be manipulated into various holes and the child learnt the nature of quicksilver. It broke up into smaller drops and then these reunited again into larger ones. It ran all over the place without wetting the surfaces and it was shining bright like silver. These toys were duly banned because they got broken and a lost drop of mercury in a room evaporated to fill the room with toxic vapour. In past centuries it was combined with tin and used to make mirrors.

Mercury evaporates easily, it is unique amongst metals in retaining its pristine fluidity at ordinary temperatures and becomes solid at −39°C. In the solid state it has high thermal and electrical conductivity. Whilst to most substances it behaves as dry, not mixing with or wetting them, with metals it mixes to form amalgams. Amongst metals only iron and its congeners remain untouched. Today we can observe the hand of mercury in all the vast industrial and commercial amalgamations as well as in the hiving off of some less profitable activities again.

Mercury, like all liquids, assumes the drop form. Placed on a table with a bit of shellac it engulfs it in a manner reminiscent of an amoeba eating its food. In this it reveals a secret affinity to life, it wants to be alive. But at the same time it is a strong poison which is antipathetic to all life, particularly to micro-organisms. It, so to speak, mediates the heavenly cosmic forces to earth on one hand, yet the killing forces of the world of Hades on the other.

In the alchemical tradition, out of which modern chemistry and psychology originated along their divergent paths, mercury stood mediating between Sal on one hand and Sulphur on the other. The ancients recognized the four states of substance, Warmth, Air, Water and Earth. The alchemists were particularly concerned with the transitions between these states and these they could see more clearly in the living kingdoms of nature than in the physical world. The root of plants was the salt pole where the fluid phase passed over into earth, the flower was the sulphur pole whence emanated the perfumes and pollens, dematerializing in warmth, whilst the leaves were mercurial, air and fluid intermixing. Today we study colloids in which these phases interplay with each other.

Mercury, then, is a guide leading from one realm to another, standing at crossroads, gateways, doors. He is concerned with distribution and re-distribution, with breaking up and reuniting. Where something or some function seeks to go its own way, forsaking its social relationships and responsibilities, he leads it gently back again into the fold.

If we search for such functions within the organism, we are led first of all to the mucous membranes, the skin and sense organs. Under the influence of mercury, the glands of the mucous membranes become overactive, catarrhs develop and may progress to ulceration. The mouth and large intestine are most affected. The upper respiratory passages become involved and this process can pass down into the larynx and bronchi. So in the corresponding therapeutic uses of mercury we find particularly *Mercurius corrosivus* of help in dysentery and inflammatory conditions of the bowel. It acts strongly also in the mouth, throat and larynx and on the bladder and kidneys. Its characteristic in the bowel and bladder is the failure of the discharges to relieve the tenesmus. *Mercurius cyanatus* proved of immense service in diphtheria when this disease was a common part of daily medical practice. *Mercurius* itself, characterized by increased salivation and ulcers in the mouth, green and yellow nasal catarrh and purulent middle ear discharges, with profuse sweating, was in its actions well known when mercury was the main treatment for syphilis. Records show how mercury poisoning was pushed to extremes in the treatment, and inflammation around the teeth led to loss of teeth and necrosis of the jaws. Often the mercurial disease was worse than the syphilis.

In all these modes of action we can see an increased glandular activity. With them there is often enlargement of lymphatic glands, and mercury could well be helpful in acute glandular fever which symptomatically resembles secondary syphilis. We can add inflammation of the eyelids and iritis in the eye and various forms of eczema on the skin. We are dealing with glandular activities but also with activities lying on thresholds of the inner and outer. Can we also catch a glimpse of the mercury process in the region of the small intestine which seems relatively unaffected by the gross mercury poisoning? Here in the small intestine the food is completely broken down in the digestive process. It is de-natured and broken down to a mineral status. After passing through the intestinal wall the nutritional stream must be re-enlivened, incorporated into the living whole of the organism. Here we again find the mercury process, enlivening, integrating. Inside the lumen of the gut the action is concerned rather with sucking the surplus life out of the cells and out of the flora and fauna. Without the mercury process (not the substance of course) the prolific cell life of the intestinal mucous membrane would always develop carcinomatous tumours.

The mercury drug picture is also above all characterized by certain modalities, styles in the manifestation of the local symptoms. All the symptoms are made worse by heat and cold, reminding us of the thermometer. They are worse at night. This relates mercury to syphilis in which the symptoms grasped and interpreted as in homoeopathy are worse at night. It is thus related also, in the great polarity of the emotions, to fear as opposed to shame. Fear is the shadow side of our thinking, as shame is the shadow of our willing. One wonders whether Hahnemann in his teaching about the Miasms caught an intimation of this great inner polarity of our psychosomatic life. Syphilis, fear and the nervous system on one hand, sycosis, gonorrhoea, shame and the metabolic system on the other. Whilst we find anxiety, as the shadow side of the love hate play of our emotions, manifesting constraint in the very rhythmic system itself, related to Psora. In asthma and angina we see the very physiognomy of angst-anxiety.

The mercury discharges, whether catarrhs, diarrhoeas or sweats, do not relieve.

Here we have a most telling modality. We are accustomed to think of disease processes working from within to without in curative gesture and here such a gesture does not relieve, it may even aggravate. Can we perhaps see in this an indication that disease, disharmony, can come about from two sides? On the one hand from the metabolic pole, the abdominal, arise the inflammatory, exteriorizing diseases and on the other from the cephalic-nerve pole the interiorizing, sclerosing processes. This mercury modality, not relieved by discharges, points then, to the cephalic pole and leads us to the mercury effects on the brain and nerves. These are usually recognized as insomnia, headache, tremor, loss of memory, depression and intense irritability — mercurial erethism — which includes reticence and timidity. There is a characteristic tremor. In homoeopathic and some other literature this is often described as similar to parkinsonism, but whereas in that condition there is usually reduction of tremor on movement, in mercurialism the tremor is, according to most books, aggravated by movement. But the rigidity of parkinsonism is not found in mercury poisoning, nor the characteristic facies. The tremor may be severe and some authors compare it more to chorea. Hallucinations and fear may develop and a marked timidity. At some stages a great restlessness aggravated by warmth of bed is characteristic. We should also recall the now extinct pink disease in children, attributed to mercury teething powders.

These together with the metallic taste and marked fetor are the main symptoms found in the homoeopathic drug pictures. In the grouping of remedies associated with the bowel nosodes, Dr John Paterson found *Phosphorus* and *Silica* and the syphilitic nosode *Lueticum* to be most closely associated with *Mercurius* and the *Gaertner* nosode. Both *Phosphorus* and *Silica* are remedies characterized in the drug pictures by fearfulness and phobias. *Lueticum* amongst other symptoms of a similar sort has in its drug picture the obsessional symptom, always washing the hands. It does seem that this group of remedies is related to phobic and obsessional tendencies in which it becomes difficult to let go of an idea or ritual behaviour. There is, so to speak, a fear of the forgetfulness of sleep and hence of the night, a fear of the realm of the unconscious, of the other world. This fear of letting go seems to represent a metamorphosis, from the somatic to the psychic plane, of the retention of air in the lung in asthma. There the air in the lung cannot be let go, here in phobic and obsessional conditions the psyche cannot let go of its content of fear or ritual.

We have here begun to touch on the organ of the lung as distinct from the glandular processes and secretions which made up the most part of the mercury drug pictures. And we have to admit that the lung as an organ presents us with problems and paradoxes.

We can watch in the tadpole the metamorphosis from fishlike swimming form into the air-breathing frog walking on land. Lungs are formed inwardly and at the same time the legs are formed on which the frog can come to land. It is as though coming to earth implies taking a breath of air as well as standing on the ground.

148

We remember at the same time the child's first breath with which the soul enters the body, echoing the Genesis story:

> And the Lord God formed man of the dust of the ground, and breathed
> into his nostrils the breath of life; and man became a living soul.

The lungs develop as an outgrowth from the alimentary canal and look, to begin with, as if they would form a gland comparable to the liver or pancreas. But then they move forwards or upwards, even as the kidney moves backwards or downwards from its cephalic position as pronephros, to meso and metanephros. With this reversal of their relative positions a further change in what could be called its original intention comes about for the lung. It gives up its glandular intentions, sacrifices them we could also say, and opens itself to the outer air. The air can then enter into the lung and pass into the blood whilst the carbon dioxide can pass outwards. A respiratory and rhythmic function is then superimposed on what was originally a metabolic organ.

This upward movement of the lungs reveals itself in another remarkable phenomenon. Many fishes have swim bladders and secrete air into them; some of these bladders have connections with the outside. In some fishes these bladders have sacs extending between many of the muscles, as in birds. Mostly it seems these organs are not so much accessory respiratory organs as concerned with balance and rising and falling in the water. In some fishes they are connected by a series of small ossicles to the semicircular canals in the head region. They thus as lung analogues have connected themselves to that region from which the kidneys fell.

The lung becomes the organ through which the organism enters into the most direct relationship with the outer world. Without the digestive processes to which food is subjected, the oxygen in the air passes directly into the blood, which opens itself directly to the outer world in the lung. Carbon dioxide excretion helps to control the balance of carbonic acid in the blood which is so intimately involved with calcium in bone formation. The bony skeleton is the expression of the earth element within the organism. Further, the breathing rhythm is closely related to the rhythm in the nervous system and cerebrospinal fluid. The lungs have moved into the rhythmic realm of the head and it is from the head that the sclerosing dynamic of the skeleton proceeds. All these gestures point to the lung as the organ through which we become earth men. It can become in this way the organic basis of the melancholic temperament, the earthy temperament which experiences the weight of matter most intensely. But it plays also a balancing role within the organism, firstly compensating for the fall of the kidney, secondly relating the metabolic realm to the nervous pole and thirdly in the breathing rhythm in interplay with the heart beat mediating between the great blood-nerve polarity of the organism.

We can now perhaps begin to see that the figure of Hermes-Mercury is a true picture of this organ system mediating between the realms of head, chest and abdomen, or heaven, earth and the underworld.

In psychiatric disorders, where the organic dynamics invade and over-determine the soul life, we can follow these lung dynamics further. In lung conditions such as asthma and emphysema we can see the head forces taking over too strongly in the lung. The lung becomes too like the head. Such dynamic disturbance manifesting in the psyche produces obsessional, compulsive and phobic symptoms. The thought life becomes too rigid and structured. On the other hand in lung conditions where dissolving processes predominate, as can happen in tuberculosis, dreamy romantic yearnings come to the fore. In the obsessional compulsive disorders mercury can prove very helpful as a remedy, bringing movement into the rigidity. The vegetabilized preparations *Bryophyllum Mercurio cultum* and *Nasturtium Mercurio cultum* have proved especially useful. Guirdham has characterized the obsessional conflict as the expression within us of the unresolved conflict between the heretic or mystic and the inquisitor. These two types would have resulted on the one hand in a formless freedom and on the other in a frozen rigid dogmatism. Do they not represent the polarity between the metabolic and nervous poles within the organism, between Apollo who can become a right-minded prig and Dionysos who can also degenerate into a drunken vandal.

The centre of the world's mercury ores is in Europe, in Spain, Italy and Southern Russia. Europe itself should be the mediating, balancing, healing function in the world, a mercurial function. In the North of Europe, Mercury became Odin-Wotan leading the Vikings, and in Italy and Spain the Church adopted the legalism of Rome into a rigid organization and dogma. Instead of fruitful polarities, confrontation arose and the true spirit of Hermes-Raphael has been lost to sight, as it has been also in medicine. Can the youthful, lovable figure of Mercury-Hermes grow up and mature in our consciousness into the genius and inspirer of true healing?

18. Silver (*argentum*)

We are all familiar with silver, whether in the form of mirrors, spoons, forks and other table ware or as ornaments, and some of us can remember when our coinage still contained appreciable amounts of this noble metal. We are also under its poetic spell and from time immemorial the moon has been linked with silver. Shakespeare has used this correspondence again and again:

> The moon like to a silver bow
> New-bent in heaven, (*Love's Labour Lost*)

But again it stands for the wisdom of older age:

> Venerable Nestor, hatched in silver . . .
> And to achieve the silver livery of advised age. (*Troilus and Cressida*)

Water, rivers and the sea claim affinity, too, as well as music:

> This little world, this precious stone, set in the silver sea. (*Richard II*)

> Music with her silver sound — why 'silver sound'?
> Why music with her silver sound?
> Marry, Sir, because silver hath a sweet sound. (*Romeo and Juliet*)

In ancient Greece, the goddess Artemis was associated with the moon and with silver; her bow and arrows were of silver, whereas her twin brother Apollo was even at birth adorned with gold and the sun was his planet.

The human soul responds to the processes and substances of our world with myth, legend and poetic imagery, and these can be understood as the revelation of the higher reality lying latent, like a sleeping princess, within the natural phenomena. They constitute, one might also say, a homoeopathic proving in a very clear and heightened form. In contemplating these images and symbols we may be led deeper into the hidden genius of the substance and its remedial actions than by confining our attention strictly to the realm of material effects and the statutory rubrics of official provings.

But at the beginning of our study we must also take note of phenomena in which the genius of silver comes to expression in the realms of chemistry and physics. Foremost amongst these, and again familiar to all of us, are the processes occurring when we take a photograph. It is to silver salts that we are indebted for our capacity to make photographic reproductions. Silver salts, particularly the chloride, bromide and iodide, are extremely sensitive to light which reduces the salt, thereby liberating metallic silver. Another characteristic is revealed in the Liesegang rings which form in concentric rhythmic circles when silver nitrate solution is dropped on chromate-impregnated gelatin. These rings form rather like the waves on a pool of water when a stone is dropped into it. A rhythmically repeated series of coloured rings is formed and when, to take an instance from yet another realm, we stand between two mirrors we can see an endlessly repeated series of reflections of ourselves. Reproduction itself is another example of repeated manifestations of an original form or species type. Silver very easily enters into the colloidal state. We know that life phenomena are dependent to a great extent on this colloidal state. The intimate relationship between the silver process and the life processes is here suggested, and relates to the connections between the moon and these same life processes.

When we turn to the occurrence of silver in nature we find the greatest part of it in the sea, where it is present in a dilution of 10 mg to a cubic metre. Today its ores occur most plentifully in the western hemisphere. It often occurs in the midst of lead ores or in association with gold or copper. Commonly it is combined with sulphur or with antimony or arsenic. The native metal occurs in two forms. In the one it is found as wire-like threads or delicate fern-like growths, whilst in the other it is also found as knobs like bunches of grapes.

These two forms in which native silver occurs lead us back to the goddess Artemis or Diana. Artemis has two very different aspects in Greek mythology, so much so that some scholars look upon these aspects as coming from quite distinct sources. On the mainland of Greece the goddess was a young maiden loving to live with her girl companions in the woods, hunting and caring for the animals, particularly in their giving birth. As Patrick Geddes pointed out, she represents a stage of girlhood when even today girls often prefer to lavish their love on pet animals rather than on pimply youths and can aim their arrows at any such who are foolhardy enough to approach them. In Athens girls from an age of about nine were apprenticed to the goddess at her temple at Brauron, where they were known as she-bears. This young Artemis has her silver bow and arrow, reminding us at once of the native silver threads and of the newborn crescent moon. But at Ephesus on the coast of Asia Minor was the great temple of Artemis, one of the greatest of the wisdom mystery centres of antiquity. There the great sage-philosopher Heracleitos lived and wrote, and there St Paul incurred the wrath of the silversmith Demetrios who saw his livelihood endangered by the new religion. Thither too, according to ancient tradition, came the Virgin Mary and St John. The statues of the Ephesian Artemis show us a different aspect, a mature and deeply moving goddess, dressed in temple costume on which hang bunches of fruit. These have mistakenly given rise to the description 'many-breasted Diana of the Ephesians'. They remind us of the knobs of native silver and of the full moon. The two forms of the goddess seem to correspond to the new and full moons respectively and also to the contrasted appearance of the two forms of native silver.

We have referred to the use of silver as a mirror. Not only is silver the most perfect reflector of light, giving nothing of itself to the image, but also when used to make musical instruments such as flutes and bells, it gives the purest sweetest tones. That the moon is a mirror we indeed all know. When the astronauts on leaving the moon fired their capsule back to hit her, the instruments left on her surface recorded her continuing reverberations for half an hour — a fine bell indeed. Yet a further strange correspondence between silver and the moon can be observed when silver is heated to melting point. It then absorbs a large quantity of air and when it is cooled again this sputters forth, leaving the surface pock-marked with craters like the surface of the moon.

We cannot, of course, take it that the moon is made of silver, in the sense that schoolboys used to maintain it was made of green cheese. But that the moon manifests processes and qualities which we associate with silver here on earth is perhaps not inconceivable. We understand that Professor V. Gutman in Vienna has been discovering that certain metals can be made, by varying the context of forces in which they act, to behave in the manner of different ones. L. Kolisko was able long ago to show by capillary-dynamolytic techniques that the patterns of silver salts on filter paper were drastically changed during lunar eclipses.

We have been touching upon the correspondences between silver, the moon and the goddess Artemis. These relationships, well known to the ancients, were perhaps directly perceived in a dreamlike clairvoyance in those days. A common theme runs through them, reproduction and reflection. That the moon is intimately related to the rhythms of reproductive life and to the romantic dreams of lovers is beyond doubt. Artemis as maiden goddess was concerned with all the reproductive powers of nature and as goddess of Ephesus with the re-creation of the human soul. We shall now have to find the connections between silver and the reproductive processes on the one hand and the reflective forces of consciousness on the other, as these come about in the human organism.

When we come to study the homoeopathic drug pictures of *Argentum* and *Argentum nitricum*, we are struck especially by a twofold affinity between silver and the processes and organs within the human realm. There is a definite affinity to the reproductive organs and the strong life processes in them. Connected with this there is a relationship with the digestive-absorptive processes through which the organism is materially replenished and regenerated. On the other hand there is a relationship to the head, brain, spinal cord and nerves. These are the very organs in which life processes are at their weakest — as shown by the early loss of regenerative power in nerve cells. But they are the organs in which consciousness is most awake. Reproduction takes place in the uterus, reflection takes place in the brain. Mankind conceives babies in the uterus, and thoughts in the head. Nor has it escaped notice that the brain floats in its cerebrospinal fluid within the membranes of the skull in a similar manner to the foetus within the amniotic fluid and membranes in the uterus.

There is an old tale from Hellas about the birth of Pallas Athene. Zeus became aware that his wife Hera had become pregnant without help from god, hero or mortal. He became so anxious about the implications of this event that he developed a bad headache. This became so bad that he sent for the Eileithyiai who were the Olympian midwives and asked them to examine him. They confirmed his suspicions that he was pregnant. Meanwhile Hera had given birth to Hephaestos, the Olympian smith, and in the manner of the immortals he had rapidly grown up. Zeus sent for him and commanded him to take his axe and cleave his skull and deliver him. This Hephaestos did, rapidly departing as Pallas Athene leapt fully armed from her father's head. Thus was Zeus's migraine cured.

A year or two ago I noticed in a medical journal a comment characterizing migraine as cephalic dysmenorrhoea and dysmenorrhoea as uterine migraine.

Argentum metallicum and *nitricum* are characterized by intense unilateral headaches, surely migraines, and by headaches with a sensation of great swelling, as if the head was becoming larger and larger, surely an excellent description of cephalic pregnancy. The pain also may build up slowly and stop suddenly (when the axe of Hephaestos accomplishes delivery by a cephalic Caesarean section).

In the genital region we find *Argentum* associated with uterine haemorrhages at the menopause and also midway between menses. Severe erosions of the cervix with leucorrhoea and a sensation of enlargement of the ovary, (usually, according to the books, left). In the male there is pain in the testicle (reported as usually the right) and impotence.

The symptoms in the digestive tract can help us get a little nearer to the inwardness of silver. There is profuse watery diarrhoea, often brought on by emotional causes such as anticipatory anxiety or shock. But characteristically there is also large and repeated accumulation of wind in the stomach. Presumably the wind is swallowed. So we have a very marked separation of the airy from the fluid element in the digestive realm, in the stool the watery diarrhoea, in the stomach much wind and gastralgia. It would seem therefore that in place of a harmonious interpenetration of the fluid, gaseous and solid components in the alimentary sphere, a loosening and separation has come about. Sometimes patients can tell how with a shock they 'jumped right out of their skin', and may add that they never seem to have quite got back inside again.

We have been touching on various pointers to the relationship between the vital processes and the fluid or watery element. It is not difficult to see that the psyche or soul is more related to the gaseous or airy phenomena. In Latin the word *animus* refers to both soul and air and in Genesis we can read 'the Lord God formed man of the dust of the ground, and breathed into his nostrils the breath of life; and man became a living soul.' Everyone can observe how with each in-breathing we wake up a little and with every out-breathing we go a little to sleep, and when we are born we take our first breath in, when we die we give our last breath out.

So if shock is particularly liable to jump us out of ourselves, and especially so in the realms of the genital and digestive functions, we can understand how *Argentum* may help to reunite the soul and body again. But we can perhaps help to bring out these connections further by taking a digression through some related phenomena.

There is a tendency in modern biology to aspire to finding a direct continuous material connection between successive, similar, entities. For instance in evolution theory it is the physical line of inheritance that is the centre of attention, and in embryology and related studies the transference of the genetic code from gener-ation to generation and from cell to cell has assumed central importance. It is of course obvious that although all the cells in the organism have the same code they develop in very differentiated ways to form the distinctive tissues and organs. And, varying at different stages of embryogenesis, there is a capacity, when faced with mechanical injury or mutilation to a part, to regroup and reform and restore what we can only call a whole embryo. How can one begin to grasp this wholeness? It is almost axiomatic for modern science to deny the possibility of so doing, and all attempts to approach this central issue of biology are sneeringly referred to as mysticism. Nevertheless, let us explore a little further.

How does it come about that from piles of building materials a building takes shape? Certainly the work of builders, aided by mechanical devices of varied complexity, is essential, but by itself this would not lead to a pig-sty, let alone a house, or factory, or temple. For this to happen there must be a plan, whether in the builder's imagination in the simplest case, or transferred to complex draw-ings in more complicated instances. From these plans or blueprints many copies can be made and many identical or only slightly varied houses built. It would not be sensible to look for the cause of the resemblances between these houses solely in the building materials. Again, a student artist can copy a great painting and the way in which the chemical substances in the paints come to lie on his canvas is not caused materially by the pigments on the original painting. By searching out the chemistry one will never discover the picture, although this could not come to manifestation without the materials as well as the artist's skill and imagin-ation. The picture represents a whole which determines all the parts and processes going into its creation. The picture, the image, is the whole which orders all the parts and processes which go to its material composition, but it does not materially determine them. But how far can such examples from the physical world help us when it comes to living organisms? In the first place, in the sphere of life, the idea, the archetype, is full of life, no longer a finished form or scheme. The

155

archetypal idea of the organism, for example the *Urpflanze* of Goethe, is a continuously metamorphosing veritable Proteus. In short, it is full of life and movement, and further it is full of wisdom. Our examples then were only temporary props and scaffolding to point the way towards the living, metamorphosing wisdom-filled 'idea' which we can only perceive with the eye of imagination, but which as reality is the wholeness which pervades and unites all the diverse processes which constitute the life of an organism in time as well as space. If we are able to grant, even as hypothesis, the reality of such an ideal entity full of life and wisdom, then the problems of reproduction and nutrition take on a new form. When the food has been broken down in the digestive process to a stage of merely chemical building bricks, denatured and stripped of the life and *Gestalt* of its original source, whether animal or plant, it has to be not only rebuilt but enlivened by the organism into which it is entering. Current thoughts look to mechanical templates as models for this process. But these could at best only produce structural replicas. To be enlivened and taken into the living wholeness of the organism, this nutritional stream passing into blood and lymph must be ordered within the living image, which in the case of a living organism implies differentiated order in time as well as space. It is not a question of restructured units, but of an introduction into the realm of activity of the living ideal entity we have been pointing to. This entity cannot be conceived in terms of a vital force comparable with other natural forces. It is an entity more comparable to a picture, but a picture or idea which metamorphoses in time. By devoted observation of the phenomena of metamorphosis in living nature we can gradually strengthen and inwardly vitalize our thinking, to perceive these living ideas in a manner similar to that by which our dead intellectual thinking grasps the abstract, rigid ideas appropriate for handling the world of dead and physical things. To such an entity the traditional name of etheric body has been given. The name is not important. Paracelsus called it *Archaeus*.

We can also extend this approach to the problems of reproduction, and look for the ordering principle which enlivens and guides the embryonic metamorphosis in this same realm of the ideal image entity which can again and again manifest itself in a new and similar organism. In nutrition, the organism constantly renews itself; in reproduction, in a more total and radical way, a new organism comes into existence.

Now how are we to approach closer to the nature of this ideal entity? We have suggested that it is closer to the fluid, watery element than to the solid, earthy. The solid and earthy element is certainly known to us as three-dimensional. We usually think of the fluid element also in such terms, but perhaps mistakenly. A study of water in movement reveals that it becomes a manifold of interweaving surfaces, planes. Only when static, stagnant, an unnatural state for water, does it begin to become subject to the lattice structure that prevails in solid ice. In the constant flow and whirl and swirl of water it loses this three-dimensionality and becomes two-dimensional, multitudinous surfaces interweaving from all directions. In the discipline of synthetic geometry, the plane becomes a reality of equal validity to the point, and the interweaving of these planes a matter of geometric study. George Adams was able to pioneer the study of the living forms of plants and their metamorphoses from this point of view, and clarify the importance of the two-dimensional leaf in the vital phenomena, as indeed the archetypal organ of the plant. In his published works, these themes are beautifully developed.

Two of the particular properties of silver from which we started are especially planar and surface phenomena, mirror reflections and photographic reproductions. We have briefly discussed the relation of photography to reproduction and we must now as briefly touch on the mirroring of events in our brains. That we can form memory images of our perceptions is our common experience, and these bear a comparable relation to the original perception as do mirror images to the objects mirrored. The images in both cases are not 'real' in the sense of the originals, they lack substantiality, touchability. It is further possible to understand our concepts, our ideas, as, in a similar way, mirror images of the creative realities amidst which we lived in our prenatal existence. Plato took it in some such way, and St Paul's 'Now I see in a glass darkly' may also refer to the same realm of experience.

We can now relate the mirror reflections in our heads and the reproductions in our uteri to the silver processes and to the younger and maturer figures of the goddess Artemis.

There remain a few further indications in the drug pictures to consider. Under the picture of *Argentum metallicum*, references are made to action on the cartilages. However, closer study brings out no evidence of any action on the cartilages as such; rather it seems that there is pain without swelling around the joints. Hysterical joints are particularly mentioned and various cramplike pains in the limbs. From the psychosomatic point of view, there are connections between the joints and reproductive processes. The word 'join' is connected with the root *gn* or *kn* which occurs in gynae, generation, know, knee, and a multitude of similar words. In Genesis we read Adam knew Eve, and Shakespeare has the expression 'In the pregnant hinges of the knee', reminding us that Homer refers to the future lying in the knees of the gods. In the old marriage ceremony of the Church of England we hear 'We are met here to join together in Holy Matrimony this man and this woman.' Enough, it is clear from the side of symbol and language that the connection between joints and generation exists, and I suggest that the action of *Argentum* on painful, hysterical joints finds its explanation here.

The larynx and voice figure in the pictures of *Argentum met.* and *Argentum nitricum* under hoarseness and loss of voice, clergyman's sore throat. Are we not here still in the same realm of connections and symbols? Speech and the word have always been regarded as creative. In speaking, we create forms in the air which 'body forth' our meanings. These forms are related to sound as the mirroring and photographic processes are related to light and bring us back to 'Music with her silver sound.'

Silver nitrate, lunar caustic, has of course a relation to irritation and ulceration of mucous surfaces. The gastro-intestinal tract, particularly the duodenum, and the conjunctivae are centres of its action. In older days it proved its worth for the eyes of infants and babies, both by local application and given in potency by mouth. The reports of suppurating conjunctivitis of the new-born clearing up in hours with *Arg. nit.* in potency seem incontrovertible. These would seem to point to some affinity with the eye organ, and perhaps yet again this is to be grasped through the symbol.

So far we have attempted to bring into some wholeness the scattered range of symptoms under *Argentum met.* and *Argentum nit.* To do this we have used the image of silver, Artemis, moon and water, and found the centres of the silver process in the human in the reproduction organs on one hand and the nervous system on the other.

Some further uses and indications for *Argentum* may now be mentioned. Foremost are all conditions arising out of shock, fright and emotional upsets. These may show particularly in dysfunction of sexual processes, menstruation particularly, and then, as the soul tries to cramp back in again after being shocked out, it may indeed cramp into other organs such as the intestine, giving rise to many bizarre clinical disturbances of function. The *Argentum* helps to consolidate the harmonious interpenetration again of psyche and soma in the genital functions and thus lay the foundation for further therapy. This may be, and often is, the basic first line in treating hysterical conditions and other psychiatric conditions when shock stands at their origin. It is out of the shock syndrome, understood in the widest sense, that the anxiety symptoms of *Argentum nit.* arise. Through not getting properly back into one's skin, the feeling of both general anxiety can come about and also the strange fears of high places, corners, not being able to find one's orientation rightly into the spatial world. Such symptoms find varied itemization in the drug pictures.

The preparations of silver first precipitated as a mirror are particularly helpful, *Argentum pr.* 6x for instance. Silver can also be used in two polar psychological tendencies. Firstly in those like somnambulism where the soul life lacks form and is open to all sorts of extrasensory influences. Here *Arg. pr.* 6x during waxing moon and *Phosphorus* 6x during waning moon have been found helpful. Secondly, in conditions where the soul life has dried up too much into rigid abstract intellectualism, *Argentum* in combination with *Sulphur* as *Silver glance* can help restore life and healthy imagination to the arid mental scene.

In tracing the silver process in these varied realms I have been trying to bring some wholeness into the chaotic pictures of *Silver* in the materia medica. I have not found either the toxicological facts or the vague and unlimited lists of mental symptoms alone much help, rather they are the problem, the riddle waiting for a solution. By grasping the image of silver in the way indicated and searching in man for the realm of processes rather than either structural end results or peculiar isolated symptoms, I am confident one can take a step forward. It is a method, of course, that rejects the one-sided reductionism of modern physiological and pathological research, and also an equally one-sided merely symptomatological approach. I am of the opinion that the drug pictures are related to the realm of processes or functions, a realm which is intermediate between structurally grasped soma and the purely subjectively grasped psyche. The fact that this is the realm of the specifically living which cannot be grasped by dead abstract intellectual concepts does certainly face us with a challenge, but not perhaps an absolutely insuperable one. Perhaps even some silver to increase our capacity of living fantasy could help us.

19. Fungi

The realm of the fungi is a strange and paradoxical one within the plant kingdom. What are we to make of plants which have no chlorophyll, and therefore live as saprophytes or parasites; have no leaves, those most essential and characteristic organs of the plant; and have a metabolism which is katabolic, in some respects more like an animal's than anabolic like a plant's? They are composed of mycelial networks which are made of fine hyphae, threadlike columns of simple cells which in the yeasts even fall apart into these separate cells. These mycelial threads may become matted together, as in the mould on jam, which cannot really be called a tissue, as the mycelial threads grow only lengthwise in one dimension. From these mycelial networks arise, in some forms, the fruiting bodies, amongst which the toadstools and mushrooms are familiar to everyone. Nowhere do they produce the two-dimensional planar organ, the leaf, and nowhere do they produce the green chlorophyll of the typical plant. They do produce some brightly coloured pigments, familiar to us in the variegated toadstools. There is something rather garish, even ghoulish about many of these, and mostly they emit stench rather than the perfumes of true flowers. They are visited mostly by flies and beetles and slugs rather than the bees and butterflies attendant on the blossoms of higher plants. What are these fungi? What element of the fully developed plant do they represent or manifest in such a one-sided specialized mode?

These fungi play a great part in our social economic life. Under their influence organic matter is decomposed into the inorganic. They can destroy the timbers of buildings, as anyone unfortunate enough to have had dry rot in his house can tell. In the forests and woodlands they bring about the decay and rotting of fallen trees and vegetation to prepare new soil. Their existence around and even within the roots of many trees and plants is necessary for their growth. Invasion of the tissues of plants by fungi on the other hand is one of the major causes of diseases in plants and calls for constant surveillance and use of fungicides in horticulture and farming. They can cause disease in animals and humans. The occurrence of the fungus *Claviceps purpurea* on rye and other grains has been responsible over centuries for many terrible epidemics of St Anthony's fire, arising from the consumption of bread made from contaminated flour. Only regular public health inspection has brought this danger under control. On the other hand yeasts play a valuable part in the production of bread and beer.

During and since the last war fungi have been a main source of the new drugs, the antibiotics, which have transformed much of medical and veterinary practice. Hundreds of thousands of different fungi have been screened as possible sources of new antibiotics and the array of rival antibiotic drugs now available for the physicians and surgeons has become bewildering. They are clearly important in the economy of nature and in the economics of man. Can we approach the riddle of their real nature?

In normal flowering plants we do find processes which are essentially parasitic on the rest of the plant. The flowering and fruiting processes are dependent on the anabolic processes in the rest of the plant. In the blossom, chlorophyll disappears and although the petal retains the planar two-dimensional form of the leaf, this almost gives way to linear form in the stamens. The fungus has no stem, its fruiting body arises straight out of the earth or earth equivalent. It can grow in the dark. So if we are to compare the parasitism of the fungus with the parasitic flowering fruiting process in the higher plants we must add that here this process has been transposed downwards to the earth and makes no relationship to the light. The normal plant develops between the dark and damp earth and the light and airy realm. We can watch this polarity of influences in the plant. The plant unfolds its true form and nature within the play of this polarity. In the fungi, the influence of light is missing, so that the fungi develop one-sidedly as earth beings. They show no influence from the realm of light, the wide spaces of the universe. They lack the true expressions of plant form, the stem and leaf. Their linear growth by cell budding at the mycelial tips is entirely an example of Euclidean geometry, knowing nothing of the planar forces and forms of negative Euclidean space. The cell principle, atomic principle, dominates, and there is a constant tendency to disintegration into spores. Their influence is towards disintegration to dead mineral substances. Chains of fungi work together to accomplish chains of chemical breakdown. Those forms and forces which lift up the dead mineral substances into the realm of life in normal plants are foreign to them. They themselves turn to dust in spore formation and turn everything to dust. They are the expression of earthly and sub-earthly forces and show us that the life and living forms of the true plant world must be looked for elsewhere than in the earth. It was indeed a clear message, indicating the true nature of the forces involved, when the atomic explosions gave rise to the mushroom clouds. Disintegration, mineralization, destruction of life forms, production of dust, these are key notes of the 'life' of fungi.

We may however get another view of the world of the fungi from the phenomena of plant galls. These abnormal growths on trees and plants are produced by fungal infestation or by the larvae of mites, gnats, wasps or sometimes by nematodes.

We are struck on the one hand by the similarity in the influence upon the host plant of the fungus and larva. On the other hand we are faced with the gall itself which often resembles a fruit or nut from some other tree. The parasite, whether fungus or larva, instigates the host to a fruiting or pseudo-fruiting process displaced from its normal position in time and space. This may result in damage to the further development of the host. But the host may isolate the abnormal process and appear otherwise unaffected. Some of these galls really imitate fruits, such as plums or cherries, to a remarkable degree and some, developing on leaves, bring about a transformation of the leaf into a pseudo-carpel, a pod. A fungus or larva therefore in touching the plant initiates a fruiting process. The fungus in this gesture again betrays its 'animal' aspect. When a plant blossoms and fruits, it is, as it were, touched by the animal world of insects hovering over it; it attains to the status of animal in its fertilization and fruiting, as Oken long ago pointed out. The particular forms of the gall are very specific to the particular larva or fungus involved, typical for that parasite rather than for the host. They may show the same character when the same parasite invades a different host. The form of the gall comes more from the parasite than from the host.

Something similar is observed in those fungus infections known as rusts. In these the fungus invades the under-surface of the leaves of grasses and other plants. They produce spores reminiscent of those produced normally on the under-surface of the leaves of ferns. Through their action the higher plant reverts to a more primitive fernlike condition, and a premature 'spore' formation replaces the normal 'fruiting' process.

We get yet a clearer indication of the nature of the fungus when we see it replacing the stamens and anthers of some plant. Then it sheds its spores instead of the plant shedding its pollen. The plant itself remains unaffected. We can see the fungi as a fructifying process which has been pushed downwards into the darkness of the earth. Or, as in these infestations, we have to understand that the telluric earthly forces have themselves risen up in the plant, affording a second dynamic earth level for the fungus to grow in.

If we now turn our attention to the realm of the lichens, we discover a fungus living in happy symbiosis with an alga. These two one-sided primitive plants come together to establish a new rank of plants, the lichens. But they are really a symbiosis. The alga which contains chlorophyll contributes photosynthesis whilst the hyphae of the fungus form a protective covering and make minerals accessible to the partnership. These primitive plants, the lichens, can survive and flourish under conditions impossible for other types of living creatures, but on the other hand they are peculiarly sensitive to atmospheric pollution. They are found under Arctic conditions of extreme rigour. Commonly we know them on rocks and the bark of trees, contributing their multi-coloured covering.

We have been struck so far by the predominantly katabolic metabolism of fungi. Their activity is largely a breaking down of organic substance to inorganic matter.

Enormously complicated processes come about through the co-operation of different fungi together with bacteria. They tend together towards disintegration, they are in the main death processes.

Does this not lead us to question the relation between this realm of fungi and the system which in the human organization carries pre-eminently the forces of death — the brain and nervous system? The nerve fibres run as threads throughout the organism. The brain and nerves live fundamentally as parasites upon the organism. Only in the embryo do the nerve cells multiply; probably after birth or early childhood they lose the possibility of reproduction. The fungi of course retain this capacity and the hyphae are composed of long chains of cells, unlike the nerve fibre arising from a single cell. In the embryonic stage of life, and even to a great extent in babyhood, we are almost all head with a small appendage of trunk and limbs. Gradually we grow down from this head, as a plant grows up from the root. It has often been noted that plant and man stand in inverted relationship to each other. A man would have to be turned upside down and planted with his head in the earth, trunk, limbs and genitals pointing upwards, for the correspondences between man and plant to become clear.

So if there is a possible relationship to be discovered between brain and nerves and the realm of the fungi, it would point again to the earth as the home of these strange forms of life. In the embryo and baby, the head is still concerned with growth, and consciousness is obviously not yet imprisoned within the witch's cottage of our head. But as the death processes gradually take over in our brains, we wake up in our heads. Historically it was only in Greek times that thinking began to be experienced as related to the brain.

Can we get any further by looking at the drug pictures and medical experiences in relation to fungi? The very nature of fungus activity leading to fragmentation and disintegration, even to atomization, is echoed in the intellectual activity based on the brain. This too in its one-sided analytical and abstracting activity leads to information of ever increasing complexity and chaos, the information explosion. So it is understandable that synthetic grasp of the phenomena is particularly difficult in this study of fungi.

In the homoeopathic materia medica we find the following representatives of the fungi:

Agaricus emeticus
Agaricus muscarius
Agaricus phalloides
Boletus satanas
Bovista nigrescens
Secale cornutum
Ustilago maydis

to use the names still used in the materia medicas.

To these should perhaps be added *Thlaspi bursa-pastoris* (The shepherd's purse)

163

a plant belonging to the Cruciferae, the family which contains Cochlearia, Iberis, Raphanus and Sinapis in the materia medica. Thlaspi is almost always heavily invaded by a fungus and O. Leeser suggested that its drug picture, divergent from the other members of the family, was in fact due to the fungus parasite, not to the host plant.

The lichens, a symbiosis of an alga and fungus, in the materia medica are:

Cetraria islandica (Iceland moss)
Chladonia rangiferina (reindeer moss)
Sticta pulmonaria
Usnea barbata

We must also consider, in broadest outline, the antibiotics. But the huge range of diseases arising from fungus invasion is outside the scope of this essay. It is worth noting, however, that poisonings and provings have been due either to eating the mushrooms or fruiting bodies or, in the case of provings, taking tinctures of these. In the case of fungus diseases, mycelial invasion of tissues takes place. The first are usually called mycotoxicoses, the second mycoses. There are also allergic reactions, such as farmer's lung.

Agaricus (Amanita) muscarius, fly agaric. This toadstool or mushroom is in appearance known to everyone as it is the one usually depicted in fairy-story books with its brilliant scarlet or orange-red cap with white patches. It has been used to prepare decoctions for use as a fly poison. It has also been used to prepare an intoxicating drink by many peoples including the Lapps and some tribes in Siberia. Amongst some of these it is said to have been used by the Shamans to help induce the trance-like state in which they utter their prophecies.

The main active principle is muscarine, which produces most of the symptoms and is antidoted by atropine. Some books claim that this toadstool also contains atropine.

In non-lethal doses it induces intoxication, sweating, salivation, lachrymation, vomiting and diarrhoea. The pulse is slow and irregular, and vomiting and diarrhoea, double vision and hallucinations may occur. Symptoms occur rapidly after ingestion and in non-lethal cases pass off again equally quickly in a few hours.

The homoeopathic drug picture which includes results of provings and clinical experiences, characterizes the emotional state under such terms as loss of emotional control, laughter, loquacity, and tendency to versifiction. Senses are intensified and appearances become very beautiful. A teaspoon may appear as a lake and other objects appear enlarged. The disturbances may intensify to maniacal dimensions.

Irregular movements, tics, blepharospasm and choreiform jerks have all been caused and cured. In earlier times, when chorea was common, it was a most useful remedy for this condition.

Many older accounts refer to 'spinal irritation' as a well recognized condition, even diagnosis. Was this a variant on the 'railway spine' which was supposed, about a hundred years ago, to manifest in extreme sensitivity along the spine, with spasms in the muscles? Frequently the patients were reduced to wrecks. Theories of meningeal irritation, of ascending or descending spinal degeneration, of meningomyelitis and so on abounded. Some of the descriptions equal those of Charcot with his 'hysterics'. The terminology gradually changed to 'traumatic neurasthenia' and later such phenomena became transferred to the categories of psychoneurosis. Today they contribute to the mixed bag of ME and post-viral syndromes.

To return to *Agaricus muscarius*, we find prominent in its drug picture, chilblains with discolouration, burning and irritation. These symptoms are worse for cold and better for heat, distinguishing them from the *Pulsatilla* chilblains and from the burnings of ergot poisonings which are worse for heat. Bunions are reported as within its sphere of action. There are pains as of ice-cold needles also relieved by warmth, and headaches with these icy needles, or as if a nail were driven into the temple. Also described are intense vertigo, worse walking in open air and in sunshine. These patients are cold and very sensitive to cold; they are also exhausted by mental work and by coitus. They tend to be owls rather than larks.

The acute symptoms are rather naturally marked by severe diarrhoea and vomiting.

So the main actions are to be found in the changes of consciousness and the nervous irritability showing itself in hypersensitivity along the spine together with tics, spasms, and choreiform movements. In addition, we find the chilblains and bunions with the marked modalities: relieved by warmth and aggravated by cold, mental work and coitus.

The question arises as to how far the changes in consciousness are brought about by changes in the nervous system itself. And how far the nervous symptoms such as spinal sensitivity arc hysterical.

The brain and nervous system normally function in adult life in an inhibitory manner. The expression 'to keep a cool head' is highly indicative. Bergson at the beginning of this century showed that our senses screen for us, as it were, the multitudinous incoming impressions, so that we become conscious only of a tiny selection, those needed for our action. It would seem then that the fungus represents the brain and nervous system at an earlier, more embryonic stage of development, before it has been overwhelmed by the death or dying processes characteristic of the adult stages. Sense impressions in our drug picture are therefore described as more vivid, more full of life, beauty and springtime. When we look back even as far as the Greek civilization we are enchanted by the freshness of their thoughts, which are still full of life and perception. They have not yet been killed off into the abstractions of modern thought life. So under the influence of Agaricus the Lapps and Siberian Shamans find it easier to re-enter states of consciousness of a dreamlike clairvoyance. They become mediums for inspiration

165

by other influences. Wordsworth's *Ode to Immortality* represents a similar idea in respect to childhood.

We may further question whether the movements of uncoordinated character also reflect in some degree the uncoordinated movements of the baby before it has learnt to still the unnecessary, useless movements and permit only the useful ones to occur.

In agreement with such an interpretation of the *Agaricus* picture would be the use of this remedy in mental retardation where there is a failure of the child to wake up in its mental functions and persistence in a consciousness of babyhood.

Older generations of homoeopathic physicians found this remedy of use in organic diseases of the nervous system such as parkinsonism, general paralysis, multiple sclerosis and epilepsy, in addition to chorea.

Agaricus emeticus has a brief mention in the materia medica for vomiting and severe vertigo relieved by copious cold water.

Agaricus (Amanita) phalloides is the cause of 90% of deaths due to mushroom poisoning. Some have suggested that it was a favourite poison used by the Borgias, because the symptoms do not develop for 6–24 hours after ingestion. By this time the guest could have been conveniently speeded on his way. In spite of its toxic qualities it has been little used as a remedy, its homoeopathic indications having been focused on violent diarrhoea with cramping pains and collapse, leading to its suggested use in cholera. The toxic properties are due to a group of substances known as the amanita toxins; they include 5-cyclopolypeptides, phalloidin, phalloin, and α, β, γ-amanitine. They give rise to the violent vomiting, diarrhoea and pain in the abdomen, with intense thirst and scant urine. The symptoms abate only to return with increased violence, and this periodic remission and return of the symptoms is characteristic. After some days coma and jaundice develop and lead to death.

The symptoms are mainly or even exclusively abdominal and in the liver and kidneys. The coma is probably secondary to these effects.

Boletus satanas together with *Boletus laricis* and *Boletus luridus* appear in the materia medica with severe symptoms of gastro-enteritis. Little else is mentioned.

Bovista nigrescens, the puff-ball, is characterized by sensations as if the head were enlarging and by distensive headaches. Also there are reports of clumsiness, dropping things, mixing words up, weakness of limbs. Skin symptoms are marked, urticarial and eczematous in type. Haemorrhagic tendencies mainly related to the uterus are also reported.

19. FUNGI

The next member of the Fungi for consideration is one of the most important. Still known in the homoeopathic literature as *Secale cornutum*, it is in fact the ergot fungus, *Claviceps purpurea*, which infects rye and other cereal crops. Poisonings by this fungus, inadvertently included in the bread, have been known from the Middle Ages at least. Thus it was known as St Anthony's fire on account of the intense burning pains in the extremities from which the saint was reputed to have suffered.

The gangrene associated with these pains is dry and due to constriction of small blood vessels. In more acute and severe poisonings, hallucinations and convulsions may occur. For centuries ergot has been known to have effects on the uterus in labour but it does not cause premature abortion. A variety of alkaloids and active substances have been separated out, each with varying emphasis of action. This has been made use of by the pharmacological industry in preparing remedies for specific uses. Ergotoxin, ergometrine, ergotamine are examples. It was in the course of studying this range of substances that lysergic acid was discovered.

In orthodox medicine, ergot and its derivatives have found their main spheres of use in obstetric practice on the one hand and migraine on the other. This relationship between migraine and the uterine pains of labour or dysmenorrhoea we have come upon before in several drug pictures. Dysmenorrhoea is uterine migraine; migraine is cephalic dysmoenorrhoea.

In homoeopathy, ergot, or secale, to use the wrong name under which it is still found in the materia medicas, has found its main use in peripheral arterial disease. Raynaud's syndrome, scleroderma, and arteriosclerosis leading to severe circulatory obstruction, intermittent claudication, and gangrene have all on occasion been greatly ameliorated. The modality of pain worsened by heat runs through the symptoms. Paralyses of indeterminate type are mentioned, with cramps and the notable symptom of the fingers being spread out wide. In the last century *Secale* found a use, as did others of the fungi, in the treatment of cholera. This builds a bridge towards *Cuprum* which proved the main homoeopathic remedy in cholera and is also a main remedy for cramps and convulsions. A certain common spectrum of conditions amenable to these two remedies can be traced. From cramps of the peripheral vessels and limbs to cramps of the uterus and intestine to cramps of the head in migraine and 'brain storms' showing themselves in temper tantrums with *Cuprum*, and full-blown hallucinatory storms with LSD. *Cuprum* also plays into the respiratory system with asthma and paroxysmal coughs. *Secale* seems to avoid the respiratory system and its slight action on the heart seems secondary to its peripheral actions. Paterson placed both these remedies in the bowel nosode group of Proteus which he characterized under the key-note of 'brain storms'. The materia medica also refers to haemorrhages, mainly uterine, but purpura is also mentioned. In veterinary practice early symptoms include the shedding of hoofs and gangrene of the tail, ears and tongue. Recently bromocriptine and several allied substances from ergot have found a use in the treatment of parkinsonism.

167

Ustilago maydis, the corn-smut, seems to have some similarity in its spheres of action to the ergot. It has, according to the provings, a strong relationship to the genital organs and functions. In women, it produced haemorrhages and has found a main use here in menstrual, climacteric and post-partum bleeding. Animals have shed their hoofs and hair, and shedding of nails and hair in humans is recorded. Headaches with vertigo and double vision and scotoma point to migrainous phenomena. So in this little known or used remedy the same directions of action as in ergot have been noted.

We have mentioned *Thlaspi bursa-pastoris*, the shepherd's purse, on account of its almost normal symbiotic invasion by a fungus. The main use of this remedy has certainly been in relation to uterine haemorrhages, profuse menstruation. It remains a most valuable remedy in these conditions.

Throughout these different pictures of the fungi used, to some extent, in homoeopathic medicine, we have found certain common features, spheres of action. Like most severe poisons they produce gastro-enteritis. This symptom might be dismissed as merely typical of acute poisoning in general, but for the phenomena resulting from eating *Amanita phalloides*. In this case the patient or victim feels perfectly well for hours after eating the mushroom. It may be up to 24 hours before the symptoms commence with severe abdominal pain and diarrhoea and vomiting. The poison must have been absorbed, perhaps metabolized, before manifesting specifically in the abdominal and alimentary symptoms.

Then there is a tendency to varying skin manifestations. In *Agaricus muscarius* this is a chilblain-like itching, burning, red-purplish discolouration relieved by warmth. In *Secale* the discolouration and burning progress to gangrene, the pains being relieved by cold. With *Bovista* there are varied skin eruptions, eczema, urticaria the most common. With *Ustilago*, loss of hair with associated eruptions of the scalp, scald-head, are typical.

Headaches run through the pictures, there are in any case few drug pictures without headache. But migraine comes to the fore with ergot and its use in orthodox medicine for this condition. In *Agaricus*, various headaches are described and the ice-cold needles are a feature. In *Bovista* there is headache and sensation of enlargement of the head. Vertigo also is a marked feature in these drug pictures.

Haemorrhages are another common characteristic, notably in *Secale, Bovista, Thlaspi, Boletus* and *Ustilago*. In *Agaricus* it occurs but is not so marked a feature.

We come to the actions on the nervous system which have been most studied in *Agaricus*. 'Spinal irritation', twitchings and tics, chorea and spasms all point to actions on the nervous system. Then there are disturbances of the senses, everything becomes very beautiful, small things appear large, and the sense of balance is disturbed. The mental faculties are retarded, the emotional balance is labile. The symptoms may intensify to mania. In ergot the mental symptoms have come under scrutiny of recent years owing to the use or abuse of LSD. Intensification of sensory impressions and dissociation come about, leading to schizophrenia-like experiences. Another group of fungi have also come to notice, the *Psillocybe* species which have hallucinogenic effects, and are used by Mexican Indians in religious rituals.

To summarize, we may point to the main spheres of action in the metabolic and sexual organs on the one hand and the nervous system on the other. The lungs seem unaffected (if we consider the mycosis caused by *Aspergilla* separately). However in the lichen *Sticta pulmonaria*, lung and respiratory and rheumatic symptoms dominate the picture.

This is indeed suggestive. The fungi, as we have noted, have no leaves or proper stems, nor chlorophyll. They lack the middle realm of the plant between root and flowering process. This middle realm of leaf is related to the lung in inverted fashion. The leaf takes in carbon dioxide, photosynthesizes it into carbohydrates and gives off oxygen. The lung gives off the carbon dioxide and takes in oxygen. They both belong to the rhythmic middle realm between the polarities of head and abdomen, or root and blossom. In the fungi this polarity is not established; flowering, fruiting have, as it were, collapsed into the root or, perhaps better stated, have not yet emancipated themselves. In the lichen *Sticta pulmonaria*, the lungwort, this middle realm is provided by the algal part of the symbiosis. What is more, we know that lichens, which are particularly hardy in respect of climatic extremes, are particularly sensitive to atmospheric pollution. They are indeed used as indicators of this pollution. The lichens therefore seem to be particularly sensitive to the realm which the fungi alone do not care about, the realm of air and light.

We have still to consider the application in modern medicine of substances derived from this fungal underworld, the antibiotics. Starting with penicillin, an ever increasing variety of these substances is available. They are used in controlling bacterial infections, inflammations. Their antipathy to certain bacteria is based on similarities in their metabolic processes, competition between them resulting in blocking the bacterial growth. This is of course a homoeopathic action on a very selective narrow front. Looking at the problems more broadly, from the periphery towards the centre rather than from the centre outwards, that is to say more holistically, what can we see? On and around the roots, in the soil, flourish the vast multitude of fungi, devoid of chlorophyll. In the upper pole of trees grows another parasite or semi-parasite, the mistletoe. This plant is full of chlorophyll even into its haustorium, the root-like processes which penetrate the parent tree. It is not subject to gravity in its growth, nor to the usual earthly rhythms. It has not come to earth. In some ways we can therefore see it as a polarity to the realm of fungi, and it has an influence on carcinomata, themselves in polarity to inflammation. From mistletoe, substances can be prepared with the unique combination of cytotoxic and immunostimulating properties. We have a polarity in disease processes between inflammations and tumours and a polarity in the sources of remedies working on these diseases.

The present essay has not attempted to review the vast realms of fungi and the almost infinite complexity of their chemical processes and actions. It has been concerned to explore whether a more holistic approach, taking its start from the simplest phenomena of fungal existence and the meagre homoeopathic drug pictures, could lead to any significant viewpoints and insights, fresh perspectives. In these fungal regions, which are particularly liable to disintegrate in the information explosion, can we begin to grasp the phenomena together, meaningfully? Can we begin to make any sense of the chaos of facts? In all regions of activity today this is the challenge to our humanity, to confer sense on the meaninglessness of mere facts.

20. Ranunculaceae

The Ranunculaceae provide us with a number of our most valuable remedies and some of them have very individual characters. At the same time certain themes run all through this family, becoming modified in varying ways in the different species. It is particularly worthwhile studying the members of this family together.

Pelikan describes the family in a very clear and illuminating manner. Its members are all herbs, with the exception of the *Clematis* genus which become climbers and lignified. The leaf is the typical organ of the family, they all specialize in the metamorphosis of the leaf. This organ, the leaf, Goethe grasped as the archetype of plant development, its varied metamorphosis giving rise to the whole plant. The Ranunculaceae leaf shows us the most wonderful transformations. (In the hellebore and the delphinium, the flower is largely composed from the sepals, showing the metamorphosis from leaf to blossom very clearly. They live in the realm of leaf and blossom.) As a family, then, it is in a very particular way a typical plant and the interplay of forces to be perceived is one of living watery forces from the earth meeting and interpenetrating the forces of air and light from above.

Just as we can watch the leaf metamorphosis in the individual plant and in the whole family, so can we follow a transformation of drug picture throughout the family.

From the medicinal point of view we can reasonably confine our attention to relatively few members of the family. Among the *Ranunculus* species, the most important is *Ranunculus bulbosus*, but there are also *Ranunculus sceleratus* and *Ranunculus acer* to be remembered. Then there is *Hydrastis canadensis*, the golden seal from Canada. Among the anemones, the pasque flower, *Pulsatilla pratensis*, is the main one from our point of view, and there is *Adonis vernalis*, the pheasant's eye. Then we come to *Actaea racemosa (Cimicifuga)* and *Actaea spicata*. *Aquilegia vulgaris*, the columbine, leads the family out of the radial symmetry of the earlier flowers into those of unilateral symmetry. The names of these already indicate animalic penetration of the blossom: columbine, larkspur, and monkshood or wolfsbane, known in our materia medica as *Aquilegia, Staphisagria* and *Aconitum*. But we should also not forget *Paeonia* before passing on to *Clematis recta* (actually still only a herb) and finishing, or starting, the year with *Helleborus niger*.

Now let us follow some of the main themes or notes through this group of remedies. Many of them produce acrid, irritating substances which can cause blisters and rashes on the skin. *Ranunculus bulbosus* is associated with burning and intense itching with vesicular eruption. It has been widely used in shingles, particularly of the intercostal nerves. *Ranunculus sceleratus* is supposed to be characterized by larger blisters and acrid exudation from these if they break. Is there really any great difference between these two remedies, and how could the question be clarified? *Pulsatilla* is more associated with urticaria and pruritus, but *Clematis* again has vesicular scaly eruptions with severe itching. *Staphisagria* was used as a local application for head-lice in pre-homoeopathic days. Hahnemann seems a little unnecessarily scathing about this, and homoeopathically it is useful for eczema, especially about the face and head, with thick scales and itching. This itching is supposed to move to another spot when scratched.

A characteristic of *Ranunculus bulbosus* are pains without skin eruptions. These pains are particularly likely to occur around the chest region, as intercostal neuralgias or myalgias and pleurodynias — sharp, stabbing pains on moving or breathing. This leads us into following another theme, that of pains. *Pulsatilla* also has pains which have a tendency to move from place to place and to increase steadily up to a pitch and then to stop suddenly. They are often relieved by gentle motion. *Cimicifuga*, or *Actaea racemosa* as it is also called, is another of this family with typical pains. These are in the back and in the large muscles of the limbs and, an unusual feature, they are worse during the menstrual flow. These pains of *Cimicifuga* are associated with nervous, oversensitive make-ups, and uterine dysfunction. The patients may be gloomy, feel shut in, under a cloud, want to escape from shut-in places. The head likewise feels as if the brain is shut in and wants to burst out. The skull feels as if it is opening and shutting. They are more irritably nervous than the *Pulsatilla* patients, but in both remedies the functional association between genital function or dysfunction and pains is clearly seen. *Staphisagria*, the wild delphinium, has severe pains, pains in the teeth, an observation which led Hahnemann to study this remedy. They, too, may be worse during menstruation. *Clematis recta* also has severe pains in the teeth which may be worse from tobacco, a strange symptom but one possibly connected with the craving for tobacco of *Staphisagria*. There are generalized muscular pains in *Staphisagria*, but most especially it is characterized by pain following cuts such as after surgical operations. But the cuts may be from cutting words, insults, as much as from the cuts of the surgeon's knife. Suppressed indignation particularly can give rise to pains of all sorts, and the headache again feels constrictive with bottled-up indignation. The sphincters are sensitive and the anal sphincter particularly, so that *Staphisagria* can help after operations on, or stretching of, the anal sphincter. This leads us to *Paeonia*.

The peony actually gets its name from the Greek god Paeon. Paeon was the physician to Olympus and it is interesting to recall that paeans of praise refer to

172

the ancient celebrations in honour of this God at his festival. One day Hades, the god of the underworld, had a pain and Paeon cured it with the root of the peony which apparently got its name in this way. That the pain suffered by the god of the underworld was rectal we may take for granted. The peony is interesting for another reason; it stands out in this family of almost perfumeless flowers by possessing perfume which even penetrates to its roots. Perfumes indicate that the element of warmth has penetrated into the plant, but this family mostly lives in the realm of the mutual penetration of water with air and light, and warmth has not yet been incorporated.

It has been pointed out that the shape of the aconite flower, helmet-like, with a domed headpiece, a vizor and a chin or lower lip, bears a resemblance to the divisions of the trigeminal nerve. It is an interesting and suggestive observation. In *Aconitum* the pains reach an intolerable level, full of anguish, fear, fear of death. Everything becomes unbearable, and neuralgic pains such as trigeminal neuralgia come on the scene. Cold fear and cold winds may precipitate a crisis. The monkshood flowering at the height of summer carries in it all the Terror of the Noontide.

Thus a certain spectrum of pain can be discerned, spread out amongst the members of this family and differentiated in quality according to the general characteristics of the individual members.

We must now follow another great theme and see how the mucous membranes react to the differentiated influence of this family. It is mainly two of these plants that are characterized by catarrhs: *Pulsatilla* and *Hydrastis*. In *Hydrastis* the catarrhs are thick, yellowish, ropy or viscous, and may occur from any mucous membrane, from the nose, ears, bronchi or urethra, always with these characteristics. *Pulsatilla* is associated more with a bland catarrh, yellowish or yellowish green, blobby rather than sticky or ropy, and often affecting the eyes as well. In contrast to these we must place *Aconitum*, in which the mucous membranes tend to be dry and hot. The catarrhal state of the eyes leads us on to the occurrence, not only of acute conjunctivitis, but of those more deep-seated inflammations, styes and chalazia or meibomian cysts. Here *Pulsatilla* is joined again by *Staphisagria*, one of the great remedies for these minor troubles.

If we grasp the catarrhs as a phase of a more general tendency, namely the tendency for the fluid organization to become displaced, or for part of it to fall out of the general circulation into, as it were, backwaters, we can here gain a further insight into the dynamics of this family. In *Pulsatilla* there is the tendency of tears to flow very easily and for stagnation to develop in the veins, both as varicosities and chilblains. On the other hand menstruation is usually diminished and thirstlessness is the rule. We can follow these disturbances in the fluid household further in *Adonis vernalis* where ascites and pleural effusions complicate the cardiac failure. In *Pulsatilla* the weakness of the menstrual flow is balanced by the catarrhs, weeping and venous dilation, whereas in *Adonis* the weakness of cardiac function leads to ascites, dropsies and effusions. These two pictures seem to belong together, as do the hollow muscular organs, the heart and uterus, to which *Adonis* and *Pulsatilla* are so closely related.

In his penetrating paper, 'The Signature of the Christmas Rose' on *Helleborus niger*, König pointed to the production of the cerebrospinal fluid as the centre of its action, and to a displacement of the fluid organism upwards to the head. With this a dullness even proceeding to coma is associated, and König pointed to a polar opposition between *Aconitum* and *Helleborus*, between midsummer and midwinter. The indications for the use of *Helleborus* in head injury seem to support this view.

The piles of *Paeonia* to which we have referred are another example of this disturbance of the fluid organism, bringing it into close relationship with *Pulsatilla*'s varicosites.

The Ranunculaceae family can unfold marked and valuable activity in the genital sphere. *Pulsatilla* leads the way here, with amenorrhoea or changeable, intermittent dysfunctions. Emotional disturbances interact particularly strongly with the menstrual functions. Leucorrhoeas are frequent, part of the general catarrhal tendencies, and are usually bland. In the male it is a remedy for gonorrhoea with yellowish urethral discharge, and though seldom called for in this antibiotic era, it is worth recalling this sphere of action. Orchitis and epididymitis, however, may need it, and in the orchitis of mumps it is strongly indicated. *Clematis recta* (nicely called the virgin's bower) is strongly related to the male sexual organs. It is a remedy for pain in the testicles and for urethral pain and discharge, with interference with micturition. In women it seems to be mostly related to the breasts. *Cimicifuga* is much more a woman's remedy. Irregular periods, profuse or suppressed with ovarian pain and pain across the pelvis, are typical. The nervous irritable fidgety nature of this remedy often seems to find its focus in the uterus. From the unstable relationship of the psyche and soma in this organ seem to stem all the other rheumaticky joint and muscular pains. The variability of *Pulsatilla* becomes much more nervous in quality in *Cimicifuga*.

When we turn to *Staphisagria* we find other disturbances of sexual function arising. In the male, sexual thoughts may cause distress and depression may follow seminal discharge. A few generations ago masturbation was a frequent cause of guilty brooding unhappiness. Whilst this is less frequently so today there do remain men in whom debility and depression follow seminal discharge and guilty feelings may easily arise in regard to sexual activity. Freud has by no means exorcised sexual guilt feelings. In women *Staphisagria* comes in when cystitis follows intercourse. This frequently occurring and distressing problem can be helped; it calls for routine hygiene which is now widely taught, but beyond this *Staphisagria* is immensely helpful in preventing recurrences. Are there psychosomatic aspects in this condition which go beyond the problem of ascending infection through the urethra and unemptied stagnant urine in the bladder? It would seem so. The old

174

expression 'honeymoon cystitis' may point to the element of trauma, emotional perhaps more than physical, that lies behind this condition.

There is another strange sidelight on the sexual side of *Staphisagria*. Some years ago W. S. Inman, consulting ophthalmic surgeon, drew attention to the emotional factors lying behind styes and meibomian cysts. Forty years' experience had convinced him that thoughts about birth were the specific stimulating nucleus. Since reading his article I have personally confirmed his observations in many cases, including my own. Now both *Pulsatilla* and *Staphisagria* are frequently successful in the treatment of these infected follicles and glands of the eyelids. I have been puzzled by the association. In some cases it seems as if the person is turning a blind eye to an emotionally unwanted pregnancy, in other cases the tumour is itself the pregnancy. It is a fascinating little realm of problems and Inman's contribution opens wonderful glimpses into the world of psychosomatic connections.

We have now traced some of the main themes which run through this family, leaving till now the striking mental features of some of these plant remedies. Like the plants themselves, they show a wonderful capacity for transformation; variations on a theme would be the musical expression.

The *Pulsatilla* patient, in whom the features we have discussed spread through the whole person and manifest not only in local symptoms but in the whole emotional behaviour and response, is well known to us. Like the pasque flower she is rather droopy, tearful, easily affected by every wind of mood and opinion around her. She is sensitive to grief and sadness which may well cause her illnesses. Easily frightened and easily offended, it is nevertheless the droopiness and tearfulness, the changeableness which centrally characterize the type — rather slow and miserable. She really does find in the pasque flower with its rather heavy coloured, bell-shaped flower, hanging down and blown about by the wind, the mirror held up to her nature.

The *Aconite* patient is full of fear and anguish and restlessness; the senses are hyperacute, tension and fear reign. There is nothing passive in these situations. On the one hand *Aconite* corresponds to the acute inflammatory diseases of childhood, on the other to fear, fright and states of ill-health stemming from severe shock and fright. Again the monkshood, growing in the mountains in high summer with its tall stem of blue flowers domed like the heavens and its substantial root process, is a mirror of the high tension in which these patients find themselves.

It is somewhat different again with the *Staphisagria* patients. With them it is more anger and indignation that characterizes the situation. They are oversensitive particularly to insults and injustices, real or imagined, and often their anger is frustrated, pent up. Their depression and gloom stem from their repressed indignation. With the eye of imagination can we not see, in the long tubular spur of the larkspur in which two tubular honey leaves reach far down inside the spur, an image of this deeply repressed emotion?

With *Cimicifuga* patients we again find extreme sensitivity, perhaps sensitivity to pain, and there is gloom and nerviness. The conspicuous feature in the flowers of the species is the way the petals fall off, leaving the multitude of stamens naked as it were. This is really a good image of the sensitive state of the *Cimicifuga* patients with their ovarian and uterine irritability.

As a sort of shadow to these hypersensitive creatures stand the stuporous, dull or actually comatose *Helleborus* patients.

We can now see that the full image of the plant in its geographical and seasonal setting as depicted by Pelikan seems to be correlated with the mental and personality aspects of the drug picture. At the other end of the scale, to understand the skin eruptions, we have to look to the acrid substances produced by many members of the family. The action of *Adonis* on the heart is dependent on the glycosides and similar active substances it produces, and *Pulsatilla* produces more volatile active substances. In *Staphisagria* and *Aconite* we already have alkaloid active principles, in the case of *Aconite* one of the most toxic substances produced in nature. This is responsible for some of the features of the drug picture, the action on the heart and circulation and probably on senses and nerves.

It seems that when the somatic and local aspects dominate the picture then the more material active principles of the plant are the clue to its action, but when the whole personality, the make-up of the patient, dominates the symptoms then the image of the plant, its whole *Gestalt* and life environment, supply the answer to the riddle of its action. But it is also clear that the active substances are themselves products of the whole plant and find their explanation out of its whole inner dynamics. Sometimes clear symptoms of a local sort such as styes or chalazia call for *Pulsatilla* or *Staphisagria* without attendant mental symptoms. Sometimes the mental symptoms occur without the local stigma. We need gradually to deepen our insight both into the plant holistically grasped and into the active substances peculiar to it and its family. Then we shall also gain insight into the remedial process which the plant can mediate through either its products or its whole image.

I have attempted in a preliminary way to indicate how we can gain certain vantage points from which we can approach nearer to the genius of the individual remedies. By following Pelikan's holistic descriptions of the Ranunculaceae and the plastic metamorphoses they manifest, individually and as a family, and then comparing them with the variations or transformations of common themes in the drug pictures I have tried to deepen insight into this wonderful group of remedial plants. In no sense have I attempted to paint full drug pictures, but my aim has been simply to help, so that the study of these pictures may be less a feat of memory and also perhaps more meaningful.

176

21. Cactaceae

The Cactaceae present a remarkable contrast to the Ranunculaceae. Whereas the buttercup family belong to the moist, even wet, meadows of the temperate zones of the Old World, the Cacti, with the possible exception of the Rhipsalis species, are natives of the semi-desert regions of the New World. They are found from Canada down to Patagonia and reach up to 10,000 feet in the Andes. The Ranunculaceae can almost be said to specialize in the development of the middle realm of the plant, the stem and leaves, and to exhibit in particularly great diversity the metamorphoses of the leaf. The Cacti show an almost complete inhibition of leaf formation. Their middle realm is scarcely developed. Only a few exceptions in this family, the Pereskia species, have managed to bring forth leaves. In the typical Cacti, merely bristles, hairs, spines indicate where leaves would grow if they were not held back from doing so.

One of the most significant differences between the geography of the Americas and that of the Eurasian continents is found in the mountain ranges. In the Americas the mountains run north and south whereas in Europe and Asia there are the east-west ranges of the Pyrenees, Alps, Carpathians, Caucasus and Himalayas. In America the polar and tropical worlds meet or confront each other, head on. It is difficult to establish a middle temperate world but in the old world the east-west mountains enable an independent middle realm to exist mediating between the polar and tropical realms. In the cacti, so typical of America, this middle realm is wanting. Pelikan characterized the Cacti as being like a fruit and yet in reality managing only to be a huge spherical cotyledon. They are stems but only that stem, the hypocotyle which unites cotyledons and radicals. This becomes swollen, in many forms almost spherical, or else it may develop into a swollen and congested cylinder. Yet another form is disc-like but a thick congested disc, covered, as are all these varieties, with bristles, hairs, spikes in varied forms. The stem may also get flattened as in the so-called Christmas cactus. True leaves are held back; the green-ness of leaves is spread over the whole stem and sometimes the form is ribbed showing the latent tendency to real planar leaf formation. The surface is thick and hard and waxed like fruit. Inside, the plant stores fluid and mucilage. Transpiration is reduced to a minimum allowing these strange plants to survive long periods of drought and heat. They show immense vitality; any portion will give rise to new specimens. Very powerful life forces work in the mucilaginous fluid which, seeking to expand, finds itself confronted and constricted by the hard, impermeable skin. Congestion within, constriction from without, characterize the plant. It seems that the form-giving forces, more characteristic of the airy realm, can only succeed in placing an armour around the burgeoning life but cannot penetrate it and give rise to all the differentiated air- and light-penetrated forms in which, for instance, the Ranunculaceae manifest. For this to happen, the middle realm between the organ of light and air, the blossom, and the organ of earth and water, the cotyledon, must come into existence, as in the Cacti it fails to do.

When eventually, often after years of slow growth, the light and warmth do manage to conjure forth a blossom then this erupts directly out of the body of the cactus. The blossom does not rise up on a stem. It is perfumed, gives rise to nectar, is brightly coloured and fades quickly. Not only insects but humming birds and bats may contribute to the fertilization process. Again we may note in passing that the Ranunculaceae are perfumeless, another point of contrast.

The Cacti are a large family, some 2,000 species, adapted to a wide range of environments, most typically semi-arid deserts. But they are also found as epiphytes in tropical forests and in the colder regions of Patagonia. Many species besides the prickly pear give rise to fruits, and in some of them the plant itself, the stem, is edible and very similar to the fruit. As we have already indicated, the fruit becomes again stem or the stem fruit.

What we see then is an immensely powerful self-maintaining vitality, affirming its life against drought and desert, a vitality which holds its own watery content, the very basis of life processes, against an outer arid dryness.

The form-giving forces are mainly confined to the periphery where they act, equally strongly as the life-promoting forces, to produce the outer skin, almost impermeable to water and transpiration. These two systems of force do not interpenetrate each other so much as confront each other.

Does this style, arising, as we have suggested, from the geography of America, show itself also in the culture and social life of the continent? The greatness of America consists largely in the self-reliance of the individuals. The rich emotional life of Europe with its family networks interwoven in differentiated social loyalties and cultures is not the mark of America. There the will, the will to survive and to conquer is supreme and in philosophy the contribution of America is Pragmatism. To Europeans the emotional life of America often seems undeveloped or again simply manipulative, in the service of the will. There is high idealism but it cannot as yet penetrate and inform this all-powerful, self-assertive will. Is not the life of America on the way to becoming a Cactus? This can indeed become the ideal of the future, self-maintained and self-affirming with self-revelation in the flowering. But the self must become a revelation of the whole, not a mere sham of materialistic self-interest.

178

There are two members of this family which up till now have assumed medical importance. Firstly there is the Mexican peyote (*Lophophora williamsii*). This Cactus has a large beetlike root, an unusual feature. Above the very arid rough terrain it inhabits it rises up only to a small smooth apple-sized lump on the surface. Some hairs represent the bristles and a flower arises from the centre. This unspectacular plant was used in cultic practices by the Aztec priests and has entered at times into the modern drug scene as Mescalin. It produces hallucinations of vivid colours and forms, in spectacular movement. The sensory display, of fascinating brilliance, is divorced from real objects, that is to say the visual and tactile senses are split from each other. A similar process has come about in some modern art; colour and drawing for instance in a picture do not correspond with each other. With this dazzling hallucinatory experience there is often a heightened sense of significance, everything seems a mystical revelation of highest meaning. But the will is inactive, there is no inclination to be other than entirely passive to the power of the Peyote unfolding within one. All the enormous vitality in the root and button of this Cactus, enabling it to survive in nigh impossible, barren, circumstances, rises up into manifestation in the sphere of the nerves and senses. The root process in plants corresponds to this system of nerves and senses in man. What is hidden, unmanifest in the Peyote rises to its expression in the hallucinations of man. That it is seductive and dangerous is obvious.

The second member of this Cactus family to interest us medically is the *Selenicereus grandiflorus,* familiarly known as the Queen of the Night. In most materia medicas it appears as *Cactus grandiflorus*. Its native habitat is the West Indies where it grows up limestone cliffs. The usual Cactus bristles are largely replaced by aerial roots with which it attaches itself to the cliff up which it is climbing. It can grow to a considerable length, snake-like but branching. Pelikan compared it to a root stock above the soil. At last it develops little outgrowths which swell, become more roundish and are covered with bristles. Then one night as the sun goes down, there bursts from this gynaecium a splendid blossom, funnel shaped, white and yellow, sweet smelling, 10 cm long, 20 cm across. This huge flower which has taken years before it could appear fades by the morning into a crumpled bag. In its 'life style' the *Cereus grandiflorus* is strongly contrasted to the peyote; it grows in long branching cylinders, on cliffs; the Peyote remains a small 'button' on the dried up desert.

Turning now to the materia medica we find congestion and constriction as the keynotes of the Cactus drug picture. This plant was introduced into medicine by the Neapolitan homoeopathic physician Dr Rubini, in the middle of the last century after ten years of clinical use and homoeopathic provings. It was quickly adopted into homoeopathic practice and has remained a valued remedy to this day. It is often regarded primarily as a heart remedy and undoubtedly it can serve very well in cardiac cases, particularly in angina. But the processes to which it corresponds, congestions and crampings, occur more widely, not only in the heart. We must look more closely if we are to come nearer to its true action.

Cramps and constrictions run through all the symptoms associated with Cactus. They may appear as bandlike sensations in the limbs, as cramping dysmenorrhoea and vaginismus, as cramping pain in the stomach and the oesophagus or a constriction in the throat. We have mentioned the vice-like cramping in the heart and there are also constricting pains around the chest sometimes with frank asthma. Headaches occur often with pressing constricting pain over the head. But with all these symptoms there will be, as well, a bursting or surging in the blood, an instability in the circulation, irregularity in the heart beat and so on.

We meet the general tendency to cramps again in the pathogenesis of copper (*cuprum*) and of ergot (*Secale*). In both, in a similar manner, the cramping or spasm may occur in different organs giving rise to a wide range of syndromes which nevertheless share the same underlying cramping process. In both these remedies we notice a spectrum of symptoms from simple cramping of muscle, or blood vessel, up to migraine and then reaching in ergot (LSD) to hallucinations, in copper to temper tantrums. In the Cacti we see a similar range of symptoms from crampings anywhere to the hallucinations of the Peyote.

If we take the extended view of the kidney function suggested by Steiner and elaborated in athroposophical medical writings, then we can begin to deepen our understanding of these phenomena. The kidney has to perform work in separating the urine out from the blood. There must therefore be a counter-thrust into the organism, to which Steiner called attention as the 'kidney radiation'. This is to be understood as a complex of forces which irradiate the nutritional stream and the organism and lift up the substance from a merely enlivened state to that of sentient and ensouled substance. We can relate such a concept to the action of the suprarenal glands which, sitting like hats on top of the kidneys, can be seen to collect and metamorphose some of this radiation. I have referred elsewhere to this theme (Chapter 16). Here we need only stress the point that if this radiation is excessive, it may not only ensoul the living, etherized substance, but its surplus force may then grip directly into the physical organism, cramping and constricting. Further, if cortisone-like substances such as are produced in the suprarenal glands are given to someone with schizophrenic tendencies then this person may easily be triggered into a fully hallucinated break-down. From the kidney system, understood in this extended sense, we can now seek the origin of the wide range of symptoms and processes we have been discussing. The forces which are also sometimes called the astral forces or soul forces stream down from the head through the spinal cord as katabolic, sculpturing forces. They are switched in the kidneys into anabolic, upbuilding ensouling forces.

Now it has been found that the level of eosinophils in the blood varies during the day falling to a minimum around 11 am and rising to a maximum some twelve or more hours later. The eosinophils can be understood as markers, so to speak, of astral type processes. But the level of cortisol in the blood rises from 3 or 4 am through the morning to a maximum around 8 to 10 am then declining again to a low point between early evening and midnight. If we put this together with the observations that for instance asthmatic attacks and cardiac infarcts occur most frequently at these hours in the early morning when eosinophils are high and cortisol levels low we reach the following tentative viewpoint. The cortisol is necessary to mediate these astral, soul forces into the living substance to awaken it. In its absence these same astral forces if excessive, grip directly into the physical structures causing for instance broncho-spasm or spasm of the coronary vessels, or again nocturnal cramp in the limbs.

At any rate in the consideration of Cactus and its symptom-picture in the human organism a possible clue is found here for one feature. It is described repeatedly how the Cactus symptoms are likely to be most marked at around 11 am to 12 noon and again at 11 pm to midnight.

These remedies Cactus, Cuprum and Secale (ergot) belong together in a group with *Natrum mur.* (common salt) and Chamomilla. (They are related to the Paterson bowel nosode Proteus). It is suggestive that Natrum Mur. has an aggravation at 10 to 11 am and Chamomilla at 10 pm. The relation of *Natrum mur* (sodium chloride) to the adrenal function is well known. So we have come upon a net of related problems.

Returning to the *Cactus grandiflorus* we can ask why it is that with all these connections to the whole range of cramping processes, it is especially in relation to the heart that Cactus manifests its action. Certainly this is the clinical impression. The plant itself offers a possible clue. We have noticed the hard constricting skin of the Cacti but also the swelling, growing, life-filled mucilaginous content. In the heart the surging life of the blood is tamed and brought into measure and order by the rhythms of the heart beat. The symptomatic descriptions of the 'Cactus heart' in the homoeopathic literature stress irregularity in the heart beat and altogether in the circulation, orgasms and flushings. These tendencies occur together with the vice-like crampings in the heart. It is this combination of the surging life which becomes congested together with the cramping and constricting grip that mark the Cactus picture. The Queen of the Night brings forth her splendid perfumed blossom at night, the time when most heart attacks occur. We can imagine that the bursting forth of this blossom relieves the enormous tension in the Cactus between bursting life and constricting skin.

Can we relate this to the functions of the heart? Are there not soul functions of the heart as language itself and all traditional wisdom indicate? How physiologically does the language of the heart arise? We must all know, from our inner experiences, that intimations from the 'other side' of existence do sometimes reach us through the heart. We may call it the voice of conscience. What does the heart, an organ with a very rich nerve supply, sense in the blood surging up into it from the metabolism and limbs? This world of the metabolism is indeed the unconscious in relation to the consciousness of the brain. It somehow is the 'other side'. The great American psychiatrist Trigant Burrow was led to contrast the cerebral consciousness, ego-centred and analytical, with the belly consciousness of the solar plexus and sympathetic nervous system, integral and whole and related to the sphere of all social relationships of mankind as an organism. Between these two he divined a structural divorce, a structural insanity in man's very nature. It is this integral collective unconsciousness which the heart must sense in the blood and which we sometimes hear as the intimations and promptings of conscience. Through them we experience the inwardness of others as distinct from hearing exclusively our own.

Our speech and communication today are dominated by the egotistical, cerebral, one-sidedness of our intellectual consciousness. Only occasionally do the promptings of the heart manage to find utterance and express a truth which is on the way to other-centredness, to all-embracing validity. Sometimes it may be that we only manage to blurt out a long held back insight, confession or a stammering shy attempt at understanding another. But it may be that this attempt is shareable and accepted and then long-held inner tension and pain are miraculously freed.

The Queen of the Night seems to me to be the picture of this. After long growth and the tension, confrontation between congestion and constriction, at night the blossom appears, the self-revelation after self-maintenance and self assertion. Today it is very difficult for our modern consciousness to listen to and accept these intimations. The abyss between conscious and unconscious is deep. It is not surprising that the heart suffers; the constriction is too powerful, the blossom cannot burst out even at night. Then the 'Queen of the Night' can help, mirroring the heart's tension yet showing the way to flowering. In open speech and deed the individual can find the way forward to the expression of values and meanings of truly human scope yet idiomatic in style and caught in the fleeting moment. Such flowerings of the human spirit come in short-lived experiences which like the blossom of the *Cereus grandiflorus* have faded by the morning. More and more we shall need courage and self-presence to catch these healing and reconciling moments when conscious and unconscious can communicate together.

22. Liliaceae

The Liliaceae is one of the largest families of flowering plants, comprising some 250 genera and 3,700 species. They belong to the monocotyledons and are very widely distributed. Most of them are herbaceous, arising from bulbs, corms or rhizomes; quite a number are xerophytic and a few are fleshy like the aloe. The inflorescences are usually racemose, but in the tulips for example are single. The blooms are regular and perfect, and with few exceptions are dominated by the number three, the six perianth segments being usually three sepals and three petals.

They avoid the alpine and polar regions and also swamps and aquatic areas, but they are found flourishing in the tropics and sub-tropics and above all in temperate zones.

They are characterized by a plastic swelling and congestion in bulb, corm or rhizome; the actual roots are mostly poorly developed. From this base, after a period of tension has built up, the plant shoots up to its flowering.

We can then see how from a globular bulb there appears at the opposite pole a six-pointed star. We can compare this with the six-pointed snowflake which falling becomes a drop of rain. This interplay or metamorphosis of the sphere or circle with the hexagon is a fascinating one. The radius of a circle is equal to the side of the inscribed hexagon. Circle and hexagon are most intimately related. The drop of water and the six-pointed snowflake belong together as do the drop-like living bulb and the six-petalled flower which shoots upwards from it.

For our purposes we can bring together closely related families. So, including the snow drop and daffodil (little used in any case), iris and herb paris as well as the agaves, we are then concerned with the following; the names are those found in the homoeopathic materia medica:

Agave Americana
Agraphis (Scilla) nutans
Aletris farinosa
Allium cepa
Allium sativum
Aloe socotrina
Asparagus officinalis

Colchicum autumnale
Convallaria majalis
Galanthus nivalis
Helonias dioica
Iris versicolor
Lilium tigrinum
Narcissus pseudonarcissus
Ornithogalum umbellatum
Paris quadrifolia
Sabadilla officinalis
Scilla maritima
Sarsaparilla
Trillium pendulum
Veratrum album
Veratrum viride
Yucca filamentosa

If we try and sketch the main spheres of action of this family on the human organization, making use of the homoeopathic materia medica, certain clear fields of action are easily seen.

Here the tiger lily, *Lilium tigrinum*, leads the way, with symptoms of bearing down in the pelvic organs, a feeling as if the uterus were being dragged out or pushed down. This sensation is felt also in the rectum. Sexual desire is usually increased and there are cardiac symptoms. The uterus and heart are often in sympathy both emotionally and functionally. Anatomically they are both hollow muscular organs and the heart, as Jaworsky showed, can be looked upon as the blossom or sex of the vascular tree. *Convallaria*, the lily of the valley, which is an important cardiac remedy, has symptoms of soreness in the uterus and bladder as well. It is interesting to contrast these two members of the lily family in their appearance as well as in their relation to the human organization. About the lily of the valley there is an atmosphere of innocence and purity, the bell-like flowers hang almost shyly down in their white dresses. Striking is the contrast with the tiger lily which flaunts its spotted orange dress and exhibits its sexual parts for all the world to see. When we turn to the drug pictures we find that the action of the lily of the valley is primarily on the heart or rather vascular system and secondarily on the pelvic and genital organs. In the tiger lily the reverse is certainly true.

Helonias, sometimes called the unicorn root, and its close relative *Aletris* are two more of this family with powerful actions on the pelvic organs. Sensations of prolapse and weakness, disturbances of menstruation, languor and melancholia which are relieved by activity, remind one also of *Sepia*.

Veratrum album which is best known for its actions on the alimentary tract is

184

also related to the uterine functions. It has been found curative in some cases of puerperal insanity and of sexual mania coming on particularly before the menses.

Trillium pendulum, the birth root, has in its drug picture a relaxed pelvis as if the hips and back were falling to pieces with in addition gushing haemorrhages which are worse on motion, accompanied by the common symptom of prolapse. The haemorrhagic tendency extends to all other orifices.

In *Sarsaparilla* the pelvic congestion shows itself mostly in the bladder with symptoms of cystitis. There are also noted bloody seminal emissions and genital herpes. In women painful periods with severe pain in the breasts are recorded as responding to this remedy.

The *Aloe* with its swollen bud of succulent leaves from which springs forth a raceme of pinkish-orange bell-like flowers is known for its rectal symptoms with a sensation of a plug between sacrum and symphysis pubis. Early morning diarrhoea with bearing down in the rectum and bleeding piles further characterize the symptoms of this famous medical plant which is characterized also by similar symptoms in relation to the uterus. In allopathic medicine it has of course been used for its aperient actions.

Colchicum autumnale, the autumn crocus, is best known for its specific relationship to gout. In its drug picture it appears to have no relation to the genital functions and organs. Yet König, in a deeply penetrating and suggestive study, gradually drew together the phenomena of gout, menstruation, the cytotoxic action and the homoeopathic symptoms, notably the sensory hypersensitivity. This hypersensitivity is especially marked in relation to smell. One may add to the evidence produced by König, relating *Colchicum* directly to menstrual function, some observations on gout put forward by Professor F. Wood Jones some years ago. On the basis of the experience of his own gout, he suggested that in the acute attack, with intense hyperaemia and hyperthermia around the joint, there was an opening up of local arteriovenous shunts. As a result of this process the deposits of urates around the joint became visibly diminished by the attack. In line with König's argument, we might describe the attack of acute gout as a substitute in the male for menstruation. We should remember also that a joint unites two members, as does marriage join together two persons and that the word join is semantically related to *gynae*, generation, knowledge (and Adam knew Eve) and specifically to the knee joint, the *genu*.

For the fuller discussions of these relations between *Colchicum*, the naked lady, and menstruation, I must refer to König's paper. One other unusual member of the lily (or very closely related) family needs mention — the *Agave*. This plant after years of vegetative growth producing a large number of long narrow leaves crowded together at ground level, suddenly sends up its tall pole-like panicle carrying the flowers. After this flowering the plant dies. From a member of the Mexican agaves the pharmaceutical industry has obtained some of the raw materials for the production of the pill.

The spring innocence of *Convallaria* stands opposite the somewhat shameful nakedness of *Colchicum autumnale*, even as the purity of the madonna lily is opposed to the spotted gaudiness of the tiger lily. Something of the whole mystery of sex lies before us in these members of the lily family.

We can now turn to the opposite pole of the human organization, the head. There the brain floats in the cerebrospinal fluid as the foetus does within the amniotic fluid within the uterus. The ancients were well aware of these comparisons as the names *pia mater* and *dura mater* given to the membranes surrounding the brain indicate.

It has even been suggested that migraine in the head is comparable to a cephalic dysmenorrhoea and that dysmenorrhoea is a sort of uterine migraine. We recall that the severe headache of Zeus was diagnosed as pregnancy and relieved when Hephaestos opened his skull, allowing his daughter goddess to leap forth. Headache may indeed be the birth pangs of a repressed or new thought trying to be delivered into consciousness.

From our foregoing discussions it is therefore not surprising to find headaches running as a strong theme through the drug pictures of this family.

We find *Aloe* characterized by frontal headaches which may alternate with lumbago or with intestinal or uterine symptoms. The eyes are heavy and there is a disinclination for mental work. *Allium cepa*, the onion, has headaches relieved by the menses and thread-like neuralgias, all worse in a warm room. The headaches of *Veratrum viride* are described as full, congestive, bursting with throbbing arteries and also vertigo and nausea. The added symptom of a horizontal hemiopia points to a clearly migrainous element and the vertigo with photophobia may also be of migrainous origin. Dr R. Cooper used to praise *Veratrum viride* for sick headaches. This is in contrast to *Veratrum album* where we find cold sweat, pale face and nausea, vomiting and diarrhoea associated with dull headaches which may be relieved by diuresis or the onset of menses.

In *Paris quadrifolia*, herb paris, which is now classified in a closely related family, head symptoms predominate in the drug picture. Great sensitiveness of the scalp, feeling as if scalp were contracted, or head feels too large and as if the eyes were too large or drawn backwards by a string. In *Trillium* too we find the sensation of the eyes being too large.

Sabadilla is best known for its use in hay fever with sneezing, running eyes and nose. But in addition we find that it relates to headaches brought on by thinking and to attacks of vertigo on rising with sensations of fainting. It has a marked tendency to periodicity and a hypersensitivity to odours, like *Colchicum*. Yet another of the lily family, *Asparagus*, is recorded as causing and curing migraines with scotomas.

Closely related to the symptoms of headache are the varied range of coryzas and hay fevers. We can approach these with the help of some of this family, notably *Allium cepa* and *Sabadilla*, both of which have a well earned reputation. *Agraphis*, the bluebell, should be known as Endymion. It has been used in cases of enlarged adenoids with mucous discharges from the nose. *Asparagus* has also a relation to coryza, nasal catarrh and sneezing.

All these conditions in the head can be understood as processes from the metabolic realm rising up and drowning the processes proper to the head region, the sensory and thinking processes. In migraine, metabolic and digestive processes rise into the head and brain making thinking difficult, confused, or impossible. Vision is often similarly affected and vertigo may arise when the organ of balance is overwhelmed. In coryza and hay fever the fluid drenches the eyes and nose in particular. We can even follow this metamorphosis further upwards into the mental and soul realm. Then in *Veratrum album* we have noted mania in connection with menses and the puerperium, together with depressed sullen indifference and delusions of impending disasters. Somewhat similar are the mental disturbances with *Lilium tigrinum*, depression, torment about salvation, fear of incurable disease and a wild hurried restlessness, with nymphomania.

Several of these plants of the lily family manifest a relationship to the heart and circulation. *Lilium tigrinum* has a reputation for irregular and rapid action of the heart and for tumultuous pulsations throughout the body. The heart is described as gripped and loosened alternatively. Certainly the impression gained from the drug picture and from clinical use is of a functional disturbance of the whole circulation felt also in the heart. Emotional forces connected with the sexual functions rise up and great restlessness, tormenting anxiety, play upon the circulation. It is reported that in men the heart symptoms seem to replace the uterine symptoms which dominate the picture in women.

Convallaria majalis, the lily of the valley, is more directly related to the heart and circulation. König in his study of *Convallaria* brings forward reasons for emphasizing in this remedy too the effect on the circulation in general rather than on the heart in particular. A general rejuvenating influence on the ageing circulation bring rejuvenation to the heart as well. At the same time diuresis is brought about, probably by an improvement in local kidney circulation. An effect on renal function is part of the general actions of this family, perhaps an aspect of the broad relationship to the genito-urinary system. The diuretic action of *Convallaria* leads on to the consideration of *Scilla maritima*, the sea onion. From very ancient times this remedy has been used. In heart diseases with dropsy it provoked diuresis and its expectorant qualities have led to its wide use in cough medicines. With the advent of modern diuretics and antibiotics the virtues of this valuable remedy have been largely forgotten. The lily action on heart and kidneys also appears in *Asparagus*, but has been little used. In *Veratrum album* the circulatory action seems to be one of collapse with coldness, cold sweat, feeble pulse. The snowdrop, *Galanthus nivalis*, and *Narcissus*, both belonging to the closely related family of Amaryllidaceae, have also been shown to have effects on the heart and circulation.

Both the onion and garlic, *Allium cepa* and *Allium sativum*, are known from common usage for their regulating and laxative actions. Both have their advocates as well-nigh panaceas. It would seem, however, that *Allium cepa* has more effect medically speaking on the head region in coryza and catarrhs, whilst *Allium sativum* is more effective in digestive disorders. This may be connected with the way the garlic raises bulbils into the region of the inflorescence. *Aloe* is related to the liver and portal congestion and *Ornithogalum*, the Star of Bethlehem, has a well deserved reputation in stomach and duodenal disorders. *Colchicum* in toxic doses brings about vomiting and diarrhoea with distension and a great sensitivity to smells is noted; there is coldness in the abdomen. Very similar effects are present with *Veratrum album*.

One can also bring into the discussion the closely related *Iris versicolor* with equally violent abdominal symptoms and migraine.

We have very briefly surveyed the main directions of the actions of the medicinal members of the lily family within the human organization. It has become clear that they represent variations on a common theme, with resemblances between them often greater than their differences. As plants they are dominated by the motives of a swelling congestion in bulbs and leaves. The bulbs are really leaf buds displaced into the earth. The leaves are often rather fleshy, as in leeks and onions. There are, typically, ill-developed roots, but out of the leafy foundation there springs forth the flowering process often on a long stem. In the *Agave* and *Yucca* this reaches a remarkable development into a veritable flag pole. When incised, enormous volumes of fluid flow from this staff, and this is collected and used as the basis of beverages. The family belongs to the monocotyledons. The eye of imagination can well see these as belonging more to the moon, whilst the dicotyledons, with the rose as typical, belong more to the sun. The polarity of moths and butterflies has a similar qualitative character, as an example from the animal kingdom.

In the old alchemical tradition the root process was called Sal or salt and the blossom process Sulphur, whilst the middle realm of stem and leaf was called Mercury. We found this in Paracelsus for instance. It is clear, using this way of looking at the living processes of nature, that in the lilies the Sulphur and Mercury processes predominate, the Salt processes are weak. The lilies have not come strongly to earth. We would anticipate therefore that their chief actions within the human organization will be in the metabolic and genital realms, the sphere paramountly of the Sulphur processes, and in the rhythmic systems of the circulation and breathing which are the realm of the Mercury processes. And this is what we have found in the drug pictures.

There is a strong relationship to the alimentary system and its functions, *Ornithogalum* especially to the stomach and duodenum, *Aloe* more to the colon and rectum, with all the others also playing their part. On the genital functions, particularly the uterus, we have again seen a wide coverage. *Lilium tigrinum* and *Helonias* lead the way, and *Veratrum album* carries the action up into the realm of puerperal insanity and sexual mania. In *Colchicum* the sexual theme is metamorphosed into the peculiar and specific relation to gout and the interference with spindle formation during cell division. The relationship of these remedies of the lily family to headaches of a distinctly migrainous type can also be understood as showing how the metabolic processes, becoming too powerful, rise up and overwhelm the nerve sense processes proper to the head during waking life. Closely allied to these phenomena are the catarrhs, coryzas and hay fevers.

It seems that the action on the circulation and heart can be related more to the mercurial aspect of these plants. An enlivening, quickening action on the failing sluggish circulation is most marked in *Convallaria* and *Scilla*. Whether the diuresis is primary, through action on the kidney, or secondary to the improved circulation is open to question.

We can in conclusion grasp these spheres of action together with the distribution of the liliaceae on the earth. They are at home in the tropics and sub-tropics, the earth's metabolic zone, and also in the temperate zone, the earth's rhythmic realm. But they cannot establish themselves in alpine and polar regions which are the nervous and sensory regions, the homes of the Sal processes. The lilies cannot root themselves there. But in the deserts when the rain does come, for a short moment, a multitude of plants including lilies rush into flower, bedecking the desert with their colour. This powerful bursting forth into flower after a pent-up period of tension characterizes the family and the drug pictures.

23. Thuja and Medorrhinum

The idea of the importance of the strange, rare and peculiar symptom is often a stumbling block to the study of homoeopathy. After a medical training in which one is largely schooled to note the general symptoms common to a diagnostic entity, it comes as a shock to have attention drawn to the individual, eccentric feature which seems diagnostically meaningless and frankly ridiculous.

Goethe, Hahnemann's great contemporary, believed and maintained that Nature always reveals, in some place, her otherwise concealed purposes. Or, to put it the other way, Nature's secret and veiled laws are always openly expressed in some special phenomenon or instance. If we seek for this instance diligently enough, we shall find the law, the idea, literally staring us in the face.

It seems to me that it is a similar way of thinking in Hahnemann when he insists that a disease finds full expression in the totality of symptoms; and further that we grasp this ideal unity best when we can find the characteristic symptom in which the wholeness of the disease, or for that matter remedy, comes to open expression. But does there not lie in this affirmation of Hahnemann a challenge? The challenge to show how the idea, the law, expressed and revealed in the peculiar characteristic symptom, really does penetrate and unite the rest of the manifold symptomatology.

Goethe sought in many realms of nature for the archetypal or *Ur*-phenomena which he understood as the revealed laws enabling him to see deeply into the relevant field of nature. Alfred Adler sought in his neurotic patients the 'lifestyle', that particular, individual way of experience and behaviour which then became the interpretative key to the whole neurotic personality. He often found this in the earliest memory.

Now if we take as a starting point this idea that it is in the strange, rare and peculiar symptom that the genius of the individual disease and remedy come to most open expression, can we in respect of these two interesting remedies, *Medorrhinum* and *Thuja*, take any step forward?

They are both essentially sycotic remedies. I attempted some years ago to show how sycosis* can be understood as the deeper physiognomy of shame — as

* Sycosis was one of the three basic miasms which Hahnemann saw as the determinant of chronic diseases. The other two he called Syphilis and Psora.

190

syphilis can be understood as the physiognomy of fear. I can now only restate the essentials, but it will, I hope, throw some light on our two remedies.

Under the impact of fear we wake up sharply into our senses and nervous system and become frozen, motionless and wide awake. The experience of fear is intensified when we are alone, at night, in the dark. We become under its influence all nerves and senses.

On the other hand, when shame seizes hold upon us we become confused, our consciousness clouds, our eyelids droop, we become covered with a blush of shame and seek to run away from the sight of others and hide ourselves. The experience of shame is intensified in front of others, in daytime, when confronted. In shame we become submerged in the blood, become altogether blood.

It seems to me that in these two miasms of syphilis and sycosis, Hahnemann grasped intuitively these two extremes of our psycho-physiological experiences and expressions. In his third miasm, psora, he grasped the failure of our inherent self-healing, self-balancing functions, which inwardly is experienced as anxiety, outwardly as congestion and constriction.

How far then can we discover in the strange symptoms of these two remedies, *Thuja* and *Medorrhinum*, clues to their special and unique actions? It has always seemed to me difficult to grasp their drug pictures in coherent form and often, so it has appeared to me, their use is dependent on evidence, actual or speculative, of aetiologial factors such as a history of gonorrhoea or vaccination, or of some other isolated but valuable special symptom. Useful as these guides can be, I have always felt that they fall short of our ideal of grasping the patient and remedy as wholes.

One of the most valuable of these peculiar indications for *Thuja* seems to be, and my own experience confirms it, the frequent or intensive occurrence of dreams of falling. We should also perhaps bring in the tendency to fixed ideas or illusions such as the feeling of body and soul separated, of a stranger by the side, of something alive moving in the abdomen, and even that the limbs are rigid or made of wood or glass. What can we make of such clues? I have puzzled long about it without coming on anything helpful. Recently I was reading a book entitled *Obsession*, written by a very experienced English psychiatrist, Arthur Guirdham. In this most interesting study he gives evidence of the origin of obsessive states, compulsive behaviour, and tics, in paranormal psychic experiences, sometimes manifesting as night-terrors. The ritualistic and compulsive behaviour arise as protective measures to ward off the experiences of evil which he maintains is or has been directly felt by many of these people. In some cases he brings forward evidence of memory reaching very far back, to the intra-uterine or even pre-uterine experiences of the soul descending to incarnate in matter. In one case this was a recurrent dream of great clarity, in which the dreamer was falling through planetary spheres to earth.

Now if we take these experiences seriously, certainly reserving judgement as to their ultimate significance, but accepting the experiences as such, they do seem to me to relate to our present problem. If the dreams of falling of the *Thuja* patient are seen in this light, as memories of incarnation or the more immediate experience of the soul entering the body on awaking and as such an echo of the more profound and distant traumas of conception and birth, then I think we can take a first step forward.

This fall into matter has always been portrayed as shameful and as the very origin of shame. Our birth amidst blood and urine and faeces must be for the soul shameful. And remembering the psychoanalytic understanding of paradise as the intra-uterine bliss, and birth as the casting out of paradise, we can understand that henceforth the serpent must go on his belly. This attitude, mimicked by the dog cringing before his angry master, marks the mythological identity of dog and snake established in regard to the cult of Asklepios as well as in wider contexts. The slave, too, prostrates himself and kneels before his master, and the *Medorrhinum* patient does the same. Are not the painful heels of *Medorrhinum* the echo of the biblical curse 'Thou shalt bruise his heel'?

I remember an asthmatic patient nineteen years old who had been on steroid treatment for many years. In his asthmatic attacks he sought relief lying on his belly or in knee-elbow position. He complained to me of a crop of peri-anal warts resistant to local treatment. A week after giving him *Medorrhinum* 200, they fell off. He certainly had much sense of shame associated with his perineum. Another patient, an attractive women in her thirties most unhappily married to an abnormal man, complained amongst other things of peri-vulval warts, masses of them; they vanished after *Thuja*. Did they not mark her shame at continued intercourse with a man she no longer loved?

The *Medorrhinum* patient is described as dreaming of events before they happen and of sensations of unreality, delusions of someone behind him and of faces peering from behind furniture and many other symptoms, including having committed the unpardonable sin. There is the tendency to fixed ideas in *Thuja*, ideas which cannot be released any more than can the air in their asthmatic lungs. They are markedly influenced by the moon. In all these tendencies they certainly show some of the psychic features of Guirdham's obsessionals and their rigid ideas and brittle limbs point to the ritualistic side of the obsessional. Do the ice-cold nipples of *Medorrhinum* point to the same protective reaction against the psychic experiences involved in suckling?

An aggravation at 3 am and 3 pm is described for *Thuja* and this would seem to point to a connection with the liver rhythm so beautifully described by König. Perhaps it is especially through the fluids of the organism, the lymph and blood movements, that this comes about. This leads to understanding of the asthma and morning diarrhoea, and perhaps could also illuminate the peculiar sweat reactions. Our organisms are not only created once and for all in the foetus, but recreated continuously through the digestion and absorption of the nutritional stream into the lymphatics and blood stream. Here birth processes continue throughout our life and at the other pole of our being, in the nerves and skeleton radiating from the head, death processes predominate and with them fear has its place in our organisms. Interest, obsessional interest in the figure of death and in the skeleton developed at the end of the Middle Ages and it was only then that syphilis manifested on an epidemic scale. Ferenczi saw individual birth as a recapitulation of our phylogenetic origin from the primeval ocean and so it is natural that the *Medorrhinum* patient seeks relief back again at the sea shore.

Dr Rawal drew my attention to the use of injections of *Thuja* in lymphoedema and I have been able to some extent to confirm his observation. Have we got to learn to see together lymphoedema and the failure of the intestinal chyme to be absorbed by the intestinal lymph and blood vessels?

We are faced with the catarrhs, paramountly of the genital tract and especially those associated with the Gonococcus. How can we build an integral understanding of these? To begin with, it is obvious that the main, though not exclusive, manifestation of syphilis is on the skin and proceeds to its assault on the ectodermally derived nervous system. The main manifestation of gonorrhoea on the contrary is usually on the mucosae of the genito-urinary tract. In this we see the polarity of syphilis and gonorrhoea further demonstrated. Further we must distinguish the constitutional or miasmatic disturbance preceding and preparing the organism for the bacterial invasion from the active inflammation and discharge of the acute attack. The mere suppression of this discharge has always, in homoeopathic circles, been regarded as intensifying the real disease. The inflammation and discharge are then grasped as curative attempts, but usually inadequate to achieve healing.

Now there are normal as well as abnormal discharges from the organism and we can interpret the abnormal ones as metamorphoses or displacements of the normal. The main normal discharges are the faeces, the urine and the genital but we must include sweat, breath and other lesser modifications of them. In the digestive tract a process closely analogous to inflammation around a foreign body takes place and the faeces, composed largely of dead and living bacteria, are comparable with the discharge from an abscess. Through the digestive process the organism is enabled to overcome the foreignness of the foodstuff and maintain its own integrity. The male genital function also displays the typical inflammatory phenomena of rubor, calor, dolor, tumor, and seeks relief in discharge. And yet can we easily find a more extreme polarity than that between the seminal fluid of man and bacterial pus which is, as it were, its caricature and shadow.

It is the fate of man to be perplexed by the use of the same tube for excreting urine and the spermatic fluid. On account of this he is confused between the sacred and profane, as the modern medical world from Freud onwards also demonstrates. From this confusion woman is largely spared. For this reason, too, it may be that sexual and dirty jokes are really only therapeutic to men and help them to overcome the inherent feeling of shame and confusion connected with the processes of sex and excretion. This confusion reaches its full physical expression in the phenomenon of gonorrhoea and thereby makes possible a full confrontation and clarification. We have to admit, however, that our present culture makes this desirable consummation and healing difficult and improbable. On all sides we can see the cultural spread of the sycotic miasm and it is definitely out of fashion to allow any feeling of shame to reach consciousness, even when it concerns the murder of unborn children. It is a natural consequence that the occurrence of cancer of the cervix is greatly increased in promiscuous young girls.

Was the name fig wart coined by the folk intuition in imitation of the fig leaves with which our first ancestors covered their shame?

I have attempted to indicate how a common idea is revealed from different sides in some of the peculiar symptoms of *Thuja* and *Medorrhinum* and how this idea is related to the sycotic miasm of Hahnemann.

24. Sepia

It is a freak of history that this remedy, so widely useful in female therapy, should have entered into our materia medica and practice through Hahnemann's observation of an artist friend's habit of sucking his sepia-saturated paint brush. He suspected that the cachetic illness from which this man suffered was due to the sepia and acting on this suspicion cured his patient and enriched our therapeutic armamentarium with this invaluable remedy.

So the first patient whom we know to have been cured by *Sepia* was a man.

I have come gradually to the view that if our discipline is not to die of cachexia we must find again how it can be related to the wider worlds of knowledge and escape from its own Sepian retreats. Homoeopathy as bequeathed by Hahnemann depends on the symptoms produced in provings and on the symptoms in which the disease reveals itself. It has consequently to a large extent been cut off from natural science and from the pathology and medicine orientated in natural science. In their pursuit of quantification and in their one-sided devotion to the principle of mechanical causation, these disciplines have largely relegated qualities and symptoms to categories of the merely subjective or of placebo effect.

The extraordinary and bewilderingly wonderful pageant of nature demands from us not only interpretation in terms of causation and mechanism, it calls to our souls for a solution to its riddle in terms of meaning and significance. All outer natural processes find themselves again within our own organisms and whereas they appear separated, externalized and analyzed outside in nature, they are to be found interiorized and synthesized within us. We are the wholes whose parts are spread out around us in nature. When we seek for significance it is the relationship of parts to the whole which will reveal it to us.

Our medicament Sepia is, of course, prepared from the ink of the cuttlefish. The cuttlefish belongs to the phylum of the Molluscs which is divided into three main classes, the Gastropoda or snails, the Lamellibranchiata or bivalves, and the Cephalopoda, to which our Sepia belongs together with octopuses and squids. We have medicaments derived from each class, *Murex* from the snail *Murex brandaris,* *Calcarea carbonica* from the oyster (*Ostrea edulis*) and the ink *Sepia* from the cuttlefish *Sepia officinalis*. The question arises at once as to whether we should disregard the origins of our substances and take note only of their chemical composition, or whether their origin is not of equal, or even greater, significance. It goes almost without saying that to our modern scientists it is the chemical constitution that could alone be considered as important. There is also a temptation in homoeopathic circles to follow this line, encouraged by the unfortunate fact that most of our materia medicas go from A to Z irrespective of the animal, vegetable or mineral origin, or of the natural groupings, of the substances. However, at once a fact comes leaping at us, to cause us to stop and consider. *Murex* and *Sepia* are reported as highly complementary remedies. Kent draws attention to the similarity in discussing *Sepia* and Wheeler states that *Murex* in low potency will often prove useful during a high potency *Sepia* treatment. Now so far as I know, there is no discernible chemical relationship between the melanin pigment sepia and the substance we call Murex purpurea, the dried secretion of the purple gland of Murex brandaris and Murex trunculus. The secretion is colourless but catalyzed in air into dibromoindigo, the Tyrian purple of the ancients. This does not appear to be active. Other constituents such as murexine also do not seem to account for the action of *Murex* and Leeser concluded it was premature to form conclusions about them. However, it is strange that these two molluscs of different classes provide remedies with such closely related symptom pictures; should Hahnemann's *Calcarea carbonica* also be included in this group, rather than be left amongst the inorganic substances?

I am personally inclined to pursue this path of significance and meaning, the more so because we are dealing with human individualities whose lives are concerned so much more with meaning and significance than with mere facts. Facts are after all that which is finished, excreted, done with, as the word itself indicates, deriving from the Latin *facio* and cognate with 'faeces'. 'Face' and 'fact' would seem to be related too, which leads us back to *Sepia*, as we shall see.

Otto Leeser built up his picture of *Sepia* starting from the melanin pigments and depicting an Addisonian state of hypoadrenalism. It is a coherent and valuable account. A very similar picture was put forward by the endocrinologist and medical historian Professor A. P. Cawadias.

Karl König, using the depiction of the molluscs given by Poppelbaum, sought to find the place of molluscs both in relation to man's organism and in evolution. The play of light and dark figure in his depiction and again a coherent interpretation emerges.

Edward Whitmont gave a fascinating account of *Sepia*, using Jungian analytical psychology to unravel the symptom complex, with the archetypal figures of the Shadow and the Anima and Animus as keys to the interpretation.

The molluscs are a very strange lot of creatures. Soft, plastic, viscous or slimy, they are non-segmented, have no metamerism and in their growth develop by steady plastic remodelling rather than by dramatic metamorphoses. In these features they are very much the opposite pole to the Arthropoda. Poppelbaum and König regard them as having remained essentially embryonic, the plastic moulding characteristic of embryos is in them retained throughout life. Poppelbaum also sees them as abdomens raised to the status of the head. Metamerism is in humans characteristic of our middle, primarily thoracic region. In the head this metamerism is overcome by the new spherical form which completely dominates the segmental. In Hahnemann's day there was of course much controversy as to the number of vertebrae contained in the skull. Goethe and Oken were prominent in these arguments. In the abdomen, too, metamerism is largely lost. So it is becoming easier for us to see the molluscs as head and abdomen without any true middle realm. These creatures are trying all the time to become brains shut off and protected from the outer world within shell. The oysters and mussels breathe in and out the water in which they lie, water full of colour and taste. The middle layer of the oyster shell from which our *Calc. carb* is taken, is formed prismatically so that were it not hidden under an opaque covering it would be on the way to becoming a compound eye. Like a retina, the mother of pearl on the inside reveals the play of light and dark in its delicate colours, gentle, like after-images. In the scallops which swim through the sea with their valves like eyelids opening and shutting, there are actual eyes along the mantle fringes, and luminous organs as well. Shy, retiring, all these creatures live within their shells, forming images of the world outside.

The gastropods or snails are characterized outwardly by their spiral shells and by their foot on which they lick or swim their way forward. They seem rather to hearken to the sounds around with their foot as the cochlea hearkens within our ear organization.

In the cephalopods the eye had become elevated to an organ comparable with the vertebrate eye, taste has developed the mouth parts, lips and tongue, into the hideous tentacles covered with suckers and horny hooks, metamorphosed from the vallate and filiform papillae on our tongue. The cuttlefish loses its shell and its body is really the skull within which the viscera are sheltered like a brain, whilst the face becomes progressively, from Nautilus to decapod cuttlefish to octopus, drawn out into a gruesome, greedy, lusting, organ. Its eye is fixed wide open so that, as König suggests, it forms the sepia ink out of the forces of darkness to counterbalance this extreme openness to the light. At the same time the whole surface of the creature is subject to a continuous play of colour changes, luminous and phosphorescent phenomena. No other creatures can match these for their capacity to change colour and patterns of colour. The whole creature becomes eye or iris, but taste combines with this all over the body and tentacles.

The strange organ, the ink-sac, lies amongst the other viscera towards the front of the creature, this is, away from the mouth end and the tentacles which lie to the rear. It opens into the mantle cavity and when it contracts the ink is expelled through the funnel, which incidentally corresponds with the foot of the other molluscs. This expulsion of the ink is closely integrated into the behaviour patterns. Mostly ink seems to be emitted when the creature is pursued, when it is frightened.

Sometimes it is described as darkening all the water round, confusing the predator, at other times it emits the ink as a distinct cloud about its own size, a blob of ink, and at the same time it changes colour and shoots off in the opposite direction.

We can now take up the mystery of these creatures from another but wholly complementary point of view. Jaworski, in his book *Après Darwin* sought systematically for the correspondences between organisms in nature and the organs in man. To him the molluscs were the exteriorized embodiment of the female genital organs. The octopus to Jaworski was the uterus, with its tentacles joined together, in many species, with a membrane to form the vagina. Other molluscs individualize various aspects of female genital function. It was not accidental that Venus came ashore in a scallop shell. Jaworski was also well aware of the appearance of molluscan features at the head pole, in ear, teeth, lips and tongue. He saw the Eustachian tube connecting middle ear and pharynx as the interiorized expression of the siphon which in some rock-boring molluscs remains their only connection with the outer world.

We can easily see that the brain floating in the cerebrospinal fluid within its membranes in the skull is the polar expression of the baby in the amniotic fluid and membranes within the uterus. In the ancient terminology so fashionable today they are like yin and yang. To the cranium is added the face and mouth and to the uterus is added the vagina and vulva. In the cephalopods we can see both these complementary pictures.

It is not then surprising that our remedy *Sepia* has such a remarkable affinity for the female organs and functions, nor that headaches figure so largely in its symptomatology. It has of course been known for a long time that headaches can be a sort of cephalic pregnancy and labour pains, indicating a new thought seeking acceptance into the conscious light of day against the forces of resistance and repression. Dysmenorrhoea can be a variant of migraine. One wonders whether a timely dose of *Sepia* from the octopus so wonderfully pictured on the vases in Zeus's own Cretan birthplace would have avoided his cephalic Caesarean section whereby Pallas Athene was born.

But whilst we are on Crete let us not forget the labyrinth, that clear symbol of the brain in whose convoluted maze our whole civilization is caught unless it remembers the thread of Ariadne's intuition. One further symbol besides the octopus and labyrinth dominates Cretan life — the double-headed axe. I could not, when there, escape the conviction that this also represented the two cerebral hemispheres. Crete was the birthplace of Greece, and Knossos certainly points to Gnosis and knowledge and, as Groddeck pointed out, to gynaecology and Homer's immortal 'pregnant hinges of the knee' or genu.

These detours are only intended to indicate the extraordinary, quite wonderful, relation between molluscs and the organs of conception, whether of babies or thoughts. There is at this point one further strange phenomenon to bring forward. In some cephalopods at the time of copulation one of the arms carrying the spermatophore is actually separated off and enters into the mantle cavity of the partner. At the beginning of the last century, the great Cuvier, seeing them there, thought that they were parasitic worms and it was only later that their true nature was discovered.

Now Jaworski also came to perceive that the male reproductive functions and organs found their exteriorized counterparts in the worms so that in a deeper sense Cuvier was not so mistaken after all. The arms, the tentacles of the cuttlefish, are a male note sounded within the female world just as the tongue is a male note within the oral cavity. Acting on this I was able to cure a case of Peyronie's disease with the worm *Hirudo med.* when *Sepia* failed.

The self-cutting-off of an organ is known biologically as autotomy. Such phenomena as the lizard leaving his tail in one's hand and escaping to grow a new one belong together with this shedding of the tentacle in copulation by the cuttlefish, as examples of autotomy. Ferenczi, one of the great pioneers of psychoanalysis, in his classic study, *Genitaltheorie*, translated in America under the title *Thalassa*, saw these phenomena repeated as aspects in the sexual act of coitus. The deturgescence after orgasm he interpreted as an equivalent to the autotomy of the phallus. In these strange worlds which molluscs and sex lead us into, worlds nearer to fairy stories than to rigid mechanical models, I hazard the guess that one of the very marked symptoms of *Sepia* in the male finds a corresponding note in these phenomena. I refer to the great depression and lassitude following coitus. Here the male patient remains identified with his cut off lost member. He feels himself castrated and has not succeeded in identifying himself with his mate into whose mantle his most precious organ has passed. He is indeed depleted, deprived and understandably depressed. The *Sepia* helps him to close the circle again, to discover the twin realities of death and resurrection and to realize that dying is only a cause of new life. It may also be that it helps him to the discovery that every one of us is male-female.

So much then, in limited space, for the aspect of our remedy which has to do with its origin from the cuttlefish Sepia officinalis. We must now consider its origin in that singular organ the ink sac. Where can we find any comparable organ in nature? The ink sac lies in the mantle cavity with the other viscera. In octopus and squid it lies against the liver. I understand that in some species it lies even within the liver. In the cuttlefish it is separated from this organ by a short distance. It empties actually into the rectum from which the ink is further ejected through the funnel. It contains the ink which is constituted of melanin granules in suspension. The melanin seems to be similar to the melanins in the skin and hair of higher animals and on the back of the eye. Melanin is believed to be formed by the polymerisation of a compound derived from tyrosine and dihydroxyphenylalanine. A copper-containing enzyme tyrosinase is found in the wall of the ink sac.

What really is all this about? Certainly the ejection of the ink is integrated into the behaviour of the creatures. In response to fear, perhaps also to anger, the ink is shot out and seems to enable the creature to escape. It does not seem to play any further part in the animal's economy other than as an excretion. The use made of this excretion in the escape behaviour seems to require for its elucidation the use of slang, of vernacular expressions. It is comparable with the vulgar 'to piss or shit over someone'. But leaving aside this behavioural use of the excretion there is yet another aspect. If this dark shadow which would otherwise poison the creature, is collected and excreted there must be a back thrust into the organism, a counter process to the expulsion of darkness. At first sight it seems to me that this counter impulse into the organism must be light as opposed to the darkness, and if this is indeed so, then it may be more deeply connected with the source of the luminescent phenomena which are so outstanding a characteristic of the cuttle-fish. In any case, we can surely see the polarity of open eye and luminescent and chromatophore organs on the one hand with the dark melanin shadow on the other.

I should like to recount again a case I reported some years ago. A woman aged thirty consulted me on account of vitiligo on the arms. This condition was causing her embarrassment, apart from the restrictions it imposed on sun bathing. There were multiple sharply defined depigmented areas over both arms. The condition had been developing for about a year and gradually it emerged that the onset followed a breakdown in her relations with her fiancé. It was obvious that she was deeply distressed and also ashamed. A further peculiarity was the development of generalized increased pigmentation of the lower abdomen from about the level of the umbilicus down, and a relative depigmentation above this level. The general symptoms fitted well with *Sepia* and she was given weekly doses of *Sepia* 30. Her general mental state improved very markedly with this and the pigmentation of the abdomen returned to normal fairly quickly. After some months the arms also showed improvement. She omitted treatment for some months and the abdominal pigmentation began to return, but again became normal on treatment with *Sepia*. At the time I commented as follows. One could not handle this patient without the impression being forced upon one that the pigmentation of the lower abdomen was a cover behind which she was hiding and the resemblance to the cuttlefish's use of its sepia cloud was inescapable. Perhaps I should express it differently today, and notice also how she was expressing openly the dark passion which dwelt within her. But it remains the most dramatic case of pigmentary changes related to *Sepia* that I have encountered.

To return to the ink sac lying against the liver and the inescapable question it raises — is the ink sac related to the gall bladder of higher animals? We have of course to distinguish the cuttlefish with its copper-containing haemocyanin blood pigment from the vertebrate with iron-containing haemoglobin. Moreover, the bile salts play an active part in fat digestion and the bile pigments are partly resorbed and excreted in the urine. Moreover, the constituents of melanin are related more to the adrenal than to the bile. But *Sepia* is certainly closely related to the liver and portal circulation as well. The *Sepia* patient goes dark pigmented but the gall bladder patient goes yellow jaundiced. My colleague Dr Marianne Harling supplied me with a suggestion which seems very well worth pondering upon. She suggested that these two are related to the Black Bile and the Yellow Bile of the ancients, that the Black Bile is not necessarily to be taken as identical with but related to the Sepia melanin-containing ink. Most certainly the *Sepia* patient goes dark and depressed, is fearful and overwhelmed by melancholy. Certainly the excretion or expulsion of yellow bile is related to anger and the fiery spirit in man, needed of course to confront the exogenous heat in the fats in the intestine. So in *Sepia* we have more to do with the polarity of light and darkness, and with yellow bile we are more involved with heat and cold. The expulsion of sepia ink is related to the emotional disturbance of the cuttlefish, fear and also anger or irritation. The expulsion of bile is related to stimulus of fat in the intestine, but also to anger, and I am convinced that jaundice can be provoked by jealousy.

In man the phenomena of melanin pigmentation are not usually regarded as emotionally determined, but I quoted a case to suggest that it may be. Where in the cephalic pole are we to find the correspondence to the ink sac? Where in the cuttlefish, which is our head, can we look? Is there any connection between the substantia nigra in the brain and our sepia. The substantia nigra contains melanin and also copper, reminding us of the copper haemocyanin and the copper-containing tyrosinase in the wall of the ink sac. L-Dopa, now used in the treatment of parkinsonism, is involved in the production of melanin. The drugs used today in the treatment of mental illness are liable to bring about parkinsonian tremors. Are not depression and parkinsonism two phases of one whole? Sometimes these phases are alternatives. There is in the cuttlefish an unblinking stare, an expressionless face, there is an exaggeration of the mouth which shows itself again in the salivary incontinence and facial prolapse of the parkinsonian, and perhaps even more in the postencephalitic child.

I am not suggesting that *Sepia* is a remedy for parkinsonism, but I am suggesting that in this whole that is the cuttlefish and its ink there are important clues for a holistic understanding of the relationship between depression, parkinsonism, and all these other phenomena.

Now one of the outstanding symptoms of *Sepia* is the sensation of the uterus being pushed down, prolapsing. It is of course interesting that this is a masculinizing tendency. In the male the testicles descend and are prolapsed. In complete procidentia the everted vagina and uterus take on the appearance of the male penis.

Another outstanding *Sepia* symptom is the flushing or blushing, conspicuous at puberty or menopause. Groddeck observed that 'Changing colour, blushing or growing pale is associated with a feeling of shame and a desire to hide. More primitive people than ourselves may have realized that in blushing a woman disguises her weakness by the show of strength, for a man who reddens in anger is terrifying to the timid, so the It of the timid woman imitates him and behaves as though it were the dangerous male'.

It is also possible to see that the outstanding *Sepia* symptoms, fatigue, weariness, depression, are also really the postcoital male fatigue to which I have referred. Here again the woman is reacting in a characteristically male way. But when the man relaxes, at the weekend, then he gets his migraine, which the woman gets more with her periods when her emotions and passions are highest.

So we are faced with the paradox that these outstanding symptoms in *Sepia* women are in reality expressions of maleness or imitations of the male. Loss of hair in women can also be looked upon as imitating men and here again *Sepia* is often of real value. *Sepia* does have strong action on the skin and we should remember that the word *hide* in English refers both to the skin and to concealment. Both the phenomena of the ink cloud and the colour-changes in the cuttlefish are integrated into perhaps one of the best concealment performances in nature, and octopuses are notorious escapologists able to slip through very narrow slits. It is then, as Whitmont observed, the shadow side of woman united with her male side, the Animus, that is helped by *Sepia*. In men it is their shadow side united with the female Anima that comes in question. How does this manifest? In moodiness, sulkiness. I well remember how as a child I was prone to bad fits of sulkiness and how I was admonished to get rid of the black dog on my back, my cloud of sepia.

Can we then begin to draw these wide-ranging observations together? The men and women who are most likely to need *Sepia* are those in whom the problem of the other sex within us and of the shadow has arisen. Jung used the term 'shadow' for that alter ego in each of us of which we are ashamed and which we try to avoid acknowledging as really belonging to us. The more our conscious personality is upright in a narrow moralistic sort of way, the darker does our shadow become. Today, when our conscious personalities have become very narrow, but very white hot with an intellectual intensity, our shadows, individual and collective, have become the enormous problems with which we are everywhere confronted. In the case of men Jung used the term Anima for the female being inside us and in the case of women the corresponding inner male being he called the Animus. It is true that to begin with these figures of the Anima and Animus are almost indistinguishably bound up with the shadow.

Now I think we would all agree that there are two periods of life when *Sepia* is most often needed as a remedy: adolescence and menopause. Are not these the moments when the problem of the other sex in us looms greatest? At adolescence we can often notice how girls for a time become hoydens, and in dress and behaviour are often more like boys than girls. It seems as if, before taking on the responsibilities of womanhood, with the one-sidedness and sacrifice of wholeness which this involves, a last despairing effort is made to hold on to the fading memory of the wholeness of childhood. In the case of boys a period of effeminacy, writing poetry, artistic yearnings and so on, is often lived through before the plunge into the materialism of career with all its competitiveness and ruthlessness.

At menopause or thereabouts the reverse problem arises. The primary responsibilities for establishing a home and family are achieved and no longer mark the road and task ahead. Career will have reached its zenith and retirement is not far ahead. A new and different task arises for us now. It is the obligation to work for wholeness, to work to redeem our shadow side which we exploited and sacrificed in our headlong search for success and achievement. The Anima and Animus must be integrated with our personalities, we must work towards wholeness. One can easily see that at adolescence we are faced with the tasks of generation whereas at menopause we must undertake the tasks leading to regeneration.

I think also, that we can all see that our whole world today stands under this sign. A great division has come about, in individuals and in society. The western world has one-sidedly developed its outer, materialistic side and the other half of the world has been left in the shadow. It is the same problem on the world scale as in our individual psyches. Civilization has gradually led to the experience of spiritual death but this is a necessary prelude to the experience of spiritual regeneration, of rebirth.

We can respond to a remedy in many ways. We can eat it and through taste and its continuation in our digestions we can prove it. But I believe that the responses of our thoughts and feelings when we bring to bear our other senses and the whole of our personality upon a remedy belong also to its fuller proving. Perhaps most of all we could discern its deepest nature in the impulses in our wills to which it could give origin. In this sense I would link *Sepia* both with adolescence leading to inevitable one-sidedness and disintegration, and with menopause heralding the rebirth and healing of our disordered state. In contemplating *Sepia* we can receive the inspiration needed to undertake the spiritual tasks of our time; the redemption of the Shadow, and rebirth, rebirth of the whole within our individual hearts and souls.

25. The leech
(*Hirudo medicinalis*)

Some years ago a case of Peyronie's disease was treated successfully with oral *Hirudo medicinalis* 12c. Peyronie's disease consists of a painful nodule developing in the shaft of the penis. In 10% of cases there is associated Dupuytren's contracture. The condition in the penis tends to spontaneous resolution after four or more years. In the case I reported, disappearance of pain was rapid in response to *Hirudo* and the nodule resolved completely in six to nine months. After stopping treatment for two months, some recurrence of pain and of the nodule was noticed, but this quickly cleared up on resuming *Hirudo* 12 twice daily. *Hirudo* is the medicinal leech.

In the proving of *Hirudo* carried out by Raeside, no symptoms were recorded in the genital organs, but there were spots and pimples on the nose and face. Raeside mentioned the work of the physician-biologist Jaworski. Jaworski was concerned to discover and verify in practical application, correspondences between organisms occurring in the outer world and the organs, tissues and cells within our own skin. He himself, regarding birds as externalized pulmonary functions, used sera prepared from birds as a remedy for pulmonary disease in man, in emphysema, bronchitis and pneumonia. Our own use of *Tuberculinum aviare* in such cases may be successful on account of the pigeons from which it is derived as much as on account of the tubercle. In any case, I have personally seen it produce excellent improvement in respiratory function in such cases.

Jaworski also pointed to the correspondence of tortoises and turtles to the liver in man, and used preparations from them in treating cirrhosis and other liver diseases. The molluscs he regarded as striking a note of female genitality. Our use of *Sepia* and *Murex* in disorders of function of the uterus confirms this insight. Jaworski further demonstrated that the worms correspond to the male genital organs and functions. The leech in particular individualizes the erectile function, it becomes engorged with blood and its locomotor activity is based on this variable condition. Having observed these creatures over some time, I am persuaded that the word lecherous must be related to leech. On the basis of this correspondence of *Hirudo* with the penis, I used the preparation successfully in the case of Peyronie's disease.

A hundred years ago the English physician Compton Burnett drew attention to the importance of organ remedies as introduced into homoeopathy from Rademacher's Paracelsianism. He seems to have used three main methods of choosing the remedy — firstly the matching of the totality of symptoms, secondly the organ affinity of remedies, and thirdly nosodes aetiologically chosen. The organ remedies are perhaps most used today in the drainage remedies of our French colleagues. I believe the use of animal remedies such as *Hirudo* represents an extension of this concept of organ remedies.

Another remedy which I have used in a similar way is *Bufo*. In the amphibia the skin is the dominant organ, and it is not difficult to see that the toad displays outwardly in its skin the mucous membrane which in higher forms is internalized in the intestine and particularly in the colon and rectum. I have used *Bufo* in proctitis and ulcerative colitis, sometimes with considerable relief of symptoms. The first time I used it was in the case of a man with radiological evidence of Crohn's disease of the terminal ileum. Gradually over 18 months the condition cleared up and the X-ray appearances became normal.

A remedy which is not very often used as far as I know is *Hekla lava*. It was introduced into homoeopathy by James Garth Wilkinson in the last century. He noticed when in Iceland that sheep grazing on the slopes of Mount Hekla developed exostoses on their jaws. *Hekla* lava has been used for various dental troubles, abscesses and tumours of the jaw. I have used it in osteoarthritis, particularly in Heberden's nodes of the terminal phalanges. These can erupt quite quickly and painfully and I have often seen them greatly helped by *Hekla lava* 6 or 12 given twice daily. The sudden development of these nodes reminds me of the way in which a few years ago a new island was formed by eruption off the coast of Iceland.

James Garth Wilkinson was a Swedenborgian and his book *The human body and its connexion with Man*, published over a hundred years ago, is still thought-provoking and stimulating. It provides a valuable look into the way homoeopathy and Swedenborgianism worked together, particularly in the United States. Constantine Hering was a Swedenborgian and the tradition ran through American homoeopathy to Kent. Although Wilkinson was an Englishman, I cannot find that Swedenborgianism was so much of a stimulus to the development of homoeopathy in Great Britain.

Another type of organ remedy exists. When an organ or tissue from an animal, suitably prepared, is given to a human being, a vitalizing action of the corresponding human tissue can be brought about. This can be of help in treating disease of tissues like cartilage or nerve tissue, where vitality is in any case low, or in intensifying the action of remedies into some particular organ. My experience with these remedies (such as the Disci preparations of Wala) leads me to believe that they can be very useful in cases where there are pathological structural changes and where, as is often the case, classical prescribing symptoms are absent or rare.

In conditions in which it may be difficult or perhaps impossible to find the symptomatic similimum, it may still be possible to find remedies which can cure or help, by resorting to various types of organ remedy. Not only can we help by these methods, but we enlarge our understanding of the action of remedies and enrich our conception of the similar remedy.

26.   The snake (*Lachesis*)

Our remedy *Lachesis* is prepared from the venom of the Bushmaster *Lachesis muta*, perhaps one of the most aggressive and poisonous of all snakes. Again, as in the case of *Sepia*, we are faced with the question whether the source or only the chemical nature of this venom is significant. The chemical nature was the basis of Otto Leeser's study and must be allowed to stand, but the serpent nature, as revealed in myth, forms the basis of Whitmont's interpretation. Both approaches convince us of their validity. H. H. Engel, some years ago, contributed a profoundly suggestive paper which included the biological physiognomy.

Let us begin with the serpents themselves which have from immemorial antiquity figured so largely in myth and legend. It is strange that these creatures, which are really rather inconspicuous and mostly rather timid and which in their outer form are so simple, should have become symbols of wisdom and of man's fall and redemption. It is strange that there is such almost universal revulsion from them. To our untutored observation they do not manifest any especial wisdom in their behaviour. Some of them are poisonous, most of them are not. The majority of them are said to live in the sea or, like the Anaconda, in fresh water, but we are more familiar with them on land. In evolution they appeared as polar opposites to the birds, both developing from primordial reptiles, but in opposite directions, clearing the air, so to speak, for the mammals and man to make their appearance in the middle. The similarities and polarities of these contrasted forms were brought out by Poppelbaum. Whereas in birds the whole trunk has been condensed into a sort of cage serving altogether as a head, in the snakes everything has become digestive. Snakes, as Jaworski also saw, are intestines merely served by other organs. Everything in them is concerned with swallowing and digesting. The digestive capacity of these creatures is staggering; they envelop their prey, in the case of pythons it may be a whole pig; they do not eat it or chew, they swallow it whole. The girth of the creature may be six times its normal size after a meal. The digestive force is so strong that practically only pure uric acid is eliminated. In this elimination of uric acid they resemble the birds. Mammals eliminate urea, with the strange exception of Dalmation dogs which also excrete uric acid. This colossal digestive capacity is true of both the poisonous and non-poisonous varieties. Snakes often eat each other and there is the famous symbol of the uroboros, the snake eating its own tail.

There are many witnesses to the overwhelming horror of the open mouth of a snake. Owing to the system of levers by which the lower jaws are attached, it is possible for them to swallow objects many times larger than themselves. In the venomous snakes the poison is secreted from modified salivary glands, in the vipers it is actually shot through hollow teeth like hypodermic needles. In one species this is so arranged that the venom is ejected to a distance of some yards in front of the creature and it can hit the eye of the victim from a distance.

We have seen in the case of the cuttlefish and molluscs that they are character-ized by a non-segmental form. There is no metamerism in the molluscs, they are heads or pelves without trunks. In striking contrast the snakes are a series of almost non-ending vertebrae, up to 400. They have lost their legs and pelvic and shoulder girdles. Their heads with attached jaws are almost just a simple continu-ation of the vertebrae, with ribs for jaws. There is no sternum, no thorax, and the jaws can move separately so that the snakes can, so to speak, walk over their prey. In them segmentation, metamerism, reaches its highest expression, but it is entirely in service to the digestive function. They have usually only one lung, the left is greatly reduced or practically absent. Here the asymmetry which governs the abdomen extends strongly into the lungs, again showing how everything has dropped backwards or fallen downwards in these creatures. Just as in the birds everything has jumped ahead, so in snakes everything has become intestine, has fallen down. It is interesting also to note how in lizards and kindred forms, as legs diminish towards limbless forms the number of vertebrae correspondingly increase.

In the realm of the senses similar tendencies meet us. The eyes of the snake, contrasting with the ever-open eyes of the cuttlefish, are forever sealed, the eyelids have become transparent but are closed. It seems, too, that the snake only sees movement. Stationary objects it cannot see. It probably has no sense for colour. The sense of sight therefore can be said to have fallen out of its true sphere into a sense of movement. The tongue, flickering in and out through a small hole in the closed lips, seems rather to touch the air around than to taste anything. The swallowing whole of the victim is against any real tasting.

The tongue, with horny tips, seems to be an extended organ of touch, not taste. The ears are scarcely developed, the middle ear, with the three ossicles, morphologically representing thigh, leg and foot, is absent, as is to be expected in creatures without limbs. Hearing has become a sense for mere vibration extended through the length of the creature. The senses also are fallen, degraded lower than their proper station. We have the impression that everything has slipped down a stage, is out of its proper place.

In the birds, a great range of colourful motifs and gestures come to outer expression in plumage, ritual dances and behaviour, and in song. In the snakes, very little of all this psychic world, which the birds have around them, manifests outwardly. No bird is poisonous. In the snakes, we are compelled to see that all this rich realm of psychic forces has entered into the very metabolic, digestive processes. It is this world of forces, penetrating too deeply into the physiological realm, that gives rise to the poison. Is it not also this occulted world of the psychic which has become concealed in, rather than manifested around, the creature, that is the wisdom of the serpent? Like the blind sage Teiresias, like the blind Homer, the snake's attention is towards an inner world in which profoundest wisdom is concealed.

But the endless repetition of the vertebrae, the inability, as it were, of the snake to put an end to it, is still enigmatic. The vertebral note sounded again and again, like the repeated nodes of plant growth, points to immense vegetative forces of life. The bringing of this to a conclusion in skull and pelvis, as in root and blossom, belongs to other than purely vegetative forces. In the snake these other psychic forces have gone entirely into the digestive realm, neither can they bring forth limbs, and proper lungs from which inner sound can come forth. The snake can only hiss.

The snake often has a sexual, phallic, significance. This again is enigmatic, seeing that its life patterns are so much more digestive than sexual. In considering the cuttlefish, *Sepia off.*, we were faced with the bipolarity of sex; the cuttlefish and cephalopods can represent both the uterus and head. Conception in mankind is predominantly female in the uterus and male in the brain, and we are reminded of how the bisexual primitive forms became divided into separate sexes as Plato indicates in the *Symposium* and as indicated also in Genesis; male-female created he them. This moment of division is usually associated with the Fall of Man and we have been seeing how much the serpent is a revelation of fallen state. Now we also saw in the molluscs how the oyster is a polar contrast to the octopus and cuttlefish, and how the oyster strikes a predominantly cephalic note, the octopus a predominantly uterine one. In the case of the snakes, we shall have to look to the birds to find the complementary form. Taken alone, the serpent represents a sexuality concerned only with sensuality and reproduction. The higher pole of sexuality concerned with knowledge and consciousness is missing, sex has also collapsed into a fallen, or partial aspect which again for this reason fills the soul with a horror, the meaninglessness of mere feeding and reproduction, the horror of the snake pit.

I think we can also glimpse the nature of the horror to which the spectacle of a feeding snake gives rise. The eating is also sexual, but wholly, appallingly, lacking in the higher metamorphosis which gives meaning and which is expressed in the gnostic writing which Holst set to music in his 'Hymn of Jesus'. 'Fain would I eat, fain would I be eaten.' We can now also glimpse an aspect of the mystery whereby man's fall came about through the Serpent and his redemption began with the Baptism in Jordan and the manifestation of the Holy Spirit in the form of a dove. The healing snakes of Asklepios are raised up vertically along the staff of the caduceus and are winged, thus indicating the nature of the healing art, the restoring of wholeness to that which has fallen and become partial and divided.

How far can this picture of the snake help us to unriddle the drug picture of *Lachesis*. The greed of the snake which compels it to swallow its victims whole finds its place in the egotism of *Lachesis*. The great emphasis on swallowing must be related to all the throat symptoms of all the snake venoms, but particularly *Lachesis*.

In the egg-eating snake this note is most tellingly expressed. Special bony knobs on some of the vertebrae break right through into the oesophagus. The egg, swallowed with difficulty, is held behind the head as a great bulge; then it is cracked against the vertebral bones and the shell sent up, the egg contents swallowed down. In the globus hystericus, which in minor degrees is a common symptom, we sense a difficulty in swallowing, a reluctance to swallow the bitter pill of truth, a fear of being poisoned.

This question of the throat, of swallowing, so central to the *Lachesis* picture, calls for our further consideration. The throat is the gateway to the world of the belly, the world of the unconscious, the underworld. When we swallow something it passes from the sphere of consciousness into the unconscious, there we digest it and absorb it and are ourselves changed in the process. We swallow not only food but experience. We are often reluctant to swallow unpleasant truths and experiences and thus they stick in our gullet, but then we cannot forget them either, nor can we grow through their digestion. The throat is a threshold and we learn from mythology that at doorways or thresholds there are guardians. These are often dogs, the most well known perhaps being Cerberus, the three-headed hound at the crossing of the river Styx.

Now in the mythology of the healing god Asklepios, snakes and dogs are interchangeable. In the Roman museum at Bath there is an altar to Asklepios and on one side there is a snake, on another a dog. San Rocco, the patron saint of the plague and a mediaeval saint of healing, is always portrayed with a dog. It is indeed strange to find that *Lac caninum*, our remedy from bitches' milk, has also this predilection for the throat and with *Lachesis* and *Mercurius* is one of three great remedies for sore throats and diptheria. The god Mercury, of course, carries the caduceus and is the psychopompus, the guide to the underworld, whilst our remedy *Lac caninum* is characterized by dreams of snakes.

The egotism of *Lachesis* may also be based on the selfishness of the snake digestion which gives so little back to the earth. In contrast we have to think of the cow, another sacred animal, which however, with its profound and mysterious digestion gives to the earth the potent restoring manure of its excrement and bestows its beneficent milk.

Does the dog gain its relationship to the snake through its descent from the mean and cowardly jackal and the greedy wolf? Certainly the dog is easily over-whelmed by shame, and then cringes on its belly like the snake. 'Upon thy belly shalt thou go.' Expressions like 'a dirty dog', 'a whipping dog', indicate the tendency to throw our guilt elsewhere. There is also widespread belief that a dog howling at night heralds a death, a crossing of the threshold.

The great sensitivity of the throat to touch in the *Lachesis* patient belongs partly to the general throatiness of snakes we have been considering and partly to the extreme sensitivity to touch altogether shown by these patients.

Bearing in mind the main features of our characterization of the snake, the predominance of the digestive function and the fall of other functions to a lower status than normal, we have to see how certain main symptoms of the *Lachesis* picture fall into place.

Firstly, there is the aggravation of symptoms during and after sleep, with waking into an aggravation of symptoms. The predominantly katabolic activity of the brain and nervous system during waking life gives way during sleep to a predominantly anabolic life. The balance tilts decisively during sleep in the direction of anabolism and those symptoms and disease processes which arise from anabolic superfluity are exaggerated. These are exactly in *Lachesis* conditions. Oversleeping can be as much a cause of illness as undersleeping, which falls more into the *Nux vomica* field of action. *Sepia* conditions can be ameliorated or aggravated by sleep, in my experience they are often ameliorated, and *Phosphorus* is usually better for even short sleeps.

Secondly, symptoms are relieved by the onset of discharges, whether nasal, menstrual or other. Again here we see how a disbalance which has developed under anabolic supremacy is restored to harmony by the excretory, katabolic functions culminating in discharges.

Thirdly there is the extreme sensitivity to touch and particularly to constriction of any form. It is a little like the *Ignatia* hypersensitivity and is more to light touch than firm pressure. It seems to be associated with hypersensitive, hysterical types of women and it may be connected with the definite tendency for hysterical symptoms to manifest more on the left side of the body. Hysterical symptoms proper reflect a predominance of the metabolic pole, in contrast to neurasthenic symptomatology which expresses the overweighting of the balance in the direction of the nerves and senses pole. This connection with the left-right polarity is also suggestive. The left side is both the feminine and the unconscious side and so here again we are brought up against the balance of conscious and unconscious which we have considered in relation to the throat. We should also bring it into relationship with the arterial-venous polarity. The left side is the arterial and centrifugal side, whereas the right side is venous and centripetal. The *Lachesis* tendency to purplish, venous discoloration is thus found to be related to the left-sidedness and sensitivity to constriction. Any constriction, more particularly on the left, centrifugal side, will result in congestion and venous distention. A firm enough pressure will also result in stopping the arteriolar flow and hence will prevent the venous overfilling. This preponderance of the venous side of the circulation may well be the basis also of the desire for air, for open windows, characterizing these patients. The aggravation from warmth with its relation to digestive and metabolic activities and its tendency to dilate the skin circulation is to be expected, as is the aggravation from alcohol. The *Lachesis* headaches of congestive type, aggravated by heat or sun and often left-sided, can be included here.

There is one further mental symptom which needs to be mentioned, the loquacity sometimes seen in and indicating this remedy. It is an endless chatter of unrelated themes in which no real expression of the personality is achieved, no real communication. Any restriction of their logorrhoea is felt as is a constriction in the physical symptoms. It reminds, too, of the endless repetition of the vertebrae, with the inability to put a stop to it, and finally the flashing in and out of the tongue, restlessly touching the air as the chatter seems to be more a feeling, a testing of the environment than an utterance from within. The snake can only hiss, it cannot sound forth its inner world.

The *Lachesis* patient may have a craving for oysters which seems indeed another telling symptom. The oyster as head puts an end to and a crown on top of the vertebral column and so it is indeed what the snake in us seeks, as a healing and completion of its exaggerated onesidedness.

Amongst the general indications for *Lachesis* we find the menopause and this seems to be related to certain features, two of them already familiar to us. The menopause marks the threshold of a new phase of existence, it marks the time when the individual can begin to take in hand his or her renewal, when the primary tasks of reproductive life are over. It is the transition from tasks of generation to those of regeneration. The cessation of the healing discharge of menstruation adds another note. The other feature of the snake which finds expression here is the changing of the skin, the renewal which it experiences every spring. We can also relate the spring and autumn aggravations to these same dynamics.

So far we have attempted to sketch the relation of the *Lachesis* drug picture to the serpent archetype, using as a help the essential features revealed by biology and mythology. It is perhaps surprising how far this can go, especially when we consider that the remedy is prepared from the venom rather than from the snake itself. It does seem that the mental and general symptoms and modalities are more understandable in terms of the characterization of the serpent as a whole than in terms of the chemistry of the venom and the acute symptoms of snake bite. However, Leeser did attempt to build up the drug picture from the known biochemistry of the venom.

The acute picture of snake bite depends on the injection of venom, usually some millilitres, into the flesh of the victim. The venom, considered as a complex mixture of enzymes, is also understood as a powerful secretion of salivary or digestive glands. The presence of such powerful enzymes in salivary or modified salivary glands again relates these glands of the mouth to the intestinal and pancreatic juices. The same note which we have observed before is again struck here and emphasized by the presence in snake venom of zinc, which is a normal constituent of the pancreas. Powerful digestive processes, normally only occurring in the secret coils of the intestine, are after snake bite unveiled to our observation. Perhaps this is one further reason for the dread they invoke. These processes should not happen to the living, intact, victim. They should be reserved for the digestion of the chewed up, masticated portions of already killed prey. Understood in this way, these phenomena find their natural place within our overall picture. They manifest clinically in the severe septicemic states which in the pre-antibiotic era were one of the chief successes in the *Lachesis* claim to fame. The crude toxic phenomena of snake bite then find their disease correlate in the toxic inflammatory states. The phenomena of provings, in which potencies are ingested, find their general correlation in the organs and regions of the body, e.g. the throat, in laterality, and in the modalities. The mentals on the whole seem to be correlated with those 'provings', as I would maintain, that are expressed in myth and legend and which are the response to the total impact made by the serpent through all the senses of the soul and not merely through the sense of taste.

We started from a comparison of the contrasting forms of snakes and cuttlefish. The contrast goes into the secretions which are the basis for our remedies. The sepia ink is an excretion used in the escapist defence ritual of the cuttlefish, whereas the snake venom is a mixture of fiercely active digestive enzymes used in attack. It is not surprising that the drug pictures are so distinct. It is also not surprising that in contrast to the highly sexually orientated action of *Sepia, Lachesis* has little real relation to the genital organs. It is more concerned with egotism and aggression.

We may conclude with the picture of the Acropolis at Athens. Two temples crown it. One, the Erectheum, was dedicated to the snake god-king Erectheus of ancient Athens. In this temple, a serpent was always kept. The other, the Parthenon, was the temple of Pallas Athene, goddess of wisdom. Behind the Parthenon in thc Museum is a statue of Athene in all her terrifying divinity, her cloak edged with serpents. She also is a serpent goddess. She is perhaps better known to us with her bird, the owl. Zeus has his eagle, Aphrodite her doves, but Pallas Athene has her owls, the birds of wisdom, the nocturnal birds, who in reversing the normal sleep rhythm of birds have become the true complement of the serpent raised up to the vertical around the staff of Asklepios, and plumed.

PART III

27. The problem of neurosis

We have to deal with a field in which the confusion of the patient is equalled by that of the medical profession. What is neurosis, what is psychosis, how are they related? What is nervousness, is it the same as neurosis or anxiety? What determines whether a neurosis seeks organic or psychological expression? You may hold that neurosis and anxiety are the expression of repressed sexual instincts or are the residue of the new-born babe's anxiety and first breath. You may hold that they arise out of inferiority feeling based on organ inferiority and later on social inferiority. You may on the contrary hold that they arise out of complex disturbances in the conditioned reflexes of our hemispheres or alternately out of biochemical disturbances at cellular or subcellular level determined perhaps by genetic disturbances. Again you may prefer to regard them as symptoms of the social disorder in which we are all involved and which you may prefer to regard in the light of historical determinism or as a symptom of the fallen state of man. In short, you may hold any or all of these views or others. But in any case, we can agree that we are in the midst of a very wide-spread epidemic, a pandemic, of nervousness, anxiety, depression, tiredness, sleeplessness and so on. When one considers that millions of sleeping tablets are taken nightly in this country, when one adds to this the tranquillizers, stimulators, antidepressant drugs and all the others, the magnitude of the problem is realized to be gigantic and quite out of hand. Moreover it seems a matter of chance mostly what treatment a patient gets. Drugs, psychotherapy, psychoanalysis, conditioned reflex re-education, hypnosis, ECT, and in the recent past leucotomy, LSD and so on — you pay your money and you take your choice.

What can be brought from the side of homoeopathy to help in this problem and can we develop our homoeopathic legacy to give us greater confidence in tackling this ocean of confusion? I confess that I have not much patience with those who think we already know how to handle these problems satisfactorily. It is of course

215

true that we all get surprised and delighted by improvements following straightforward prescribing in this as in other fields of clinical medicine. The improvement can be so remarkable as to whet one's appetite. Should it not be always possible to cure simply by a simple prescription? But when one reviews one's own cases and enquires gently of colleagues as to their experience, not being put off by the anecdote of the wonderful case, it becomes obvious that it is not always so easy.

The handling of these patients is, of course, not simply a matter of careful case taking and prescribing, rather is it a matter of bringing wisdom and insight and kindliness to bear on the complex human situation. Within the whole handling of the case remedies play their part, sometimes a very important and at other times a less important part. These cases bring one up against the realities of our human situation, the social influences mostly chaotic, the cultural values mostly distorted, the family problems often ghastly and wellnigh hopeless, and the final questions as to 'What is it all for, anyhow?'

Hahnemann already distinguished amongst mental patients between those who could be treated by kindly encouragement, sympathy, understanding and so on and those who remained inaccessible to this approach. Obviously this is no sharp distinction although it reminds one of the distinction between neurosis and psychosis; one doctor might reach and heal a patient by personal approach who would remain inaccessible to another. The personality, or rather the depth of soul experience, from which the physician can speak is all important. However the distinction points to a useful observation. In practice healing can come sometimes through a talk. The patient can be and can feel understood and can be restored from a broken to a whole existence. Usually today this is when the soul injury is not too severe and has not sunk down too far into the organism. Then a lucky meeting, a lucky word, can heal. Often however the original trauma, the shocks, griefs, strains, angers, fears and so on, have become fixed in the organic and we do not any longer have access to them. Perhaps they may still be accessible to psychoanalysis and sometimes their discovery and acceptance can heal. Often it seems today they have become really fixed in the organic and are manifesting in organic disturbances, functional at first but later structural. Sometimes again these disturbances are reacting again upon the soul and give rise to mental symptoms which are no longer amenable to direct personal approach. Then we must approach the problem with deepening insight and with remedies to help.

It is all very well to say that the similia will heal, but when the symptoms which would lead to the prescription were buried thirty years ago the statement becomes academic and unverifiable. Neither should one be misled by a superficial resemblance between two cases into thinking that because in the one case one could prescribe easily and successfully one's equally obvious prescription will work in the other. It may not.

It seems justifiable, therefore, to open the discussion wider.

Hahnemann drew attention to mental diseases or syndromes as examples of 'one-sided' disease in which the physical phenomena have escaped attention or have dwindled into insignificance. He also drew attention to the phenomena of alternation between mental and physical manifestations of a disease, an example of what today is referred to as 'syndrome shift'. It seems to me that here one has a jumping-off point for the attempt to grasp the phenomena of neurosis and psychosis in a psychosomatic and holistic spirit and for developing a methodology for study and research in this field.

Before coming to a closer study of the subject there are several viewpoints which seem to me to be helpful and in full accord with the spirit of homoeopathy. First, I believe one must take the soul as real and as operating in a real and demonstrable sense in the living ensouled body. One cannot accept the current dogma that the soul impinges in some inconceivable manner on the cerebral cortex alone or even on the brain and nervous system alone, whilst the body like a mechanical marionette dangles on the nerves (a crude legacy of a Descartian dualism still bedevilling everything). Garth Wilkinson, who became an inspirer of Kent, himself wrote in 1851:

> In a similar manner the body answers to the wants of the soul, being the soul's wife, the soul's friend, the soul's house, the soul's office, the soul's universe. It is engaged to the service of the soul; shaped into usefulness by the soul's ministrations. As the hand shapes the pen and then writes with it, so the soul forms the body and then makes use of the properties resulting from the form. The connexion between the soul and body is not more mysterious than the connexion between the pen-maker and the pen, excepting that our knowledge of the pen is so much more complete than our knowledge of the body.

One must take it that the soul ensouls our whole body and transforms it, it is fully incarnated and enfleshed, not just titillating the cortex. In other ages also men have accepted this. Father Victor White in his most valuable discussion on whether the soul of the theologians is the same as the soul of the psychologist draws attention to the fact that for Thomas Aquinas the soul had organic functions. At the summit of European philosophy Eduard von Hartmann likewise recognized the organic functions of the soul under his conception of the unconscious Will and Idea.

Let us take it then as Garth Wilkinson took it that the soul builds its body as its instrument and then learns to use it, and that a functional correspondence exists between the soul and the organs. I believe it will depend to a great extent on our understanding and discovering these correspondences how we are able to grapple with the problems of mental illness.

Secondly and following on this, one must come to study the natural arc of human life from childhood to maturity and old age and to observe the quite different psychosomatic relations and problems at different ages. During the ascending arc the soul, the individuality, is involved in constructing the organism and organs and only gradually emancipates and unfolds its conscious inwardness; the soul gradually awakens out of the organic slumbers. On the descending arc from maturity to old age and death it depends on the free, self-guided activity of man whether the emancipating soul can develop further or whether it will degenerate with the body. In this latter case the now regressive soul forces will impinge destructively on the organs from which they were emancipating, giving rise to disturbances of function and even ultimately of structure. Many functional disturbances of digestion and respiration which are so common are recognized today as expression of neurosis and of anxiety and one must add to these vasomotor disturbances, many allergic phenomena and on throughout the vast range of functional disturbances. In so far as these conditions arise from a failure to develop the emancipating soul forces consciously and satisfactorily it is certain that no ultimate cure can be produced by medicine alone whether allopathic or homoeopathic in type.

In connection with this I would mention in passing the following facts. It is estimated that since 1980 more scientific work has been done than in the whole previous history of mankind. More scientific papers have been published, more scientists occupied, more man-hours devoted to scientific research than in the whole of previous history. It is a rather, a very, terrifying thought. Further, a great deal of all this work, certainly what is new in it, is done by people under thirty years of age. By the age of thirty, it is accepted, one is no longer capable of original scientific research. In so far then as our whole modern world is under tutelage to science it is dominated by the mental efflorescence of people in their twenties and it is or should be obvious that such tutelage is inherently incapable of wise guidance for the developing soul in the thirties and later. Almost all this research, over 90% of it, is devoted to the study of chemistry and physics and their ramifications and even in biology most of it is pursued by chemical and physical methods which are not concerned with the realities of life but only with how much of death and corpse there is in it.

One can then understand the particular relevance of the famous statement of C. G. Jung to the effect that in his vast experience he had never met a patient over thirty-five whose neurosis was not primarily centred in the failure to establish satisfactory relationship to the world of religious values. It is the traditional function of religion and religious symbols and rituals to afford the means by which the further development of the soul as it emancipates from its organic functions can be achieved. Today, of course, our individual and social relationships to these traditional symbols are in the melting pot and consequently enormously many people find themselves, round about thirty, grown beyond the age at which our current scientific activities satisfy and without usable guidance for their future. Faced with the failure to carry human development further or even to achieve an ideal of a human being more worthy than that of an omnipotent computer, the fever of scientific research is redoubled in a kind of despairing frenzy. One must note in the growth of nervousness, anxiety, restlessness of our time a failure, on a colossal scale, to carry through the metamorphosis of soul development called for in the thirties of a person's life. The great interest in psychology and in many sects today is a symptom of this situation. One can also see that the entirely suppressive methods employed on such a gigantic scale — tranquillizers, thymoleptics, ECT and so on — only intensify yet further the real problem.

Now it is not my aim to suggest that homoeopathy can deal with the essentially cultural and spiritual issues which are raised by the problems of neurosis and psychosis. In so far as an individual physician succeeds in the tasks of his own life development he will be able to help others. As there are very many types of human beings many types of development and physician are needed. However in a modest way I do believe that out of careful observation and study of the phenomena of clinical medicine connections between the psychological and physiological realms can be perceived, and that our homoeopathic ways of thought and our drug pictures can contribute both to this needed insight and to practical therapy.

Now let us turn to the question of nervousness, bearing in mind that all these terms are very loosely used and that we can easily lose our way in mere verbal confusion. In the field of life, realities interpenetrate each other and one cannot reach mutually exclusive definitions. I personally think that there is a reality concealed in the often abused term nervousness. Today our senses are so over-stimulated, the tempo of our life is so exaggerated, we so seldom sit quiet to ponder, to digest, to ruminate on our experiences. Everything in our civilization rushes and presses on us, emotions are subjected to continuous shocks and we cannot develop deep emotions or sustain them when they arise. The capacity for strong powerful decisiveness is rare, and mostly life is so organized that decisions are not taken but things, events, dictate and individuals give up the unequal struggle and a mood of depression settles on everyone. The life of will and emotion is overwhelmed and shattered by the nervous excitement and stimulation and one can understand and sympathize with men like D. H. Lawrence who tried to react against this too cerebral life. Should we not learn to study in a psychosomatic manner at least some aspects of our problem as definitely connected with the one-sided development of the life of nerves and senses which have become too autonomous and sensitive in relation to the life of our blood and metabolism? This problem is the same problem as the conflict of science and religion and art. They used to work comparatively harmoniously together, today they have become three mutually incomprehensible and independent activities.

Closely connected with these phenomena of nervousness is the experience of anxiety. Anxiety is regarded as a common undercurrent in all the neurotic states and it is often a matter of an individual psychiatrist's terminology whether a patient is primarily regarded as suffering from anxiety state with obsessional or depressive aspects or vice versa. So let us take up some of the clinical circumstances in which

219

anxiety arises and see whether anything of value can be discovered. Perhaps the most devastating anxiety is that associated with cardiac disease. In the anginal attack and in coronary thrombosis the anxiety can be extreme and the patient can often tell one afterwards that it was an extreme fear of death, of imminent destruction. The gripping, strangling, constricting sensation appears here very strongly as the keynote of anxiety or *angst*. Other types of cardiac failure are also often associated with great anxiety and restlessness often nocturnal in occurrence. One thinks of *Aconite* and *Cactus*, of *Aurum* and *Spongia* as well as of many other remedies for this heart anxiety, and one may in passing suggest that the effect of being tied up in endless lengths of bureaucratic red tape is a similar experience to many of us and may indeed contribute to the incidence of coronary thrombosis.

The anxiety associated with disease of the lungs is of a different quality. One has seen often in cases of bronchiectasis and asthma an anxiety associated with more obsessional and compulsive traits and with specific phobias. A person becomes gripped in an idea or ritual and cannot escape from it, somewhat as the breath cannot escape from the asthmatic. There can be extreme anxiety associated with for instance dirt, resulting in compulsive acts and ritualistic behaviour. Minor forms of such disturbance are widespread and can be of use in some professions as for instance to the airline pilot and perhaps also the surgeon. The treatment of severe forms of this neurosis is amongst the most difficult of problems and I would suggest that we should explore the possibility of helping them through the treatment of the lung function. Lung disease can also manifest in a more romantic attitude such as is usually associated with tuberculosis. Could it be that the obsessional ritual of treatment which marked the old TB sanatoria was an unconscious attempt to balance the romantic traits and could it be that the swing in our cultural and social life from romantic to obsessional attitudes is behind both the compulsive ritual of cigarette smoking and of cancer of the lung itself? In any case, the fears and anxieties of the lung are directed to things in the environment and in this one can also see the close relation of the lung to the brain and senses, a relationship well known to Garth Wilkinson and Kent and based on Swedenborg's demonstration. In the allergic processes in asthma it is frequently impossible to separate the phobic and psychological from the more chemical antigen-antibody aspect of the process. Often too, mental disease will alternate with asthma and allow one to study the traits which arise in connection with disturbances in the lung function.

Another mode of anxiety arises with disease of the liver. One can often see in cases of jaundice that the depression is greatest before the jaundice appears, one more example of alternation of mental and physical aspects of disease. Depression does seem in many cases to be connected with the liver as folk tradition also has it, and a peculiar form of anxiety arises with this depression. Many of our remedies known to have an affinity for the liver are characterized by both depression and anxiety and phases; modifications of the main theme can be studied in the drug pictures. There are for instance *Nat. sulph., Nux vom., Lycopodium, Sepia, Pulsatilla, Ars. alb.* and, as Dr Fergus Stewart put it, 'Poor Maggie Muir was uneasy and sad.' One could mention many others. Depression can be regarded as a paralysis of the will and as it is the will which leads us into the future it is not difficult to see that the anxiety of the liver is more a fear of life. The hangover feeling comes into it and our livers seem to have become reservoirs not only of modern chemical poisons but of disappointments, frustrations, insults.

There is, I think, yet another group of anxieties of distinctive quality. In thyrotoxicosis we have a picture and experience of anxiety resembling almost completely the 'anxiety state' of a psychiatric textbook. So close is the clinical resemblance that often a thyroid function test is the only means by which they can be distinguished. The anxiety in these cases is not a phobia, a fear of death or a fear of life; it is an organic fear, a state of anxiety and nervousness and excitement arising out of the organism itself. Somewhat similar, I fancy, is the anxiety experienced after an injection of adrenalin. This leads us into all the maze of vasomotor disturbances and disturbances of sympathetic function as well as into the realm of stress and of the suprarenal cortex as well. Much of modern psychosomatic medicine has to do of course with these protean disorders. Can one perhaps distinguish three levels of nervousness, using the word in its popularly accepted sense of excitability and hypersensitivity? There is the nervousness proper where the life of the senses is overstimulated and a feeling of being hurried and harried, of time pressing on one, with a loss of power of concentration, and so on, an *Argent. nit* picture. There is the thyrotoxic state, the *Iodum* picture, and there is a state arising out of the whole suprarenal function in its widest sense. I think that *Nat. mur.* has a great deal to do with this as one might expect from its relation to adrenal function and Addisonism, from its value in conditions of stress, hyper- and hypotension. Its clinical use in thyrotoxicosis I suspect bubbles over from the suprarenal. I would draw attention to the frequency with which hypotensive patients are over busy, always being driven by an inner anxiety or restlessness, and how excitable they often are rather than deeply emotional.

Now what I am driving at is this — in dealing with the host of neurotic symptoms which patients present we are often lost; it is a chaos, and so long as we stick on the individual symptoms we cannot easily discern the pattern. But if we begin to discriminate the quality of a mental symptom and relate it to disorders of various organs we begin to see daylight. The more excessively one-sided a case is, the more it manifests entirely in a mental symptomatology for instance, the more necessary is it to grasp by a comparative method the organ disturbance on which it is based, and one must look for disturbed processes, functions, rather than ultimate structural end results. In this way I believe we can deepen our therapeutic capacities and build bridges across the chasm which divides homoeopathic from modern scientific medicine, without endangering our essential position.

28. The liver and depression

There are to be found in Hahnemann's work ideas which appear to me to be still full of untapped potentialities. One of his most valuable indications is the concept of one-sided diseases. Whereas, he points out, most disorders have some local or somatic aspect intermixed with mental or emotional disturbances, there are cases in which the symptomatology is so one-sided that it is almost completely either local or else mental. There are cases in which even severe disease, gross pathology, occurs in some organ whilst the personality remains to all around normal. It is not uncommon to find patients with quite advanced malignant tumours of some organ who yet still feel in themselves well and manifest no change in behaviour or emotional balance. Again in the so-called mental diseases, such as the schizo-phrenias, the symptomatology is one-sidedly in the mental sphere and it is not easy to localize it in some organ, even the brain. In such cases physical health may continue over many decades whilst the personality becomes progressively crippled. These two polar extremes of one-sided disease set, as it were, the limits of a spectrum of psychosomatic and psychoneurotic disorders spread out between them.

In 1963 the Bahnsons, working on the psychosomatic aspect of malignant dis-ease, put forward a disease spectrum. On one side they pointed to a progression from conversion hysteria through hypochondriacal conditions and psychosomatic disturbances to the somatic diseases and ultimately to cancer. On the other side of the balance the progression indicated was from anxiety hysteria through anxiety neurosis to the phobias and obsessive and compulsive neuroses, and then to the paranoid and deteriorated psychoses.

The similarity of this attempt to Hahnemann's seems to me obvious and in need of no further development here. They both however demand that we should attempt to build bridges from one side of the psychosomatic, psycho-neurotic balance to the other. One particular instance of this immensely demanding task is the problem of the psychic connections of particular organs. It is the liver which is the centre of this consideration.

Now where can we look for clues from which to start? Two come immediately to hand. Firstly there is the common experience of infective hepatitis. Whoever has experienced this disease can usually tell of the intense depression which commonly ushers it in and which is often somewhat alleviated when the frank jaundice manifests. Secondly there are the varied symptoms of illness which manifest in the early hours of the morning. In 1958 Karl König published an important paper entitled 'At Four o-clock in the Morning' in which he explored the connections between the twelve-hourly cycle of liver function and the somatic symptoms like cough, asthma, sweating, diarrhoea coming on at this time of the day. He pointed out that remedies related to these symptoms are those with a definite organotropic relation to the liver. We can instance *Ars. alb., Lycopodium, Chelidonium, Nux* and *Mag. carb.* König emphasized the somatic symptoms arising around the time of 4 am and traceable to disturbances in the cyclical change from the assimilative to the secretory phase of liver function. He did not draw attention to the equally conspicuous symptoms arising in relation to depressional states. It is well known that it belongs to the picture of endogenous depression that the sufferer tends to awake in the early hours and to remain awake for some long period, usually in a distressed and deeply depressed state.

Now we must characterize more distinctively certain mental-emotional states. There are sorrowful moods, the emotion of sadness as distinct from joy, the melancholic temperament and depression. There is certainly something common to these, a colour or tone of life, and yet they surely are not the same. The emotions of joy and sorrow belong to the middle realm of soul life. They tend to come and go and pass into each other fairly easily, casting sunshine or cloud shadow on the landscape of our soul. Unless the sorrow is so deep that it imprints itself right into the physiology and metabolism, no lasting impairment of health results from the play of the emotions. But the melancholic temperament is not an emotion. The temperaments belong more to the physiological level of our being and characterize the tone of the bodily instrument on which we play and through which we act into the world. The melancholic is in fact strong and persistent in his actions, often to the point of becoming obsessionally fixed on one specialized pursuit. Sorrowful moods again are something distinct. They are more persistent than an emotion, and often need more effort or shock to change them.

But would it be right to call depression an emotion or a mood or a temperament? It obviously would not. The character of depression is really quite another phenomenon. It is better approached through the nature of the will rather than the emotional life or the life of thinking. It is the state which arises when the will is paralysed to a greater or lesser extent. Our thinking is directed to the past, we look backwards and study how things came about, it is bound up with memory and produces clear pictures. Our feeling and emotional life, however, lives in the systole and diastole of the present, in the ever-changing movement of the 'now'. It stands between the past and the future into which we walk with our will. We cannot think the future or intellectually plan it, we will it. Paralysis of the will therefore is one way for describing that state in which we experience being cut off from the future and thrown one-sidedly upon the past. If we can relate only to the past and to the inevitable continuation of the past which mechanism implies and which intellectual thought can alone grasp and accept, we cannot escape overwhelming guilt and despair. We are saved from the burden of guilt for our past misdeeds or the one-sidedness of our deeds by our determination to make good in the future these incomplete actions. When through the paralysis of our will we are cut off from the possibility of making good in the future our errors, we are exposed without defence to the one-sided burden of the past. This, it seems to me, is the real nature of what we call depression. It is not emotion, mood, temperament, it is a disorder of the will.

And here we come up against one of the obstacles presented by the dogmas within current physiology. The vast majority of the medical and allied professions still probably believe that the soul, the psyche, our personality, call it what you will, has mysterious access to our bodies only through the nervous system. It would seem that they try to believe, for instance, that when a pianist plays the piano, he does not do so but rather plays upon a keyboard on the motor cortex. His body is then supposed to dance on the ends of nerves almost like a marionette and move the keys of the piano. The most serious workers in neurology know that this is not true, but have no idea as to what is true.

Rudolf Steiner and his followers have sought to show that only our thinking is related to the system of nerves and senses, that our feelings are related to the rhythms of our organisms, mainly the rhythms of our breathing and heart beat, whilst our will is based upon our metabolism and limbs. Our thinking is a sort of reflection in the mirror of our brains, and our thoughts are images lacking reality, though they may be true images of reality. But we are awake in this experience. In our feelings, however, we only dream and come and go on the to and fro of our breath. 'We are such stuff as dreams are made on.' Still more obscure and difficult is the realm of the will, in which we are asleep. Here the soul submerges itself in the metabolic processes, and in bringing about real objective changes loses its consciousness. When we search out the metabolic processes we find of course the liver as the central organ of metabolism. And so if this, which we can treat as a hypothesis, is true, we might expect to find evidence of disorder of the liver in depression. It is to be expected, however, that the more endogenous the depression the less overt the evidence of liver pathology will be. One can see in some cases that deep sorrow which is not psychically digested and metamorphosed into wisdom can sink down into the liver. It becomes not transformed but buried and then may become later the basis of endogenous depression. The symptomatology has become one-sidedly mental, emotional.

Confirmation can perhaps be gained by using the homoeopathic remedies as research tools, in addition to their usual therapeutic use. *Nat. sulph.*, *Nux vom.*, *Sulphur* and *Sepia* all relate to different aspects of liver function. We must also mention in particular the metals *Stannum*, *Ferrum*, *Magnesium* and of course *Aurum*. Kent related the depression of *Aurum* to the heart and liver. It seems to me that its function can best be described as helping to lead the ego which has become imprisoned in utterly material goals and possessions, whose loss is the cause of the depression, into new relationships with more universal spiritual ideals and aims. The grief buried in the liver is then led up through the heart and metamorphosed into wisdom and compassion. In this way our remedies can help us to heal not only the individual patient but the deep divide, the split which exists in modern medicine between the body and the soul.

29.   Hysteria and neurasthenia

The origin of the term hysteria seems to date back to at least Greek times. The uterus (*hysteria*) was thought to break loose from its anchorage and wander through the abdomen causing trouble. The Greeks were not fools and it is unlikely that they understood by this that the physical organ wandered but rather the forces related functionally to the uterus were the cause of many varied symptoms. It cannot have escaped notice that emotional and bodily symptoms were often related to the menstrual cycle. For a long time hysteria was regarded as exclusively a disease of women and only in quite recent times has it been accepted that men too can suffer from this condition. Today there is a widespread tendency to get rid of the word from medical diagnosis because no-one seems to know what to do with it. There tends to be the hint in this diagnosis that the disease is unreal, make-believe, blameworthy, a moral weakness and so on. Hysteric patients are most disturbing to any physician or therapist who tries to take their symptoms seriously. No sooner does the doctor think he has grasped the problem than it, chameleon-like or octopus-like, changes colour and vanishes, only to reappear in changed form. That the octopus and other cephalopods, those masters of colour changes and escapology, are so to speak externalized uteruses relates to the old idea. The problem is intensified by the way in which in hysterics' emotional problems manifest as somatic symptoms, and what appears at first as straightforward physical disease is found to be the expression of psychic problems. Nowhere are the problems of the psychosomatic relationship so obscure as in these problems, and we also become perturbed as to whether such patients are really as morally blind to their motives as they appear to be.

We shall, I think, be well advised to put the realm of hysteric processes in polar relationship to what used to be called neurasthenic symptoms. This term was first used in the United States by G. M. Beard in 1869 to describe a state of physical and mental exhaustion with the impossibility of performing any physical or mental work. It was characterized by headaches, neuralgias, hypersensitivity to all sensory stimuli, noise, light, changes of weather and so on. Often loss of appetite and other functional disturbances of digestion were added. Beard came to regard the symptoms as brought on by the American way of life but earlier than this in

England James Johnson in 1831 described 'the wear and tear syndrome' or 'English disease'. This was attributed to the ravages on natural life brought about by the industrial revolution. Apparently sanitoria were erected throughout America and Europe to cope with this disease of civilization. Weir Mitchell, the foremost American neurologist, instituted a strict regimen of isolation, bed rest, splendid food, and regular massage and tender loving care. This could last months and even years.

Though the term neurasthenia has passed out of fashion the underlying constitutional condition seems to continue to worry both lay and professional circles. It is difficult not to associate the current interest in the post-viral syndrome or myalgic encephalomyelitis (ME), or any of the dozen other names currently applied to the syndrome, with the neurasthenia, or equally 'railway spine' of a century ago and with the English disease or wear and tear syndrome. According to changing fashions in scientific theories so do the names change but the condition of extreme fatigue and hypersensitivity persists.

Faced with such patients it is natural for those around, whether family or friends or professional advisers, to want to discover what is wrong. According to our personal prejudices or mental type, the search for cause follows psychological or physical directions. Present fashions lead to biochemical or trace element or vitamin deficiencies and viruses on the one hand, and on the other to emotional conflicts, buried psychic traumas such as childhood sexual abuse, or to conflicts in the family dynamics. These two conditions, hysteria and neurasthenia, do seem to be phenomena calling for what we can term a constitutional approach. By constitution in this case we should mean the way in which the bodily and soul elements are related to each other. This again demands that we understand the soul as a real entity that acts into the bodily organization. We can be helped by the concept of the soul-body, sometimes called astral body, as that inwardly existent organism of soul forces which particularly play into and contribute to the form of the bodily organization proper. In addition we must also grasp the Ego, the individuality, not as just a passive subject of awareness but as the powerfully directive moral core of our being.

Now in the hysteric constitution these soul forces which flow through the nervous system, acting the while in a katabolic and sculpturing manner, then tend to flow on out through some organ into the outer world. Normally they should be switched through the kidney and suprarenal system into anabolic upbuilding forces in the metabolism. In the hysteric however some organ leaks these forces away. It is with these forces that the hysteric penetrates into the unconscious of other people, divining their secret intentions before they know them themselves.

Before attempting to characterize the hysteric make-up further let us contrast the neurasthenic constitution. Here, these soul forces are cramped into the brain and spinal cord so that only to a reduced extent can they reach to and penetrate the metabolic organs. If in the hysteric these forces are seen to leak away through their organs then in the neurasthenic, cramped and imprisoned in the brain and spine, they cannot rightly arouse the whole metabolic world which remains unable to cope with and nourish the organism. The soul of the hysteric lives semi-consciously in the environment so that everyone feels bathed in, even swamped by the continuous surges of sympathy and antipathy, love and hate which are leaked all around them. The problems of adolescence are the problems of hysteria. Hysteria is the norm of adolescence.

We can group the somatic manifestations of hysteria around the phenomena of anaesthesia. We may find an area of the body to have become anaesthetic, we can stick pins into it painlessly, and so on. The area involved does not correspond to any nerve distribution, or for that matter to blood circulation. It corresponds to a mental image. So we may get the typical glove or stocking anaesthesia. The left side of the body, the side on which the arterial circulation goes out, centrifugally, is more affected than the right, on which the venous blood returns centripetally. One can add, the left side is the female side, the right the male. In these cases the soul forces or soul body flow out, and it is of course the soul which feels, not the body.

The hysterical paralyses can also be understood as a further development of anaesthesia in which the 'sense of movement' is lost. These paralyses affect mostly those movements which have been achieved by the individuality, standing, walking, arm and hand movements, and speech. Inability to phonate, hysterical aphonia, occurs in spite of the movements of the vocal cords being intact as in coughing. It is the capacity to phonate in speaking that is lost. The ability to speak properly again can be restored in a short time by a confident and competent doctor, often ear, nose and throat surgeon. The hysteric cannot incarnate certain motions, the 'idea' of the movement does not sink down into the region of the will. It hovers and enjoys itself in the realm of the feelings without putting itself to the test of reality. It remains uncommitted.

If the anaesthesia penetrates more inwardly still it may affect the 'sense of life' and the appetite for instance may be lost. I believe this is one aspect of the complex phenomena of anorexia nervosa. It may also lead to constipation and menstrual disturbances.

Lying at the back of hysteria is shock. The hysteric could almost be described as allergic to shock. When someone is suddenly severely shocked, terror stricken, he or she may say 'I jumped right out of my skin' and sometimes may add 'and never seem to have got right back again'. What they describe is true, the soul was shocked out of the body. From which part of the body or from which organs is the soul most easily dislocated? I think experience points to the genital region and organs. Amenorrhoea can easily follow shock and dysmenorrhoea and other irregularities may arise from these shocked-out soul forces trying to get back and cramping rather than incarnating smoothly into the function. Shocked from the uterus and genital organs, with frigidity as a symptom, these forces may also cramp

228

into other organs giving rise to spastic colons, asthma and many other symptoms. In this way the primary leaking out of the soul or sudden dislocation may be followed by a secondary reaction and abnormal cramping back again.

The question is bound to arise as to whether shock, particularly childhood shock, predisposes to the later sensitivity of the hysteric or whether an innate sensitivity allows the ordinary and inevitable shocks of life to penetrate too deeply. Perhaps shocks to the mother during pregnancy also contribute to the whole condition. We can however affirm that the hysteric is abnormally sensitive to shock and made worse by shocks. We can also point to a tendency to extravagant behaviour and reactions, originating in the soul living too freely and uncontrolled in the outer world. This also helps us to understand the normal hysteria of adolescence. At puberty the soul-body begins to be set free to some extent from its organ building functions. The adolescent is then exposed to the free play of soul-forces playing between love and hate and all the pairs of opposites. The ego-individuality is not really born till the coming of age at twenty or twenty-one and is not therefore yet able to undertake the task of holding the balance and establishing a true middle ground and objective relationships.

Hysteria should become less frequent from twenty onwards, which it does. Adult hysterics therefore are stuck in adolescence and remain younger-looking than their years. The childhood hysteric on the other hand is precocious and behaves provocatively as if already adolescent.

From all these considerations it should be clear that constitutional medical treatment is needed in order to draw in, as far as maybe, the leaking soul forces. The potentized forms of *Argentum* are a mainstay in the anti-shock treatment and the plant *Bryophyllum* a main vegetable remedy. But many other remedies may be required according to the particular organ weaknesses. It is clear that the ego function, related to Janet's function of psychic synthesis is weak. The ego is drowned in the tides of pleasure and pain, sympathy and antipathy and only with difficulty can be educated to objectivity of judgement. But the hysteric can find a useful outlet for his or her over-sensitivity in the caring professions provided professional discipline is maintained. In a similar direction the hysteric can be said to yearn for religious instruction and this makes them an easy target for all the bogus sects which now as always, but particularly nowadays, abound. All efforts at objective religious teaching will be ever and again subjected to assault from the unconscious wish-world of the hysteric. It may well be that the teacher in the end learns more than the pupil.

In contrast to all this colourful, soul-filled phenomenology, the neurasthenic presents a meagre picture. Constant headaches picture the cramped-in soul forces in the skull. These are the 'tension headaches' of today's nomenclature. Over-sensitive eyes and ears, no bright lights or loud noises can be tolerated. These are hypersensitive spines, always 'going out', and tendon reflexes are usually exaggerated. Digestion is weak, very little can be tolerated, and patients are the opposite of robust. Fatigue as already mentioned dominates the picture and neither physical nor mental work can be tolerated. Sleep is shallow, there is difficulty in getting to sleep, the soul cannot escape from its cramped prison in the skull. Often sudden starts re-awaken at the moment of falling asleep. The cramping may extend from the spine to be experienced in the heart and chest.

On the whole neurasthenics look prematurely aged and are understandably prone to hypochondria and obsessions. They are mainly introverted in contrast to the predominantly extroverted hysteric. It must be obvious that the currently popular post-viral syndrome usually belongs to the neurasthenic rather than the hysteric pole.

As with hysteria constitutional medical treatment is needed. When 'wear and tear' of modern city life is an important factor *Prunus spinosa* is invaluable and *Phosphorus* preparations are usually required. But these cases now as in the past call for patient, kindly and continuing care.

The issue is not whether such conditions are psychogenic or physical in origin. In such constitutions the katabolic soul forces work too strongly in the nervous system and senses. The 'wear and tear' picture of two centuries ago is a fair description but it is the soul forces themselves which bring about the wear and tear in neurasthenics and all of us. Normally these ravages of daily waking life are repaired during sleep but in the neurasthenic sleep is short, interrupted and shallow.

The thinking becomes too strongly fixed on the brain and senses. Such people are not imaginative whilst the hysteric is over-imaginative. They therefore need to be surrounded with an artistically imaginative sense environment rather than with the strident matter-of-factness of today. They need to be helped to live into the worlds of myth and fairy story which help the soul escape its prison in the witch's cottage of the skull.

A nervous system worn out and disintegrated in the manner indicated will become a happy culture medium for viruses, which we may look upon as indicators or results of, rather than causes of the nervous exhaustion.

It is important to grasp this polarity of hysteria and neurasthenia under whatever names we choose. Otherwise we can pursue endless hypothetical causes and get caught in an endless web of the patient's symptoms. In the case of the hysteric, it will end in the patient manipulating his treatment and the doctor or therapist as well. In the case of the neurasthenic it is probable that he will find further medical advisors in an endless search for help.

In conclusion we may add that all diseases and individuals tend more to one pole or the other of this polarity. Hysteria tends more to the inflammatory pole and neurasthenia more to the sclerotic pole of illness. These terms are not therefore moral judgments on people but attempts to grasp the constitutional basis of symptoms with a view to discovering how to help them. It will also be apparent from what has been said already that the reactionary cramping back of the loosened or leaking soul forces in hysteria may produce hypersensitivities rather than the anaesthesias more typical of hysteria. It is not usually too difficult to sort them out. The imaginative pictures of this polarity of disease tendencies can illumine many of the most difficult problems facing one in therapeutic activities, difficulties in which one can easily get lost. This is nowhere more important than in traditional homoeopathy. Here the emphasis on the symptoms can lead to 'symptom chasing' with the patient's hysteria calling the tune. If the diagnosis of hysteria is made it will be clear that the ever changing-symptoms are simply the 'common' symptoms of the disease and of no importance therefore in the task of prescribing a remedy.

30. Migraine

The word migraine derives from the Greek Hemicrania signifying a half-head and thereby pointing to the tendency for migraine headaches to be one-sided. The descriptions of migraine dating from classical times show the same features as are recognized today. Migraine seems to belong amongst those disorders which persist throughout long periods of historic time as distinct from those which occur mainly or only at certain times or places. Migraine can and does manifest also at all ages of the individual from childhood to old age. In spite of immense interest and research many problems remain in relation to the phenomena of migraine and so it may be worthwhile to look again at these in a physiognomic way.

We can start with the characteristic feature of one-sidedness. Of course migraine may be two-sided but usually it manifests on one side. It may, in a particular sufferer, always come on on one side. It may start on one side and then move to the other, or again it may alternate in different attacks from side to side. What does this marked asymmetry point to?

The human bodily organization is not fully symmetrical; left and right do not fully mirror one another. Where does the twist come from? The brain is initially symmetrical; the distinctions between left and right are built into it from the use of the limbs. In early childhood it is still possible to determine left or right-handedness by appropriate exercises. One gains the impression that the symmetry of the body stems downwards from the head. If we were only head we would be symmetrical. Logical head-bound thinking wants to have everything and all arguments balanced and symmetrical. This is the typical male sort of thinking and it finds the twist in things difficult to put up with. Nature however is always twisted, even in crystals we find dextro or laevo rotatory forms, and Einstein spent a great part of his life trying to reconcile the bi-polarity of forces like magnetism and electricity with the apparent unipolarity of gravity. The spirit of levity escaped him. If symmetry stems from the head, whence emanates the twist of asymmetry? Our abdominal organs show the twist early in embryological development. The alimentary tract begins to coil, the stomach moves to the left, the liver to the right, the spleen and pancreas to the left. The kidneys retain a symmetrical relationship, consistent with their origin as the pronephros in the head region, but the suprarenal glands sitting on top of the kidneys show asymmetry, the left being semilunar, the right triangular in shape. This twist builds itself upwards into the thorax where the heart comes to lie slightly to the left and the left lung has two lobes whilst the right has three. Moreover the blood vessels develop so that the aortic arch in mammals and man persists on the left, the right arch atrophying, whilst in birds on the contrary it is the right aortic arch that persists. In this way the arteries in man come to be centrifugal to the left and the veins centripetal from the right. In the brain it seems that the functional distinctiveness of left and right hemisphere is built into it from the use of the limbs. In this way we have come to be a wonderful balance of two spatial principles and we can find these two aspects sculptured in the inner ear. The semi-circular canals, at right angles to each other, manifest the tendency to symmetrical order, right-angled and right-minded regularity of the three dimensions of space. The cochleae, the snail shells within our ears on the other hand are spirally formed.

The one-sidedness of the migraine headache seems, then, to point to processes arising in the metabolic, abdominal pole of our organization and overwhelming the true nerve sense processes in our head pole. For consciousness to wake up in our heads, the life processes must withdraw. When the constructive, up-building forces of the metabolism push up into the brain we lose consciousness as for instance when we fall asleep. During waking life, when we can think and reflect, the dying processes in the nerves predominate. The brain is only functionally a true brain when we are awake and thinking. We wake up in our sense organs when the metabolic life processes withdraw from them and allow the outer world to penetrate.

We can now begin to unravel the tangled skein of the migraine phenomena. In the attack the senses are disturbed, most dramatically in vision. The loss of half of the visual field, usually left or right but sometimes the upper or lower half, is fairly common. Central scotomata and varied dazzling displays of peripheral light are also common. Tunnel vision and effects like snow storms add to the bewildering and varied phenomena of the visual aura of migraine. Hemiplegias, to be interpreted as loss of the sense of motion and position, vertigo, disturbance of hearing or smell or taste may also herald the onset of the attack. Most sufferers from migraine would also agree that during the attack thinking is disturbed and, when circumstances permit, the best thing to do is to sleep. Some attacks of compulsive sleepiness seem to bear the signature of migraine rather than narcolepsy. Could we also approach Ménières syndrome, as another aspect of the same process?

The great Swedish philosopher-scientist of the eighteenth century, Emanuel Swedenborg, drew attention to the peculiar way in which the arteries lead into the skull. Both the vertebral and internal carotid arteries supplying the brain enter the inner sanctuary of the skull with a sort of 'S' shaped twist. In this way, Swedenborg suggested the full drive of the pulse-beat is held back and the brain can take its blood in freedom. Altogether the head rises poised and balanced freely on the top of the vertebral column, it should not be held rigidly as a mere appendage like an animal's head. Many migraine sufferers have stiff or stuck necks and one wonders whether the success of osteopathic manipulation of the neck in some of these patients is due to the freeing of the head from the trunk, freeing the brain from the surging forces of the blood. The liberating action of the serpentine entry of the arteries into the skull becomes frozen in these necks until it is again released.

So far we have been considering the one-sidedness of migraine as an expression of the upper, cephalic, pole being overwhelmed by the dynamics of the lower, abdominal pole. Processes which should be fulfilled in the digestive and metabolic organs may for various reasons be incomplete. Then the brain may be called upon to complete vicariously the digestive and metabolic processes, functions for which it is not suited. Certain foodstuffs are not, in some individuals, overcome in the digestion and then pass as foreign and still undigested foreign substances into the brain: chocolate and cheese are well-known examples. These food sensitivities are not really allergic but rather poisonings. They may arise on the basis of specific enzyme deficiencies.

We can now more easily pass on to the migraine phenomena related to menstruation.

It has been said in an aphorism that migraine is cephalic dysmenorrhoea and dysmenorrhoea uterine migraine and in psychoanalytical circles migraine has sometimes been understood as symbolic labour pains. The old Greek story of the birth of Pallas Athene from the head of Zeus expressed this in the pictorial language of mythology.

We are here faced with the polarity of the uterus and skull. In the one the brain, in the other the embryo-foetus floats. Whereas in the one case man conceives thoughts in the head, in the other woman conceives babies in the uterus. These features again lead us to look at the architecture of the human organization. From the top cervical vertebra to the lowest lumbar one the architecture is predominantly segmental. Each segment is based essentially on a vertebra with posterior spine, two transverse processes and two ribs, a fivefold star, such as we find imaged in the star-fishes amongst the echinoderms. In the neck and lumbar regions, the ribs appear lost but they reappear, in metamorphosis, in the limbs. The five suppressed ribs coming to visibility in the fingers and toes. But in the skull and pelvis the segmental character is almost completely overcome by the spheric form. The radial, segmental architecture of the spine is replaced by the dome of the head and the head of the foetus fits almost perfectly into the containing dome of the pelvic cavity. The sea-urchins among the echinoderms echo this metamorphosis.

In nature we find two animal phyla in which these architectural principles find expression. In the arthropoda, with its highest expression in the insects, we find segmentation carried to its limit. The body is rigidly divided into segments, the appendages are segmented; even the life history is divided into segmented stages, egg, caterpillar, chrysalis, butterfly or imago. These stages are sharply separated from each other. At another level of animal organization, the snakes carry segmentation to another extreme, up to 450 vertebrae. The great contrast to these articulated creatures is found in the molluscs and again amongst the reptiles the tortoise stands in polarity to the snake.

Both Poppelbaum and Jaworski have in their own ways seen the interiorized correspondence of the molluscs in the head and pelvic organs. Poppelbaum emphasized the molluscs as corresponding to the head whilst Jaworski emphasized more the molluscan note in the female genital organs and functions. The same note which is sounded in the formation of the uterus and vagina sounds again in the realm of the cephalopods in the squid, cuttlefish and octopus. From this region of the animal kingdom homoeopathy has prepared the remedy Sepia from the ink of the cuttlefish. Sepia, is one of the outstanding homoeopathic remedies for migraine headaches and it also exercises an immense influence on the uterus and gynaecological functions. Is there not something wonderful when we find nature as it were mythologizing?

Most migraine attacks in women are associated with menstruation and *Sepia* helps not only in the treatment of these patients but in understanding the dynamics of the condition. Jaworski further traced the asymmetry, as a female note, so marked for instance in the spiral of the snail-shell, right back to the asymmetry in the process of oögenesis. In the divisions of the oöcyte leading to the formation of the ovum, the cell divisions do not lead to two equal cells but small so-called polar bodies are cast off. The cell divisions lead to unequal cells, ovum and polar bodies. In spermatogenesis, on the contrary, the cell divisions result in equal-sized cells of the next generation.

There are other homoeopathic remedies for migraine which have been found to have a tendency to left or right sidedness. *Lycopodium* and two members of the Papaveraceae family, *Sanguinaria* and *Chelidonium*, have a marked right-sided action and they have all been recognized as having a relation to the liver and gall systems. On the other hand *Spigelia* works mostly on the left side of the head and has strong affinities with the heart.

These instances help us to see into the way in which, in migraine, the processes of the lower genital and metabolic organization come to obtrude into the head organization. Can we characterize these polarities any further? The distinction mentioned between the conception of babies in the uterus and thoughts in the head points to another aspect of this polarity. In the womb real, live babies are conceived but in the head only those shadowy images we call thoughts. These thoughts have more the quality of mirror images; they are not substantial but image-realities. It is within the world of images which arise in our heads that we can wake up in freedom, they do not compel us. But we live into the realm of substantially real metabolic activities and metamorphoses found in our lower functions and then actively transform these processes. In doing so we lose our awake consciousness, we enter the realm of the unconscious, a sleep consciousness.

235

We can, even if at first only as a guess, begin to see how here we enter the realm of the will over against the awake life in that hall of mirrors we call our head, the realm of the image life of our thinking.

Leaving these considerations for the moment, let us look at another of the very typical features of migraine, the periodicity. It is true that all life activities have a rhythmic quality; night and day, the lunar month, the seasons of the year and many other rhythms come to manifestation in living organisms. Migraine often obtrudes into ordinary life, interfering forcibly with our consciously held wishes and intentions, and does so periodically. In between the attacks life proceeds normally. We have already mentioned the association of migraine with menstruation and in women the monthly rhythm usually comes to dominate the migraine periodicity. In other cases particularly in men the periodicity seems more related to stress. The weekend headache comes on to spoil the pleasures of recreation after a heavy week's work dominated by the objective demands of outer duty. The nightly renewal of the brain during sleep cannot keep pace with the accumulating deposits, débris of our over-concentrated waking activity. The attack comes as a weekly spring-cleaning. It can come on when the repressive force of conscious concentration on a task is relaxed. But again in others, attacks are more associated with some special occasion or event. They nicely come to prevent the fulfilling of the arrangement, duty or other obligation. A certain hysteric element here enters into the attack whose occurrence may certainly seem purposive and useful.

In these phenomena we meet with a polarity between those cases, on the one hand, in which excessive digestive, metabolic processes overwhelm the nerve sense processes; these include the hysterics and on the other those cases in which an over-exertion of nerve and sense activity leads to the need for a periodic curative clean-up and renewal in the brain and senses. Our conscious waking life is purchased at the expense of katabolic, break-down processes in the brain. If these are not cleared up during sleep and periods of recreation, they build up until a crisis point is reached. The migraine attack is curative. In the former type of cases a surplus of incompletely digested metabolic substances breaks through into the nerve sense processes. These two types of migraine phenomena often today play into each other.

At this point we can approach the conditions sometimes known as migraine substitutes. If we can grasp in a sort of picture, if we can begin to approach the archetypal process in migraine, then we can hope to find this same archetype in related phenomena. We can proceed to grapple with the riddles of migraine by the methods of amplification rather than by reductionism. This is not to decry the researches which unearth the fine mechanisms which play their part in illness and health. But just as a study of the chemistry of ink is only an aspect of the deciphering of the written page and must be complemented by the studies of the letters of the alphabet, of spelling, of the building up of sentences and paragraphs until with a leap we reach the very heart, mind and soul of the author, so must we try again and again to read the meanings of symptoms in addition to the chemical mechanisms in which they are written.

We have already considered migraine and dysmenorrhoea as substitutes, and other problems of menstruation can throw light on related aspects of migraine. Fluid retention is common, almost universal before menstruation and it may assume importance in severe cases of premenstrual syndrome. In many cases of migraine a similar fluid retention builds up before the attack which passes off with diuresis. Some decades ago this led to the treatment of migraine with *Urea* which was used to promote the diuresis. In homoepathic literature the remedy *Gelsemium* is often mentioned in connection with migraine ending in diuresis. *Gelsemium* relates to anticipatory anxiety and confusion and to paralytic and anaesthetic phenomena pointing to the hysterical pole of these conditions. No doubt hormonal influences are integrated into these manifestations.

A quite different condition occurs in gout. Here deposits of urates occur in the cartilage and tissues particularly round the joints. From time to time attacks of acute gout come on, the joints become red, swollen, hot and exquisitely painful. After the attack the deposits, in tophi for instance, may be reduced in size; the attack has been curative. Some years ago Professor F. Wood Jones contributed some interesting observations based on his own experience. He came to the view that in the attack arterio-venous anastomoses around the joint opened up and brought about a greatly increased blood flow. One might describe such phenomena as vicarious menstruation, particularly when one remembers that gout is mostly a disease of men, female menstruation protecting women from it.

In children various aspects of the periodic syndrome are fairly common and tend to develop at puberty into frank migraine. But quite typical migraine also occurs in childhood. The periodic syndrome may present as recurrent bilious attacks with vomiting and abdominal pain or as recurrent fevers, sometimes with inflamed throats. In adults we find so-called abdominal migraine, in which recurrent attacks of pain, nausea and sometimes vomiting occur. Sometimes these may be accompanied by headaches and the diagnosis is easy. Often however it is only the overall picture of the recurrent attacks which leads to a diagnosis, together with the exclusion of so-called organic disease of gall-bladder, kidneys and pancreas in particular. Pseudo-angina in the chest has also been recognized as a migraine substitute.

Some years ago I had occasion to record and comment on some cases in which the migraine process seemed to appear in a limb. One of these cases was a woman who had had a cancer of the left breast for ten years. She had refused treatment for it. It had now reached the stage when multiple skin metastases were present over the left breast and shoulder and upper arm. She told the story of how, over the years, at periodic monthly intervals she would have an attack which she called her fever attacks. One day she would feel particularly well and she came to expect next day to pay for it. Then next morning she would wake with a high fever (up to 31.5°C, 103°F) and the whole breast and arm area red, swollen angry. On occasions when doctors had seen it, they had wanted to give antibiotics, but she had always told them not to be silly and go away. Next day she was quite recovered. These attacks always came together with a severe left-sided migraine. It was as if one could actually see the same process both in the head as pain and in the trunk as an inflammatory reaction. If we relate this to the conception that a cancer is a misplaced sense organ we may guess that these attacks were indeed curative processes. Incidentally she also said that after radiation therapy for a metastasis in the cervical spine the attacks stopped for six months. Did the radiation suppress the curative reactions?

We have suggested that the unilateral aspect of migraine points to an origin in the metabolic processes and organs. In the homoeopathic tradition of medicine various remedies have been observed to have particular relationship to migraine. These remedies often point to disturbances of other organs and functions in addition to the headache. Can we use these empirically discovered correlations to extend our insight into these conditions? We have mentioned that *Chelidonium* and *Sanguinaria* both act on the liver and gall and tend to right-sided headaches, we also mentioned *Spigelia* with its cardiac action and left-sided headache. Sepia has its relationship to uterus and headache and *Pulsatilla* likewise often points to this connection. One of the most valuable migraine remedies is *Iris versicolor*, a remedy introduced into homoeopathy from North American Indian usage. Now *Iris* is found empirically, in cases of poisoning and in the course of provings, to have a profoundly irritative action on the gastro-intestinal tract. Clinical intuition led our predecessors to suggest an action on the pancreas as well. In any case wide use of this remedy in cases of migraine with nausea, vomiting and abdominal pain have shown its value. It produces intense salivation and this action on the glands of the alimentary tract may relate to its action on the pancreas. *Sulphur* works on the whole metabolic process and particularly on the liver. It is another important migraine remedy.

We must now consider the kidney system in so far as it relates to migraine. Following the anthroposophical school we can take the kidneys and suprarenal glands together. Sitting like caps on the kidneys these two organs catch to some extent the kidney radiation and mediate it into the circulation. Swedenborg discussed these two glands and he was historically the first to attribute to them endocrine functions, actually the first description of any endocrine gland. He also showed their close connection with the kidneys. This connection has been developed in anthroposophical medicine. The kidneys perform a lot of work in separating the urine from the blood and as a consequence there is a backthrust into the organism. Steiner discussed this back-thrust under the term kidney radiation. It works to arouse the organic processes from vegetable to animal existence. The relationship of the kidney to nitrogen metabolism indicates this, vegetable life is based on carbohydrate metabolism, animal life on protein and where protein enters into vegetable life it indicates that this has been touched by the animal level of existence. Protein has interiorized the nitrogen processes. It is probably significant that caffeine and the barbiturates are closely related to urea in molecular structure. The one acts to awaken, the other as a hypnotic. The kidneys are also involved in the blood pressure control through the renin, angiotensin and related processes and the suprarenal glands reach a high polarity of action in the contrasted pictures of Addison's disease and Cushing's syndrome. In Addison's disease the patient is hyperalert, restless, florid with high blood pressure and raised sodium level relative to the potassium. Sodium is characteristic of animal, and potassium of vegetable physiology.

When we turn to the empirical experience with homoeopathic remedies we find a group of remedies which Dr John Paterson demonstrated to be associated with a particular bowel organism, Proteus. He found a common thread running through the drug pictures of these remedies which he expressed as 'brain storms'. The main remedy in this group is common salt, sodium chloride, and it is one of the outstanding homoeopathic remedies for migraine. I have no doubt that this group is related to the kidney as the group associated with the Morgan bacillus was related by Paterson to the liver and the group associated with the dysentery organisms with the heart and epigastrium. These were empirical clinical findings. Now in this group associated with salt, *Natrum muriaticum*, we find ergot (*Secale*) copper (*cuprum*) cactus together with *Ignatia* and *Conium* (which brings in attacks of vertigo as well). In the picture of *Natrum muriaticum* we find long exhausting periods of strain followed by sudden outbursts of disease manifestation such as migraine or even herpes simplex. Paterson also included the sudden perforation or bleeding of peptic ulcers without warning, the peripheral vascular spasms of Raynaud's phenomenon, cramps, and temper tantrums in children. We are in a realm of nervous instability and irritability when a slight stimulus can result in reactions of undue proportion. The emotional instability of *Ignatia* and angioneurotic oedema of apis are also included. With ergot (*Secale*) we find the whole range of action from peripheral arterial spasms and gangrene through cramps of smooth muscle in uterus and other organs to migraine and in LSD to the hallucinated schizophrenic-like symptoms. Can we understand these trips as psychic migraine?

The evolutionary origins of the kidney as pronephros from the cephalic pole already points to a close connection between this organ and the nervous system. It is interesting to find these empirical confirmations and the whole range of symptoms of these remedies share a common style. It is this style, which Paterson called 'Brain storms', which is important. The style of the attacks points to a common ground in the kidney and related nervous disturbance. A feature of some migraine attacks, already touched on, may find an explanation in the kidney dynamics. It is not uncommon for patients to refer to the feeling of well-being, a high, the day before an attack. Sometimes it takes the form of ravenous hunger and then the headache is attributed to the orgy of overeating, whereas in reality the overeating is the first symptom in the whole ritual of the migraine attack. Starting with a general exhilaration arising from an overactive kidney radiation the process goes on to the overwhelming of the brain function and the typical migraine headache. *Belladonna* and *Hyoscyamus* in homoeopathic potency given at the commencement of these attacks can sometimes abort them as can also *Chamomilla*, particularly the preparation from the root of the plant.

In those cases where the senses are weak or exhausted, unable to defend themselves against the battering of the modern world, *Silica* and *Prunus spinosa* and *Phosphorus* become helpful. We are then led to consider the middle term between the nerve sense pole and the metabolic pole which we have mostly been considering so far. Migraine expresses itself as a confrontation between these two poles, with a failure of the rhythmic system in its function of healing mediation. The form-giving upper pole cannot succeed in informing the turbulence of the metabolic processes. The nourishing metabolic pole cannot refresh the dying nervous system but erupts against it as a pseudo-inflammation. In the natural rhythm of sleep and waking we can see the healthy inter-working of the two poles mutually interpenetrating and balancing each other. In the meeting of the breathing rhythm and pulse beat these two again work into and through each other, the breathing rhythm leads the nervous and the pulse beat the metabolic processes into harmonious relationship with each other through the interplay of these two rhythms.

Ferrum, the metal iron, in potency works healingly in the three functional realms; it is healer and strengthener of the nervous tissue, it is related to the gall-bile system and restrains its overexuberance, and it finds itself working especially in the rhythmic dances. The to-and-fro of taking up and giving up oxygen by the haemoglobin is an archetypal example of this rhythmic activity of iron. It is not surprising that, even in the still rather weakly developed homoeopathic drug picture of *Ferrum* and its salts, something of all this is visible. We find instability of the circulation, orgasms of blood, flushings, which are combined with sensitivity of the senses particularly of hearing, and indigestion, vomiting and an intolerance of eggs. All of this with hammering headaches and marked right-sidedness in the symptoms show the relatedness of iron to the whole migraine disturbance. In the anthroposophical remedy for migraine, *Bidor*, iron silica and sulphur are combined and it addresses itself archetypally to the range of dysfunctions we have been considering.

In conclusion, we can try and find the position of migraine in relation to other diseases. On occasion in a migraine attack, heralded by a prodromal hemiplegia ordinarily resolving in half an hour, we find the hemiplegia persisting and permanent. The migraine has passed over into a stroke. It has sometimes occurred to me that one can see historical parallels to this. Circumstances occur when rigidity of social structures prohibit all new impulses from enriching and renewing the social life. Bureaucracy and rigid hierarchical organization in Church and state

240

allow no influx of new life. The nerve system is the hierarchical principle in our physiology, the blood system the egalitarian and gregarious. History tells us how in old Tsarist Russia, repeated attempts were made to enliven the autocratic, bureaucratic rigidity, repeated migraine attacks. They failed and then came a bloody revolution, a cerebral haemorrhage, leaving the victim perhaps worse off than before. The blood tries to rejuvenate the sclerosing nervous system but only overdoes it and destroys it. Many such instances paralleling in social life the disturbances in our organisms come to mind.

The dynamics of migraine as they have been presenting themselves to us can be found again in the more serious and tragic condition of multiple sclerosis. Here the dying of the nerve tissue, which paradoxically can almost be called the life of the nerve processes, gets too advanced. It provokes the blood to an inflammatory response, in an attempt to reincorporate and re-enliven the disintegrating myelin sheath.

In so wonderfully plastic and ever-changingly varied a functional disorder as migraine it is not surprising that innumerable therapeutic regimes and remedies can be effective in different patients. We have indicated how migraine can relate to the hysterical process but also to that opposite pole of disease which used to be called neurasthenia and its hypersensitivity of the senses. These aspects bring the physician personally, psychotherapeutically, into the whole programme. It is only too easy for the physician to get caught in the maze of these phenomena. Today painstaking researches seek out detailed mechanisms involved in migraine, but it is also necessary to try to take first steps in a wider understanding of the significance of this archetypal disorder. The meaning of disease and of particular diseases must be sought along different paths from the mechanistic researches of present-day science. It will of course be a long time before this meaningful understanding of disease can grow up and mature but even primitive steps in this direction open up possibilities of an art as distinct from technology of healing. Art can only arise through an artist. If one aspect of today's crisis in medicine is how to restore humanity to the patient, then the other aspect is how to rescue physicianship and the person of the physician to active participation in the healing process.

31. Multiple sclerosis and parkinsonism

During the last fifty or so years multiple sclerosis has become, in most developed western countries, the commonest disease of the nervous system, replacing in this respect neuro-syphilis. This latter has become a rarity, presumably because of modern treatments. Most observers seem to agree that MS has increased absolutely in frequency during this century. Its cause is not known and many epidemiological features, such as its geographical distribution, remain unexplained. It appears to be mainly a disease of temperate climates and high civilization. It seems to merit description as a disease of the age and accordingly an attempt to understand it in relation to the character of our present times and out of the inherent nature of the nervous system seems justified.

The nervous system which arises almost as a continuation inwards of the sense organs arises early in embryonic development from the ectoderm by invaginations. Soon the future head region comes to dominate the picture in the embryo and in the foetus the head remains large out of proportion to the developing body. Even at birth the baby is almost all head with an appendage of a body and limbs. The cranium, containing the brain, enlarges relatively very little after birth, the trunk and limbs can be said to grow down from the head, as a plant grows up from the root. This gives us a first impression, the head and brain form early and growth soon stops, death intervenes and no new nerve cells are generated in the brain after birth. Indeed it seems that even before birth, nerve cells are dying in huge numbers and continue to do so throughout life. There is no regeneration of nerve cells after birth. Generation and regeneration belong to the lower, metabolic and genital pole.

We do however find in the brain a most intricate inner architecture and the more sophisticated the techniques of studying it become, the more remarkable this inner structure is found to be.

The main unit in the nervous system is the nerve cell with its nerve fibre growing from it. This may be two feet or more in length. Throughout our bodies these fibres ramify and it is estimated that if all these fibres were joined together into a single thread they would go around the world twelve times. The nerve man then is a web of nerve fibres and even the apparently solid nervous organs, the spinal cord and brain are composed of these fibres. One-dimensionality dominates; there are no leaves, no real membranes or surfaces. We are forcibly reminded of the world of fungi whose structure, even of the mushroom, is composed of one dimensional fibres, at the most matted together. Fungi are mycelial threads and at the ends they may turn into spores or dust. The fungi, too, live parasitically off decaying vegetable and animal matter reducing them also to dust. But the fungi can of course grow and multiply whereas as we have mentioned nerve cells cannot reproduce after birth. The brain has a very rich blood supply, not because it is a very vital organ but because this rich blood supply is needed to preserve it from dying completely. The brain and nervous system live parasitically upon the rest of the organism.

When we look back over human history we find that thinking was once much more alive than it has become today. In Plato we find that his profoundest thoughts are often expressed in the form of myths and pictures. Further back in the Vedas of ancient India, the thinking is still so living that it is extremely difficult for most of us to follow it at all. Gradually, from Aristotle on, thinking has become more abstract and intellectual until today it is dry as dust and capable only of grasping mechanisms and the world of the dead things.

When we look in the embryo at the growth of the brain, whilst it is still young, growing and plastic, it appears like an image of that still plastic, creative thinking of ancient times.

The brain in its inner almost infinitely complicated architecture must have been formed by equally complex forces. It is not absurd to suggest that a cosmic thinking created the brain as its image. Having created it, then it could emancipate from it and use it as a mirror to behold itself as Paul says 'in a glass darkly'.

But the head and brain show every sign of being old, stemming from early phases of evolution, and death forces now predominate in them. If our thinking models itself still, exclusively, on this dying organ it too becomes abstract intellectualism, life can no longer be found in it. As Hamlet says 'sicklied o'er with the pale cast of thought'.

We can however look at the brain from another side. It can be seen as a larval form, embryonic, lying in the cerebro-spinal fluid within the Dura, Arachnoid and Pia Maters as the embryo does in the amniotic fluid in the uterus and membranes. It can be seen that the whole body and limbs are represented in the head and brain in a synthetic mode, whereas this head and brain are displayed in analysis in the body and its organs. This larval form, the brain, foregoes its higher organic metamorphosis through which it might have become a bird or butterfly. The forces which, so to say, might have transformed the lateral lobes of the brain into wings, puffed them up, are set free so that we can fly on the wings of thought. The brain therefore shows in its 'form' early larval or embryonic features, whilst at the same time it is dominated by dying processes. The life forces of cosmic thinking have abandoned it and have become available for memory, imagination and thinking.

The baby and infant have of course still retained something of the paradise experience, the intra-uterine bliss of the psychoanalysts, and only as childhood becomes boyhood or girlhood do these life forces become really freed for head learning. Wordsworth's 'trailing clouds of glory do we come' is relevant to our attempts to understand these issues as are the poems of Traherne.

The brain, then, we are trying to depict as embryonic in form but arrested early in its development. Death processes have come to dominate. But the inner architecture reveals itself as a most intricately woven thought structure and the living forces which have woven this structure become gradually freed from their organic building tasks and available for mental activities. These mental processes can then see themselves in the mirror of the brain and become consciously awake. The physical brain offers the necessary resistance so that our thinking can become conscious. From this point of view it is obviously a mistake to regard the electrical and chemical activities in the brain as the essential nerve function. They can rather be seen as shadows cast or evoked by the real thinking activity.

There is a Greek myth about Perseus which throws illumination on the role of the brain. When Perseus is commanded to bring back the Gorgon Medusa's head, he is faced with the problem that to look at her is to be turned to stone. Medusa is a symbol for the other world, which to gaze upon is so overwhelming that one is frozen, in fear, into stone. Athene gave Perseus a shining shield, to use as a mirror, so that looking only in the mirror at the image of Medusa, Perseus would in freedom be able to use his sword to cut off her head. This he then kept in a satchel, also a gift from Athene, taking it out only in dire crisis to turn enemies into stone. Is this satchel perhaps an image for the unconscious in which we keep the realities concealed, looking only at the mirror images in our brain, which, devoid of reality, leave us free to act?

We can also extend the picture of the architecture of the brain as itself stemming from the activity of still living thoughts and look for the source of the sculpturing forces which must be active in the whole embryo and foetus, in the brain and nervous system, that is to say in forces radiating from this system. The moulding and modelling of the human form is then seen to arise in the play between a formless multiplication of cells at the metabolic pole full of reproductive life and a dying highly-formed cephalic pole radiating sculpting forces. These can be understood as acting tangentially, rather like a potter's hand when he throws a pot on his wheel. It is one-sided to look for the origin of form in differential reproduction of cells alone when the very gestures of developing form indicate planar tangential forces. In sculpture excess marble is chipped away until the pre-existant statue stands revealed. Death forces from the nervous system are constantly breaking down, katabolically, the growing burgeoning anabolic life from the metabolic pole.

An unopposed head pole would turn us into a marble statue, an unopposed abdominal pole into a formless mass of living multiplying cells. But this polarity is resolved in the middle realm where rhythm constantly mediates and heals. This rhythmic centre is not just a resultant of the opposition between upper and lower poles, it must be considered a third principle along with the other two.

So far our considerations have led us to characterize the nervous system as a centre from which radiates katabolic, sculpturing, therefore paralyzing, forces.

What light does this throw on the problems of sense experience on the one hand and of movement on the other? In the first place can we justify a look at these questions which will run counter if not to the facts then certainly to the interpretation of the facts as presently taught? Everyone agrees that there is an insurmountable abyss between the chemical and electrical changes studied in the sense organs, nerves and brain on one hand and the actual experiences of colours, tones, tastes and so on which are our sensory experiences. This abyss is no doubt traceable to the Cartesian guillotine. But it does entitle us to look again and try to understand rather than give in to resignation before the apparently insoluble. The accepted views about the movements of our limbs circle around the concept of motor nerves which mediate impulses originating in the motor cortex of the brain to the muscles. A pianist is then supposed to play upon the keyboard of the motor cortex and his hands, dangling rather like a marionette's on the end of strings, play the piano. It is of course no easier to explain how the pianist can play the cortex than play the keys of the piano. The whole idea when placed in the context of real life as distinct from laboratory experiments is really ridiculous. In passing one may recall that these problems have largely arisen from, or in any case have been fuelled by, Galvani's observations of twitching frogs' legs strung up on wires. It looked as if the electrical current must be the life force in the nerves, and that stimulus to the nerve caused the muscle to contract.

Rudolf Steiner repeatedly attacked the doctrine of motor nerves as absurd and even those who are opposed to his views would be hard pressed to show that he was ill informed or ignorant about the matters on which he spoke. As attempts to solve the body-soul problems within the currently accepted paradigms of science come up against a brick wall, we may be allowed the attempt to reach at least preliminary understanding from another viewpoint. From within the neurological profession itself some voices have been raised drawing attention to the fallacies and shortcomings in the accepted teachings. Dr J.A.V. Bates has focused attention on these, showing that the still commonly accepted view of voluntary movements originating in the motor cortex is untenable.

So let us first of all look at the embryo in which movement appears first in the blood in the small blood vessels, before the heart is included into the circulation. William Harvey himself observed this in the chick embryo and it led him to state that it was not the heart that moved the blood but on the contrary the blood that moved the heart. Again we can observe very easily in the simple protozoa Paramecium how the inner content of this unicellular creature moves in a figure of eight path of its own accord. Motion arises spontaneously in the fluid elements;

the static parts of the organism, most typically the nerve and bone, are almost, we can say, precipitated out into fixed structures. The archetypal movement is paralysed into rigidity.

Now when we watch a baby in the cradle, its arms and hands, legs and feet are in constant movement. The movements are all over the place, without apparent purpose. Movement, as it were, flows into them from outside. Gradually out of this undirected or universally directed movement, simple movements directed to an aim become isolated. Could we not say, the superfluous unnecessary movements are paralysed, leaving just the wanted one? It is rather like the sculpturing process when, as we have mentioned, superfluous marble is removed, revealing the statue. We can also see how the trained professional actor achieves the desired gesture with the minimum of movement, whereas the ham actor makes clumsy gestures all over the place. The role of the nervous system is to select the wanted movement by paralysing all the other potential motions.

Now we can ask: is not something similar the case in the sense organs? Out of all that flows in to the sense organs we become conscious of very little. If we think for a moment of the overwhelming richness of impressions reaching our eyes, and of how very little reaches consciousness, it is obvious that a selective process goes on. We notice, as Bergson pointed out, only what we need to notice and this is reflected whereas all the rest passes unnoticed into the nervous system. Consciousness always depends on reflection which produces an image. Like Narcissus of old we become conscious of ourselves when we see our image in a mirror. It is a surprising fact that the rods and cones, the sensitive elements in the retina, do not face outwards to the world but inwards towards the rich blood supply of the choroid. It is as if in a camera the film were put in so that the paper backing faced the lens and the sensitive film looked into the back of the camera. There is activity in looking. When we look at something we seem to reach right out to the object and we finger it with a delicate tenuous ethereal touch. Looking is not just passive, it is a willed activity and we have to look for that activity coming in the blood. The retina paralyses the unconscious perceptions and will activity into images.

The phenomena of so-called after-images present many problems. When we gaze for a time, fixedly, at a light, or a coloured form on a sheet of paper, and then look away to a neutral surface, we see the same form appear. It is more fleeting, insubstantial, than the original and it usually appears as a complementary colour. But if we continue to look, the colour changes and changes again if we cover our eyes. A coloured halo may appear around the central coloured form and these can then spontaneously change places. These visual displays may continue for some minutes and only gradually disappear. From where do they come? And are they not constantly intermixed with our normal vision although unnoticed? They are certainly more dream-like than the 'awake' sensory images. Most of our perceptions remain unconscious or in a state of sleep consciousness. They are gradually woken up and only become fully awake when they meet the concepts.

246

The living reality of the outer world is paralysed into sensory images. Nature, who for the Greeks was still a divine being, who nourished and formed us, has in our modern sensory experience been killed off. We can see, for instance, how the embryo is shaped like an ear, it is all ear, hearkening to the music of the spheres. But is it not also all eye, all organ of warmth and so on? The senses are still alive and utterly interwoven. And we have to think of them acting formatively into the embryo. Only gradually have they become separated from each other and almost only physical instruments. Through our separate senses the unity of nature is analysed and her life paralysed into static, rigid, images. Nature for us has become a corpse. In so far then as our thinking bases itself on our sensory experience it too becomes mechanistic and atomistic. One thought occurs followed by another unrelated to it. One has only to look at a newspaper to see the juxtaposition of unconnected items, no synthesis is attempted; analysis into isolated bits and pieces rules the day. Our thinking is scatter-brained and impotent to take charge of the realities of life. So our life of will is not informed with life purposes and goals. It becomes impulsive, driven by instinctive forces and unable to relate immediate aims to the wider, universal human needs and values.

From this state we are all suffering but we also come to a first characterization of the state of multiple sclerosis patients. For them it is even harder to hold a consistent line of thought, to relate one thought to another, than it is for others. Their senses are more dead and atomised, particularly the eye. We can observe this in the comparative weakness of their capacity to produce after-images, which is easily demonstrated. The active will element in the senses is weak. They find difficulty in grasping an object with the eye, rather are they grasped by it. The power of actively projecting an image is weak. Instead of the pictorial grasp of the whole they become prey to a bits and pieces jumble, a mosaic or jigsaw puzzle.

However the most conspicuous feature in MS patients is the progressive disability in movement, which may proceed by fits and starts or by slow steady decline. How can we form a picture of this disability, this paralysis, unless we accept the currently held mechanistic picture of messages down nerves, rather like telephone wires, which have become interrupted, broken?

When we learn to handle a new instrument, for instance to drive a motor car, at first our attention is fixed on each pedal and lever. We think each detail and are clumsy. Gradually we forget these details and our attention stretches out to the road ahead and the sign posts, other traffic and so on. The instruments of the car have become incorporated into me, have become an extension of my limbs. This is so to an even more perfect degree with the musician and his instrument. Now in paralysis we can see that the limb has become foreign to me. I try to handle it as the apprentice tries to handle his tool. The sense experiences have moved inwards into the nerves away from the periphery, whether from the sense organs in the skin and tendons or from those in the muscles usually called muscle end-plates. In the artist on the contrary they have moved outwards and embrace his instrument.

The different forms of paralysis such as flaccid spastic, ataxic, arise from the differential withdrawal inwards of distinct sensory impressions, and the extent of the withdrawal from the sense organs into peripheral nerve, spinal cord or brain. We can distinguish to begin with, sense of position, of balance, of movement. Are the nerves which end in the muscles really sensory nerves serving the sense of movement rather than motor nerves as ordinarily understood? Movement and music complement each other. In the great dancer the whole muscle system must become a musical instrument, through which the music, even the cosmic music of the spheres, plays. Dance and music give rise to form and the form and modelling of the body arise from the muscles. When dance rises to ecstasy, the music is not heard. And this is probably true both of the religious experience of dervishes and other ancient cults as well as of the degenerate caricature found in modern discos. When we want to listen to the music, inwardly hearken to it, then we sit still, we paralyse the incipient movements of the limbs. I have the impression that the so-called motor nerves are sensory for the whole world of movement or music which comes to expression through the muscles. They are therefore perceptions of a time element of movement itself and not just of a changed spatial position.

In multiple sclerosis lesions occur in the brain and spinal cord. They consist of smallish areas in which the myelin sheath of the nerve fibres degenerates. These areas become the seat of an inflammatory reaction from the blood. Blood always seeks to bring back damaged or dying parts into the living organic unity. But of course it may overdo it and the inflammations can then bring about even further damage. As the inflammation subsides the damaged areas become rather pearly, translucent in appearance. Treichler has compared them to displaced eye formations. One of the earliest manifestations of multiple sclerosis is often in the eye, or rather just behind the eye in the so-called optic nerves, which in fact are outgrowths of the brain itself. The so-called retro-bulbar neuritis develops here in the tract leading backwards from the eye into the brain. Treichler sees this as a sort of archetypal phenomenon in the development of multiple sclerosis. A process which is normal when confined to the retina and choroid is pushed back into the nerve tracts of the brain and spinal cord. These lesions are understandable as displaced eye formations and occur predominantly in the tracts in brain and spinal cord which are related to movement. Conventionally they are considered motor tracts, upper motor neurones. Here we are trying to understand them as in reality sensory nerves mediating the sense of movement. The appearance of these 'sense-organs' in the spinal cord results in the withdrawal of the movement sense from the muscles into the spine. The limb becomes in respect of movement a foreign object, which is moved clumsily and with conscious attention, as when learning to drive a car. Normal movements are performed unconsciously with the attention not on the limb but on the goal. Other lesions occur in the tracts connecting the cerebellum with the movements and result in the typical ataxias of MS, such as the tremor which accompanies movements and makes drinking a cup of tea difficult.

At this point we can also mention the polarity between MS and parkinsonism which is today almost as frequent. Parkinsonism occurs mostly in the age group over fifty, MS in the younger, usually starting in the teens or twenties. In parkinsonism there develops a mask-like face, expressionless, with unblinking eyes, and a great slowness in, for instance, a smile working through to the face. In MS the emotions often play rapidly between tears and laughter. In parkinsonism a tremor frequently develops, notably in the hands, which is most marked at rest and ceases on movement, the opposite to the intention tremor in MS. In MS further we find a strange irresponsiveness on the abdomen.

The abdomen can be likened to a face, a fact observed by surrealist artists. Normally a slight scratching of the skin of the abdomen results in a reflex twitching and movement of the umbilicus, the so-called abdominal reflexes. In MS these reflexes are lost and we can describe the abdominal face as becoming masklike.

What does this mean? The elderly parkinsonian becomes more immobile than is natural in old age. Consciousness of the surroundings is maintained but both the emotional responsiveness on the face and voluntary movements are severely slowed. These patients do not want to move but prefer to sit motionless. A certain mood of resignation seems to pervade them. There is no point in moving to do something; emotional response will bring about change, it is better just to sit, be aware of the surroundings and not to interfere. The will does not become active, even when the limbs can act. When told to do something they often can. The 'pill-rolling' tremor ceases when they do move. The will is inactive, the thinking remains but the will does not work into, to enliven, the thinking. It remains passive. The mood is melancholic. Melancholy derives from the Greek 'Black Bile', one of the four humours. There is an area in the brain called the substantia nigra containing black pigment. It degenerates in parkinsonism. This black pigment is practically the same as the ink, the sepia, in the ink-sac or gall bladder of the cuttle fish and octopus. Is it not the black bile of the ancients?

But the multiple sclerotic responds over-quickly emotionally. Changes of emotion follow each other, reverse into each other with bewildering rapidity. Tears and laughter alternate, but somehow these emotions seem on the surface, mere ripples on the water of life. Thinking too lacks any consistent line. It is all over the place. They want to do things but the limbs don't work. The impact of sensory impressions, so enormously increased as a consequence of technology, works shatteringly into the nerves and brain and the thought life becomes atomistic, scatter-brained as we have mentioned. These disconnected sense impressions are not digested, there is no time, and the emotions also become trivial and unable to carry will impulses into incarnation in movement and deed. The young person today is torn apart by the multiplicity of impressions and the accumulated mountains of mere facts, devoid of meaning. He cannot develop the deep life of feeling and he is forced to withdraw from the realities of life. We live life through a filter of abstract ideas and cannot get into it.

Parkinsonism appears in the second half of life. The thought life does not appear scatter-brained as in MS. But I have the impression that the life of thought has tended to become conventional, caught in habitual traditional moulds. These no longer have the capacity to arouse the will to enthusiasm. One sees the world through clichés of thought and feeling. No ideas enlivened into ideals come to consciousness to enthuse purpose for the future. The old ideals are today grown stale. The repetitive tremor of thumb and fingers are symbolic of a life gripped in the repetition of social conventions and ideas. The life of the blood, in which our willing ego lives, has not succeeded in nourishing the life of thought. The goals which can give meaning to the second half of life, goals concerned with wholeness, redeeming and including one's inferior functions, dealing with the shadow side of one's personality, these goals have not been awakened.

In parkinsonism it appears to be the nerve cells in the substantia nigra and corpus striatum which have degenerated whereas in multiple sclerosis it is the myelin sheaths of the nerves rather than the nerve cells as such. Now Treichler has argued that the nerve cells and the axis cylinder, the central core of the nerve fibres, serve a centrifugal function whereby the concept arising centrally is conducted to the sense organ. The myelin sheath on the other hand he regards as the 'true' nerve sending sensation, centripetally from sense organ to brain.

We must now then make clear, what has been implicit so far, namely that it is the soul and spirit and not the body in which sensations and impulses to movement arise. A mere body, a machine, can obviously not experience anything or initiate anything. The point of the nerves with their dying, disintegrating, nature is that they are withdrawn from the life of the organism. It is their organic non-existence, if one may so express it, which makes way for the soul-spirit being to enter. Steiner also pointed to the interruption between one nerve and another, the synapse, as providing entry for the blood process into the nerve function.

We can now attempt a tentative classification of the difference between multiple sclerosis and parkinsonism. In the latter the degeneration of the nerve cells and axis cylinder interferes with the transference of the 'idea of the movement' to the motor-end plate. The impulse to movements does not wake up. In MS it is rather the consciousness of the movement itself which is obstructed, not the impulse to move.

The whole character of our external civilization conduces to MS. Technology has resulted in a continuous bombardment of our sense organs, often with merely technical, soulless stimuli. These increase the already natural disintegration of the sensory organs which then feed the brain with increased dying forces. The thinking which then models itself on or reflects itself in this disintegrating organ is itself one-sidedly atomistic and this thinking will duly invent yet more disintegrative

250

technology. A vicious spiral comes about, disintegrative brain leads to atomistic thinking which creates technological environment which in its turn works disintegratively into the senses and brain.

We seem caught in a veritable labyrinth and need Ariadne's thread to lead us out again. We can also say that thinking, from Daedalus onwards, having created technology to overcome poverty and the compulsive need for slavery, has remained at this same materialistic and atomistic level. It has not succeeded in raising itself to the imaginative and intuitive heights which are now open. Only a very few pioneering spirits have so far led the way.

From these considerations the directions in which therapy should aim become clearer. Thinking and the senses need to be enlivened and warmed through by the feelings and will which itself needs to be informed with purpose. The cephalic and metabolic poles of our being which at present tend to confront each other need mediation through the middle rhythmic processes. This middle realm, the bearer of our feelings, has grown shallow or conventional. The whole realm of artistic activity offers immense therapeutic possibilities. Not only the feelings but the senses can be nourished and renewed. The formative, paralysing forces from the head become tempered by the breathing rhythm, and the upsurging metabolic forces are brought into rhythm by the pulse beat of the heart. These two rhythms can interplay. In more specific medical terms we need to find medicaments to bring healing especially to the spinal cord in MS. The spinal cord which is the middle brain of the nervous system between the head brain and the solar plexus, the brain of the sympathetic or abdominal nervous system. It is probable that iron is the centre piece of remedial substances and *Ferrum meteoricum* supports the nervous system in many states of exhaustion. Treichler has suggested the use of two antimony salts of iron, *Katoptrit* and *Berthierite* preferably given subcutaneously in 20x to 30x potencies. Cyanic acid and cyanide salts, perhaps the Ferrocyanates are also indicated and *Prunus spinosa* in which the cyanic process is strong. The Weleda preparation Bidor which contains iron together with sulphur and silica supports and harmonizes the blood and nerve processes in the nervous system. It has been used extensively for headaches and migraine and it is worth noticing that the dynamics of migraine on the functional level are really the same as those of MS on the structural. Fuller indications are available in homoeopathic and anthroposophical literature. In parkinsonism one is struck by the fact that manganese poisoning mimics this disease. Hauschka depicted manganese as one of the 'brothers of iron'. *Sepia* has obvious connections with the substantia nigra and its clinical picture, including the expressionless face, bears a resemblance. Organ preparations from the substantia nigra as well as the spinal cord are available.

But apart from these possibilities and many others the main intent of this chapter is to indicate that these diseases are characteristic of our current cultural situation. We all suffer from them. Those whose disability breaks through into manifest structural disease hold a mirror up to all of us showing us the cultural and character disabilities we all suffer. Ultimately it must be, not by therapeutic efforts limited to the actual patients with these diseases, but by the transformation and healing of our whole social and cultural world, that these diseases can be rendered unnecessary. They will no longer be needed to hold the mirror up to us. This particular crisis in human development will have been surmounted.

32. Asthma

Asthma is a condition which is familiar to almost everyone. Not only physicians but the relatives and friends of sufferers will have met with it often and there must be few who have not come up against it in acquaintances from school days onwards. In spite of the very varied features to be met with in different patients, there is a recognizable archetypal phenomenon which unites all these variations. Can we approach this entity with a view to unravelling the tangled skein? In treating asthma one is in danger from two directions. Firstly, one may adopt with obsessional strength a certain routine and regime of treatment, opposing to the patient's anxiety an exaggerated self-confidence in the treatment. Secondly, one may be diverted from consistent treatment by ever-changing symptoms and the pursuit of food and other sensitivities. In these wild goose chases, patient and physician can find themselves in a *folie à deux*. We need a compass to help steer a middle course towards healing.

Asthma is characterized by a disturbance of breathing rhythm. This disturbance may come on in fairly sudden acute attacks or it may become more constant and chronic. The disturbance is marked by airways obstruction with, usually, greater relative obstruction of out-breathing with a prolongation of the expiratory phase. The chest therefore tends to become more and more inflated, with short inspiratory gasps followed by difficult slow wheezy expirations. The obstruction to breathing is due to contraction and spasm of the bronchioles leading to the lung alveoli. This is accompanied by the secretion of a viscous mucous squeezed into these small tubes so further obstructing the air-flow. The contraction is greatest during expiration. The patient often feels that he cannot get enough air into his lungs but this is due to his chest being already fully distended. He cannot get the air out, he is fixed in inspiration and so cannot get any more air in. We can also find in the viscous mucous secretions spiral formations, known after their discoverer as Curschmann spirals and often in addition Charcot-Leyden crystals. The walls of the tubes and the secretions show a multitude of eosinophil cells. When the attack passes off the mucous becomes more fluid, softens, and can be coughed up.

Can we try to read these gestures as the physiognomy of the archetype and so approach a bit nearer to an understanding of asthma with which to supplement the ever-increasing knowledge of facts and detail? Out of this knowledge we have gained many techniques and powerful drugs for the control of asthma but at the same time we are liable to lose sight of the whole and its significance. Can we read the gesture itself, or at least take some first steps towards such an interpretation? Can we also follow the tracks of the conditions leading to asthmatic breathing, the circumstances under which it comes into being? When at birth we enter into our earth life with our first breath we fill our lungs and cry but we also wake up a bit into the sensory world. When we die we let out our last breath, we expire. We can also fairly easily notice that with each in-breathing we wake up a little and with each out-breathing we go a little to sleep. With the waking up into the senses and nerve processes we also experience an undercurrent of fear. When we are suddenly full of fear, as in sudden fright, we take a breath in and our senses become very wide awake whereas in the contrary experience of shame our senses become clouded over, our thoughts lose their clarity and become confused. We lose our presence of mind.

When we experience fear we become still, rooted to the ground, very wide awake in our senses, and our breathing becomes shallow and rather high. Indeed with sudden fright when we jump out of our skins, we take a deep sudden inspiration and may find ourselves unable to let our breath go again. Asthma can come on with such a sudden shock and it is worth considering whether repeated shocks to a mother during pregnancy may not enter into the causes of subsequent asthma in the child.

The gesture of inspiration points to the dynamics of the head and senses, to an awake or alerted consciousness. In the stuck inspiration of asthma we could also describe the state as one in which the normal awake function of the head has slipped down into the breathing in the chest. It is normally in the head that we hold a thought, follow a line of argument, concentrate on an object, and that is where we like to produce crystal clarity in our thinking. These tendencies come to dominate the breathing in asthma even to producing the Charcot-Leyden crystals. Normally in our breathing and other rhythmic processes we live in a consciousness intermediate between sleeping and waking, in a dream-like consciousness in which we also experience our emotions, our life of feelings. These feelings play in the rhythms of sympathy and antipathy, of love and hate. When our breathing is rather high and shallow, our chest rather full of air then we find ourselves constrained and anxious. In an uncongenial atmosphere we may notice this constraint in our breathing and when we find ourselves amongst friends again we say 'Oh I can breathe again'. Our breathing sinks lower down to the abdominal pole, towards the pole of sympathy whereas our upper breathing inclines towards the pole of antipathy centred in the head.

It is of course well known that in the hyperventilation syndrome with all its anxiety symptoms and fear the ventilation is focused in the upper chest. With diaphragmatic breathing the syndrome does not develop.

This helps us, as well, to understand the head as the focus of the hardening, sclerosing, form creating processes in the organism, which arise with the forces of antipathy and hate, as distinct from the softening, form dissolving processes arising from the sympathetic abdominal pole. To make of a living reality a thing, an object, is to kill it. Our intellect is always killing, objectifying, analysing, it is based on our nerves and brain. From the head the skeleton itself stems and radiates the image of death. But we can also see how in the metabolism and blood new life is always springing up. The whole nutritional process is a continuous inner reproduction and renewal of the organism.

We have noticed how uncongenial circumstances leading to a constraint in the breathing, an anxiety, are a 'coming into being,' a nascence of asthmatic breathing. We can also induce a state of bronchiolar spasm by artificially breathing in an asthmatic pattern for 10 minutes or so. By deliberately prolonging the expiration with a deliberate contraction in the larynx, a temporary asthmatic state can be induced which takes some minutes to wear off after resuming normal respiratory rhythm. It seems as if in this case anxiety arises out of the induced abnormal breathing whereas in the previous example anxiety led to constraint in the breathing. Anxiety itself is experienced as a constraint in the breathing rhythm, it can also be experienced in angina pectoris as pressing, constricting, constraint in the heart rhythm. It seems that anxiety belongs to the rhythmic processes in the same way as fear does to the nervous and shame to the blood and metabolic processes. When anxiety rises more to the cognitional pole it inclines towards fear but when it sinks into the volitional we experience rather shame.

Another aspect of the asthma process confronts us in its association with eczema, hay fever and urticaria in the allergic or atopic complex of disorders. Here we come up against the extreme sensitivity that some people develop to specific stimuli such as horses, cats, dogs or pollens and house dust. Most of these specific stimuli are either themselves proteins or have become fixed to proteins. For instance the lacquer-like substance in the poison ivy of America (*Rhus toxicodendron*) becomes quickly fixed in some ten minutes to proteins in the skin on contact. If it is not immediately scrubbed off after contact it may lead to sensitization and then further contact with the Rhus Toxicodendron the poison ivy, will lead to eczema. People vary in their tendency to develop sensitizations; some on further exposures become desensitized again, whereas others develop increasingly violent reactions even to anaphylactic shock and death. People with a tendency to become sensitized usually develop sensitivity to more than one substance. The techniques of specific desensitization do not change this constitutional tendency and further 'allergies' are liable to develop after specific treatment of one.

Modern researches are revealing ever more detailed mechanisms in these allergic and immune reactions. We can also try and approach them by finding the 'normal' range of such phenomena, the sphere of activities where we can regard such 'allergies' as normal or reasonably so. This may help us to understand the meaning of such bizarre phenomena. Everyone must be aware of how we can become emotionally sensitized to someone else. We may fall in love and then, proximity to or even thinking of the beloved stirs up all the emotional responses together with somatic ones as well. But we also know how we can become 'allergic' to someone, in the sense that any mention of them or having to meet them results in irrational reactions out of all proportion to the real facts as seen by others. These are reactions of extreme love or hate and of course they may change into each other. It seems reasonable to assume that first contact with another does not call forth emotional response of love or hate. Memory of a previous meeting, pleasurable or painful, must be there in order that love or hate, the desire to be nearer or further apart, can arise. In the case of love or hate at first sight there may be associations with other familiar persons. But when these experiences are strong they often give rise in people to the conviction that they have indeed 'met before'. However that may be we can suggest that the laws of such emotional responses are the archetypes of the allergic reactions. These allergies can be seen as the manifestations of psychological laws pushed down into the physiological realms. They are displacements.

Asthma belongs with eczema, urticaria and hay fever to the group of so-called atopic diseases. They may occur together or alternate with or replace each other. Similar mechanisms underlie each of them but in terms of experience they are very distinct. In hay fever or rhinitis water pours from the nose and eyes, it is difficult to clear the mind and think; one drowns in the rising tide of fluids and has to fight through it to air and light. But in asthma the experience is almost wholly the polar opposite. Now one is full of air and anxiety and can in no way let go of it and sleep. One has to battle with the air. Again in eczema the burning itching can be overwhelming, intolerable; one is caught in the fires of hell, at war with the element of fire. These three phases of the atopic phenomena represent the three elements of fire, air and water still unmastered by the individuality of the organism. Can we find the fourth, the element of earth? Not so long ago it was common to call the spastic colon, asthma of the bowel. In many ways it is an excellent description and here one has the battle with that which in India is called the 'night soil'. It is indeed strange to come upon these four elements of the ancients in relation to phenomena such as the atopic diseases.

We are now led to consider the cramp or spasm which plays a big part in asthma and the irritable bowel. We can notice a common gesture underlying a range of conditions from cramp in the extremities, cramp in the digital arteries in Raynaud's phenomena, cramp in the small arteries in hypertension, cramp in the uterus in dysmenorhoea, in the stomach and intestines in various alimentary disorders, in the bronchi in asthma, in the heart in angina and probably in the blood vessels of the head in migraine. The same spectrum is found in the homoeopathic drug pictures of *Cuprum* and *Secale* (the ergot) and points to the sphere of the kidney. In cramp the forces of the psyche become too directly fixed into the physical

256

organ. In the case of asthma we have seen how this gesture expresses itself in organic phenomena; it can of course equally express itself psychologically in the obsessional and phobic traits.

The presence of eosinophil cells in the walls of the bronchi and bronchioles and the secretions into them, can also be read as a gesture of the soul forces pushing down too strongly into the realm of the life processes. The invasion of the organism by foreign proteins and parasites can call forth a response from the soul forces and this tends to express itself in eosinophilia. Lymphocytes are more the expression of the 'life' forces as distinct from the 'soul' forces. The general picture is that processes which would be rightfully experienced as conscious sense phenomena become displaced into more physiological realms.

In some asthmatic patients another range of factors becomes of importance, the meteorological, geological and temporal. There are patients who are particularly sensitive to the weather. In some it is damp, in others more dry weather which disposes to asthma. Again, cold and hot weather in combination with wet or dry conditions may be the important factors. Many homoeopathic remedies have become related to these conditions. Some patients find that they are helped either in the mountains or at the seaside and these polar tendencies have become established in homoeopathic experience as related to the syphilitic or sycotic types respectively (see Chapter 23). I have sought to relate the syphilitic type to the physiognomy of fear and that of the sycotic to shame. The third of Hahnemann's miasms, the psoric, is related to anxiety. Fear we have been relating to the head pole, the focus of the cognitional processes. When we are in the high mountains, amongst the eagles, our thinking finds it natural to rise into wide vision, surveying broad sweeps of time and space in all comprehensive ideas. Our fear finds its right place in giving rise to vision and all-surveying thoughts. In contrast, shame we have discerned underlying our metabolic and volitional processes, centred more in the belly. All our pursuits, all the aims we set ourselves to win, carry a worm of shame, they are less than we ourselves are, in winning them we become less than we were. We are ashamed and seek to return to the great mother to wash away our guilt, to *La mer*. There is a strange symptom in the homoeopathic materia medica calling for a physiognomic interpretation. It is in relation to the sycotic remedy *Medorrhinum*. The patient in his asthma seeks relief lying on his abdomen or in the knee-elbow position, an unusual symptom. But these are positions of prostration before a potentate, a begging for mercy or forgiveness, such as a cringing dog assumes.

The consideration of meteorological factors has led us into the controversial field of the homoeopathic miasms. Allied to these factors are the temporal ones, the times of day or night when the asthma is liable to come on or to be worse. There is a well-established tendency for asthmatic attacks to come on in the early hours of the morning. The homoeopathic materia medica specify different remedies for different hours. There is however a wide overlap and the evidence does not support a too pedantic adherence to precise hours. Midnight and soon afterwards are anxiety ridden times and often find their remedial correspondence in the arsenical remedies. Three, four, and five o'clock usually point to the liver as the source of dysfunction and it is important to observe the close relationship between the liver and climate as an additional factor. *Natrum sulphate* has strong affinity to the liver as well as sensitivity to cold and particularly damp weather, five o'clock in the morning is its time. Its liver affinity is also expressed in its depressional symptoms and morning diarrhoea. *Kali carbonate* is a three o'clock remedy, related to cold dry weather and also to the liver. Another liver remedy with a cold dry weather sensitivity is *Nux vomica*. Earlier in the early evening children in particular may start wheezing and *Pulsatilla* comes into consideration as the remedy.

The liver as a metabolic organ has pointed us in our survey of the factors entering into the genesis of asthma to the opposite, the lower pole of the organism. Asthma can arise as a complication of chronic bronchitis and pneumonia, inflammatory processes developing in the lung and bronchi. So we find constraint in the breathing can come about from both poles of the organism, from sensory processes slipping down from head to chest and from inflammatory processes pushing up from the liver and metabolism into the chest. In the same way angina pectoris can develop from above in the asthenic type and from below in the pyknic type. In so-called cardiac asthma, really a pulmonary oedema, we are dealing with a failure of the heart's balancing function, usually in face of the liver crisis in the early hours of the morning.

Asthma can arise from the most varied causes. These causes are paths along which we can enter into the constraint and spasm in breathing which we know in its full development as the asthmatic attack, in lesser degrees as airways obstruction. From the homoeopathic viewpoint the remedies which have been found useful in treating these patients seem to be related to these different paths rather than to the final condition. The so-called modalities, the times and other circumstances of onset or aggravation of the dyspnoea, when read physiognomically, point to these paths of functional disorder. We should aim to discern as well, the inner relatedness of the respective remedies to these functions. The homoeopathic similarity should be found between the remedy and these functional paths we have attempted to grasp.

In cases where asthma follows shock and fright we have to do with a particular expression of the reactions which follow these events. In a severe fright we jump out of our skins and do not always get back in again harmoniously. Our soul gets most easily dislocated from the organism in the genital functions. This can be seen in the frequency of menstrual dysfunctions which follow on shocks and also in the case of men there can arise impotence and a host of other functional disorders.

258

The soul forces then seek compensatory entry back into the organic processes elsewhere, for instance in cramps in the alimentary system or in the bronchi in asthma. Silver as *Argentum pr.* 6x is an archetypal remedy in the therapy of such cases. Opium, also an obvious moon remedy, in higher potencies is often very helpful, as of course are *Aconite, Ignatia* and *Pulsatilla* in particular in such cases. Susceptibility to shock and fright is a characteristic of the hysterical make-up, which is 'allergic to shocks'.

Anxiety which is so central a feature of the asthmatic experience leads us to arsenic as a remedy, as *Arsenicum album, Cuprum arsenicosum* and *Kali arsenicosum*. Arsenic acts in the physiological processes in a destructive manner in a similar way to that in which the soul forces can work. It can therefore help to release the soul again when it gets imprisoned in, for example, the chest.

Anger can also give rise to asthmatic attacks and then looks rather like those fish which puff themselves up with fury. *Chamomilla* is probably the best remedy in such cases, usually in children. But *Cuprum* also relates to these problems of cramp and spasm and temper tantrums.

The allergic aspect often relates to arsenic but here homoeopathic potencies of the allergen may also help. In those cases where eczema and asthma succeed each other arsenic and sulphur will probably be called for. The fastidious anxious chilly arsenic standing as a polarity to the gregarious untidy warm blooded sulphur in the same way as do the nervous and metabolic functions to each other.

With sulphur we move into the sphere of the liver with *Nux vomica* and *Natrum sulphate* and *Kali carbonicum*. With the wheezing chests of children *Ipecacuanha* is often indicated and *Sambucus* can be useful. *Rumex* is helpful when the wheezing is sensitive to cold air. *Spongia* can be dramatically helpful and again there is sensitivity to cold dry air and the attacks may awaken from sleep as indeed they do with *Sambucus*.

In anthroposophical medicine a treatment for the asthmatic constitutional tendency is based on subcutaneous injections of three remedies given successively. On the first day *Prunus spinosa* 6x is given subcutaneously in the neck, on the second day *Nicotiana tabaccum* 10x in the renal angle and on the third *Gencydo* 1% is between the scapulae. The interval can be every second day and the course repeated after a few days. The *Prunus spinosa* restores the vitality, the *Nicotiana* brings order into the air element, the vehicle of the soul forces and the *Gencydo* (lemon and quince) helps with the allergic processes in the mucous membrane. This treatment can help to bring order into the disordered balance of the organism and enable other remedies to act more effectively.

Needless to say, the acute attack of asthma must be stopped as quickly as possible and antispasmodic inhalants should be used if necessary. Sometimes subcutaneous injections of *Lobelia* 6x will terminate an attack as will an injection of *Arsenicum album* in homoeopathic potency 10x or 30x.

It used to be said that to treat asthma successfully one must have absolute confidence in the treatment that one uses, and that one should use a new treatment whilst it still works. The danger of this approach lies in the consequence that the already anxiety-ridden sufferer is made ever more dependent on the physician and treatment. The opposite danger experienced in homoeopathic treatment is to fall into symptom chasing, every new relapse, accompanied by fresh symptoms, leading to new prescriptions. It is therefore necessary to deepen understanding of the processes involved both in the condition and in the remedies. Then treatment can be conducted reasonably, not fanatically, and with consistency rather than in a haphazard manner, dictated by the unconscious manipulation by the patient. Experience teaches how difficult this can be, but the above discussion can perhaps be helpful towards keeping one's head in the maze of symptoms and opinions.

33. Rheumatoid arthritis

We all know, to some extent, how diseases change over the centuries. Not only do acute diseases manifest as epidemics of relatively short duration, but chronic diseases as well can be regarded as invading communities in great tidal waves. In the last four or five centuries, our own civilization has undergone successive epidemics of syphilis, tuberculosis and today cancer. We could also describe multiple sclerosis and coronary infarction as becoming epidemic during this century. It seems that rheumatoid disease was unknown before 1800. So characteristic are its appearances that it would have been difficult indeed for it to have escaped the attention not only of physicians but of the observant eyes of writers and artists, not to mention the absence of skeletal evidence in cemeteries. In contrast 20% or thereabouts of the skeletons of the soldiers of Alexander the Great have been described as suffering from ankylosing spondylitis. Here is a feature which we must endeavour to grasp in our conception of rheumatoid disease; it has appeared as a scourge since 1800 when it was first described by Landré-Beauvais.

Another important feature is its occurrence four times as often in women as in men. Again this contrasts with both ankylosing spondylitis and gout which are predominantly diseases of men.

Rheumatoid disease tends to commence in the joints of the hands and feet and then to spread centripetally to wrists and ankles, to knees and elbows and then to hips, shoulders and spine. Although this is of course by no means always the case, it does seem to be so characteristic that we must bring it into our total view. We can again, without overemphasizing the point, note the contrast to ankylosing spondylitis.

We can at this point bring into our consideration two quite striking clinical observations. Firstly there is the tendency, in about three out of four women with rheumatoid arthritis who become pregnant, for the disease to remit during the pregnancy. In the remaining case it may get worse. Secondly there is the tendency for a remission to occur in the course of intercurrent infective hepatitis. It seems to me that these two clinical observations can offer us a launching pad for our homoeopathic considerations, together with the frequency with which the onset follows shocks of various kinds, and the fact that the disease manifests predominantly in the joints and in the connective tissues which might also be called joining tissues.

Let us then start with the remission of the disease in pregnancy and in hepatitis. Are we here in that realm of disease phenomena which led Hahnemann to the formulation of homoeopathy? He had noted how a disease would often remit during an intercurrent illness and return when this had passed. He therefore was led to give a new drug-induced disease to suppress, neutralize and wipe out the original natural disease, adding that the more similar the drug disease was to the natural one the more likely was the neutralization to take effect. Our problem then is to discern the similarity of hepatitis on the one hand and of pregnancy on the other to rheumatoid arthritis. Both considerations may lead us along unusual tracks.

Infective hepatitis is characterized on the emotional side by depression. A paralysis of the will is the essence of the depression. I feel that it is often helpful to see endogenous depression as a hepatitis in which the jaundice and physical aspects are reduced to vanishing whilst the emotional side comes fully to expression. How are rheumatoid and depression related? In both conditions there is a severe interference with activity, with the manifestation and expression of the will. In depression the will is itself paralysed inwardly, in rheumatoid the instruments of its expression, the limbs are damaged and made obstacles to, rather than instruments of, the will. In both cases the will is paralysed to a greater or lesser extent.

Has mankind always been subject to depression? We must, I believe, learn to differentiate between the emotion of sadness and the melancholic temperament and to distinguish both from what we nowadays call depression (with its boredom, inner emptiness, sense of meaninglessness, uselessness). Now I personally am of the opinion that whereas sadness and the melancholic temperament have been always with us, depression as a widespread pandemic is a comparatively new experience. Are rheumatoid patients depressed? Mostly I have not found them to be so. On the contrary they often seem, in spite of their pain and disability, to be remarkably cheerful and equanimous. They seem to have succeeded in keeping intact a somewhat limited personality by the sacrifice of their capacity for physical action. Somewhat similarly the appearance of frank jaundice is often the reliever of the more intense depression of the prodromal phase. These phenomena can be grouped with the alternation of mental and physical symptoms familiar to both schools of medicine as well as with those disease metamorphoses called, in psychosomatic medicine, syndrome shifts. They do, I believe, belong to the homoeopathic idea of the similar though we must deepen our concept of the similar to grasp this. When we observe the wonderful range of metamorphoses in nature and watch how from the egg grows the caterpillar which then within the cocoon or chrysalis undergoes the transformation from which emerges the butterfly, we are at pains to see the likeness of caterpillar and butterfly. Yet they are differing expressions of the same archetype. Perhaps in some similar way we can look upon depression, jaundice and rheumatoid as differing metamorphoses of one archetype.

Now if I am at all justified in connecting depression and rheumatoid in this way, as modern phenomena, and in the case of rheumatoid regarding it as really only coming into being since about 1800, we have to try and understand this fact. That was the time when Hahnemann was beginning his life's work; it was a time of great geniuses, Beethoven, Goethe, Napoleon, Kant, to name but a few. It was the time of the aftermath of the French Revolution and of the beginnings of the industrial revolution. The age of natural science had been developing since the fifteenth century and the thoughts of this natural science were crystallizing out of theory and observation into machines, into technology. This mode of thinking which quite explicitly regards mechanism as the ultimate model of truth was now bearing fruit in technology. It was also beginning to overwhelm the older religious view of things and those older, more primitive modes of science such as astrology and alchemy. By insisting that only the outer aspects of experience, which could be grasped quantitatively and mechanistically, were objective and real whilst the qualitative aspects were secondary, merely subjective, really illusory, this mode of thought opened an inner emptiness in the human soul, a veritable doubt in the soul's existence. Here I believe we come upon the ground of the modern malaise of boredom and depression. Only if we ourselves become inwardly active within this emptiness can we hope to overcome our crisis. The paintings of Kandinsky, one of the most significant artists of the twentieth century, show that he understood this present century as utterly dependent on the development of real innerness, and its true culture as consisting only in this inner activity. It is a message still sorely needed and largely unheeded.

The appearance of machines in industry and the enslaving of millions of human beings to these machines also marks a quite new influence in human affairs. Up till this time human beings were certainly involved in labour, often heavy and burdensome. But the rhythms of this labour were part of the natural world, they were dominated by the seasons, the climate, the rhythm of day and night. The machines available did not dictate mechanical rhythms to human beings. Women worked, but again, whether in house and home or field, or in producing materials and so on, their activities were full of spiritual and emotional impulses. Suddenly they found themselves tied to machines and the mechanical movements and rhythms of these machines passed over into their fingers and hands and from there into their feelings and thoughts. Times of work, too, became dictated by the clock and factory whistle rather than by the everchanging rhythms of day and night and of the seasons. What had started in the regular hours of monastic ritual here found its death knell in the factory whistle, as Lewis Mumford pointed out. Now I would draw attention to the following. Whereas men with their male intellect created, and were to some extent at home in, the world of the machines and could always find fascination in their working, women experienced the machine much more passively through their fingers which were tied to these products of the male intellect. For only exceptionally are women really interested in the working of these monsters.

Could it be that here we can begin to gain an insight into how it is that rheumatoid arthritis affects women more than men and attacks first into fingers and hands, from outside inwards? It is naturally not only the actual women working on the machines who are influenced in these ways. We all, through the levels of our being which Jung called the collective unconscious, participate mutually in these influences and it may well be that the individual working on the machine is not the one in whom the results are first experienced.

We must leave this question in order to enquire into the other problem, the similarity of pregnancy to rheumatoid, which could afford a homoeopathic understanding of the remission of arthritis during pregnancy.

Rheumatoid arthritis is predominantly a disease of joints and of those joining tissues we call connective. What are joints? We all know the words 'To join together in holy matrimony', and if we may follow for a moment the genius of language we may gain some insight into our problem. Already we have landed into the middle; genius has the same root as *join* and perhaps points to the role of the genius in joining the worlds of conscious and unconscious together or, if you prefer it, the spiritual and material worlds. Other words with the same root are gynae (woman), genesis, generation, genu the knee, gnosis and knowledge. In Shakespeare we find the wonderful expression 'The pregnant hinges of the knee' and in Homer, 'The future lies in the knees of the gods' (often translated as the lap of the gods). Everywhere we find in this root the idea of generation. Knowledge was originally a living experience, Adam knew Eve, and the word origin contains the same root. To know is to discover the origin. Now we also use the word arthros for a joint, as in arthritis. Here we come across the root *rt* and suddenly we have passed from the woman's to the man's role in sex, rod, root, radius. The word heart contains the same root and points to the strange connexion between diseases of joints and of the heart. The heart is of course the organ of love and is closely related functionally to the uterus which again has this, *tr*, *rt*, in it and heart and uterus are both hollow muscular organs. Need I remind you that gold has an affinity for hearts, uteruses and joints and is in addition a major remedy for depression. In arthritis the joints swell and become pregnant. Is it surprising that during the swelling of the uterus in pregnancy, the joints may be relieved?

There are other remedies with affinity for joints as well as heart and uterus. *Pulsatilla*, the pasque-flower, with pains which flit from place to place, is also characterized by menstruation which may be suppressed by shock. *Pulsatilla* has affinity for the veins whereas its close friend amongst the Rununculaceae *Adonis vernalis*, the pheasant's eye, acts more upon the heart. It is to the heart what *Pulsatilla* is to the uterus. *Sepia* with its great affinity for the female organs of generation is also profoundly related to depression and to disease of the joints, particularly of the knee. *Caulophyllum* is related to pregnancy and labour but also to the small joints of the hand. *Mandragora* which I find invaluable in the local treatment of arthritis is in myth and legend and ancient usage associated with sexual function. Another remedy from ancient times, *Colchicum*, the autumn crocus, is in addition to its action in gout a powerful mitotic poison interfering with cell division. *Kalmia*, one of the Ericaceae, acts upon heart and joints, the pains progressing centrifugally, whereas in *Ledum*, another member of the same family, the pains move from feet and hands upwards. With *Ledum* we have a strange connection, through its action on insect stings, with *Apis*, another powerful rheumatic remedy, and with *Formica* from the ants. Yet another member of the Ericaceae deserves mention — *Rhododendron* which in addition to its rheumatic symptoms has pain in the testicles, as of course do *Pulsatilla* and *Aurum*.

In mentioning these remedies which relate such unexpected realms of our functions and organs I hope to suggest that they can also become research tools with which we can open up hidden connections and processes in diseases.

Among the remedies related to the liver and often of value in treating cases of rheumatoid we must mention *Sulphur*, *Calcarea* and *Lycopodium*, the great antipsoric triumvirate. *Phosphorus*, *Silica*, *Arsenic* and *Causticum* can all be of great help as well.

In the homoeopathic treatment of depression there are three metals of outstanding importance and they can all play their part also in rheumatoid treatment. Gold, *Aurum*, is the best known homoeopathic remedy for severe depression. We know it also as a valuable heart remedy, and at least in the form of Myocrisin it has undoubted relationship to rheumatoid disease. Tin, *Stannum*, is the second metal which I have repeatedly found useful in depression. It is related to the liver and to the fluid organization over which the liver exercises a sort of imperium; it acts as far as into the muscles and cartilage, but not into the bones. The third important metal is iron, *Ferrum*, which in homoeopathic forms can fire the will with resolve and is quite as important as the other two in depressional states.

I mentioned earlier the importance of emotional stress and of shock in the onset of rheumatoid disease. It is commonly observed. I know of a patient who first had rheumatoid arthritis in her early twenties. The disease went into remission and caused no further trouble until near her retirement at sixty. Then one day, whilst she was sitting stationary in her car, it was run into by another. As she said, she was for some moments frozen with shock and fright. Next day her joints were all actively swollen and painful. How do shocks of this sort act? One is liable to feel, when shocked, that one is, as the saying is, frightened out of one's skin. Sometimes people do not get back quite inside their skins again. They feel this. Now where in our organization is this psychic dislocation, this separation of body and soul, most likely to happen? On the whole, women are more liable to this sort of trouble than men, their psyches are more loosely united with their somas than is the case with men. We all know how easily menstrual function can be disturbed, even suppressed, by shock. But we should also notice how impotence in men is easily determined by emotional factors. I cannot help feeling that the genital organs and functions are more exposed to the effects of shock than any other. I can only hazard the guess, remembering the relationship between pregnancy and rheumatoid disease, that in those cases where the disease is set off by shock this is secondary to the dislocation in the genital functions. What happens is comparable with the processes in conversion hysteria. The hysteric is incidentally almost allergic to shock.

I have seen quite a few cases in young women where the onset has followed quickly upon marriage. There has not been in the cases I have seen any openly expressed shock or distaste for marriage. They remind one in a way of what used to be called honeymoon cystitis, and point towards the use of another member of the Ranunculaceae, *Staphisagria*. They indicate to us, I suspect, the profoundly hidden resentments and the bottling-up of emotion and aggression which have been revealed in psychological testing. *Aconite, Pulsatilla* and *Staphysagria*, three members of the buttercup family, seem to correspond to aspects of what I have attempted to describe — fright, uterine shock, resentment.

There are, however, other cases in which more sustained grief and unhappiness and stress have been the emotional background to the onset and here of course we think of *Natrum muriaticum* with its relationship to the adrenal gland and the stress disorders, and to the bowel nosode Proteus.

I cannot leave the problem without mentioning some observations. Acting on the idea that there is a sort of fulcrum of life's seesaw at twenty-eight years of age, so that events so many years before this date find a compensatory event the same number of years after it, I have enquired of patients in whom rheumatoid arthritis came on fairly suddenly after twenty-eight years of age. I am indebted for the idea to Rudolf Steiner who stressed this age of twenty-eight in the unfolding of individual destiny. Now obviously this can relate to a limited number of these patients only, to those whose arthritis commences between twenty-eight and fifty-six years of age. However let us take a few out of many cases to illustrate the idea.

There was a woman whom I saw, aged fifty-seven. Her severe rheumatoid had started suddenly the previous year at fifty-six. Going back to twenty-eight and the same number of years again we reach birth and infancy. To my enquiry as to what befell her in infancy she at once replied that she was born illegitimate and her well-to-do grandparents had arranged for and paid for her to be brought up by an austere but competent spinster. The new home was a model of efficiency and cleanliness but without warmth or love.

Another woman developed rheumatoid at thirty-six, I therefore asked what happened when she was twenty. 'I got married.' Why? To get away from home.

A woman came to see me having developed carcinoma of the breast at forty-four, followed by dermatomyositis at forty-seven. At nine she had been sent home from India. She was miserably unhappy with resentment and a sense of deprivation. Her dermatomyositis has improved whilst she has had Iscador treatment for her carcinoma.

Another woman developed acute rheumatoid at forty-four following a severe fall. Asked what had happened at twelve she looked puzzled, as if I was mad, then suddenly said: How strange, that was when I had my first bad fall down a staircase and was on a water bed for three months.

These are only a small selection from cases where the same pattern emerged. One other case I will mention. A woman developed interstitial cystitis at forty. At sixteen she had lost a very dear sister and her parents would not or could not tell her. She found out accidentally some months later and was deeply enraged and distressed.

I have been looking for these cases and obligingly they have turned up. Maybe I have attracted them. But if there is something in it, as we say, then it extends the psychosomatic field of observation considerably and we shall have to learn to live into the organism of time, observing more widely the ways in which cause and effect, or perhaps better said event and compensatory event, are related. In these observations, the earlier the traumatic event the later its compensatory outcome appears.

There are other aspects of this disease which deserve discussion and which could lead to further insights. There are the contrasting ways in which it can begin, quite suddenly on the one hand and slowly and insidiously on the other. What do these contrasting styles of onset signify? There is the inflammatory nature of the disease process and the contrast between acute inflammations, usually leading to healing, and the chronic inflammations which never seem to be able to achieve their object. And how are the immunological phenomena related to the inflammatory?

In practice, in attempting to treat so complex and variable a symptom complex an elastic approach seems desirable. I have found it useful to pursue the treatment on different levels at the same time, using lowish potencies for local symptoms at the same time as high potencies for the more general and mental factors or apparent precipitating factors. I am relieved that none other than the late C. E. Wheeler thought such approaches justified. He also considered the use of compound remedies legitimate. I have over many years made use of subcutaneous injections of *Apis* and of *Formica* for the local manifestation and also of the preparations of *Cartilago mandragora Cps.* (Wala), and *Disci c. stanno* (Wala). They were often very useful whilst at the same time high potencies were given for the general condition.

In trying to take some steps towards grasping the bewildering clinical and epidemiological aspects of this disease in a meaningful whole, I am well aware that what I have written is tentative, but during the course of working at this approach I have myself gained certain insights, glimpses of meaning and relationship between bizarrely different phenomena for which I am very grateful. The first thread through the labyrinth was found in the remission of the rheumatoid process during pregnancy and hepatitis, phenomena belonging, I believe, essentially to Hahnemann's basic realization and observation. The second thread was found in the remedies which play upon the processes of this disease. Used as research instruments, these reveal and confirm the insight won with the first thread. I believe we should use our remedies much more in this way. It will require increasing study of the way they occur in nature, as well as in the human realm in the processes of disease and healing.

This is only a short step towards an understanding of this disease and there are many other aspects of the pathology not touched upon. On the basis of homoeopathic ways of thought I have tried to put forward an approach which may be of use or at least understandable to the other two main medical schools of our time — the mechanistic school of the laboratories and the psychoanalytically derived approaches through the emotions and instinctive forces. I believe it is very important today to try to understand each other and to build bridges between rival standpoints but it will be difficult and need all our goodwill and effort to achieve this end.

34. Cancer

The disease phenomena occurring in the course of cancer are very disturbing and not simply because of pain and other complications of a chronic progressive illness. There seem to be no valid reasons for the development of a malignant tumour. Unlike inflammatory diseases which can be understood as the organism's reaction to and defence against invasion by foreign agents, the tumour seems a meaningless breakdown in the integrity of the organism. Meaninglessness and chaos face us here as they do in so much of modern life and they demand of us that we combat their evil and transform it into higher meaning. As an aim it is not enough to extirpate the evil; it is necessary to redeem it and restore again into its place in the sun that which has fallen out of the human estate. In this sense we can hazard the guess that overcoming cancer depends really on achieving a higher, more whole and inclusive level of existence than was ours before.

We can make a start by trying to place the tumour diseases in their relationship to other conditions. We can for instance establish a spectrum of diseases between two polar opposites as has been done by the Bahnsons. At one pole we can place cancer and at the other insanity, perhaps more definitively schizophrenia. Neither of these two are of course clear-cut entities but they do stand usefully for two extreme tendencies in disease.

In the cancer disease the disturbances in the bodily structures, the organs, tissues and cells predominate, whilst the changes in what we can call the personality are minimal. Somebody with cancer does not cease to be himself, he is not beside himself, he remains interested in the normal life around him. Deeper psychological testing can reveal abnormal traits but they do not prevent normal human communication. Probably the embarrassment of friends and family and often of the doctors too, are more of a difficulty than the patient's own troubles.

In contrast to this we find in the psychoses and in schizophrenia in particular, a deterioration and disintegration of the personality whilst the body retains a surprising health. It is difficult to localize the disease, a point which comes out when we remember that for over two hundred years controversy has continued as to whether mental illnesses are diseases of the brain or not. In schizophrenia the personality disintegrates whilst the body remains intact; communication can become wellnigh impossible. In cancer the body disintegrates whilst the personality remains sane. Cancer patients only exceptionally commit suicide. Schizophrenics are to a great extent protected from developing cancer and even the families of schizophrenics have been shown to be less liable to cancer than the rest of the population. These considerations raise important issues in relation to the body-soul problems. The old adage, *Mens sana in corpore sano*, is utterly inadequate.

The Bahnsons proposed a spectrum of diseases between the cancers at one extremity and schizophrenia at the other. Hysteria as a mid-point could move to one side into mental symptomatology, through anxieties, phobias, obsessions, depressions, manic-depressive illness to paranoia and schizophrenia. On the other side it could move into physical symptomatology through conversion hysterias, anaesthesias and paralyses to so-called psychosomatic conditions such as migraine and allergies. Then on to more somatic conditions such as peptic ulceration, rheumatism and arthritis, diabetes and other metabolic disorders to the extreme of the cancers. There is a similarity between such a proposal and Hahnemann's characterization (150 years earlier) of one-sided diseases with an intermediate range of conditions in between. What did he mean by one-sided diseases? He said that most presenting illnesses had both mental and local disturbances. An asthmatic patient has both local breathing trouble in the chest and usually anxiety as well. But some conditions present entirely as local disturbances with no obvious mental symptoms whilst others show all the disorder in the mental realm with no discernible local symptoms. It seems to me that cancer and schizophrenia in the sense described fit quite well into this polarity of one-sided diseases.

From another point of view we can try to find where processes comparable to tumour formation can be found in the healthy organism. Diseases can be approached as normal processes in the wrong time or place. Many people have been struck by a similarity between tumour formation and pregnancy. Psycho-analytical investigations have long been familiar with the pregnancy symbolism of many diseases and particularly of the tumour diseases. The gesture of pregnancy is an interiorization whereas the gesture of male genitality is an exteriorization. The phenomena of male sexual function are inflammatory in nature and polar to the tumour forming nature of pregnancy. Male sexual behaviour is also characterized by excitement which can easily culminate in mania. We must also notice that the carcinomata start upon a surface and grow inwards into the centripetally flowing veins and lymphatics. They do not invade the centrifugally flowing arteries, nor for that matter do the sarcomata, although these do not arise from surfaces. Inflammations on the contrary easily penetrate into the arteries and their tendency is always to exteriorize, to discharge to a surface.

But even if we can accept such a correspondence between a pregnancy and a tumour there are obviously great differences. Can we trace some aspects or steps in the metamorphosis from pregnancy to a cancer, albeit a retrogressive metamorphosis? We can starting from a normal pregnancy, move to twins and

then to Siamese twins. One of the Siamese twins may be deficient in some organs
and so only a partial not a whole organism. It can be said to be parasitic on the
other. But we also know of teratomata, tumours which may consist of a limb or
part of a limb, or of mixed tissues of varied type, and some of these become
invasive and malignant. We also have benign tumours in which the tissues resemble
the normal tissue from which they arise. But a metamorphosis towards more
malignant and invasive character is usually attended by the tumour tissue becoming
increasingly distorted from the normal. In anaplastic tumours it may be impossible
to determine the origin, so de-differentiated have the cells and tissues become. In
benign tumours the tissue structure is normal but the tumour itself does not
conform to the normal form of the organs.

In a normal pregnancy the gradual orderly differentiation of cells, tissues and
organs takes place in the embryo. The primitive undifferentiated cells, omnipotential, become specialized into nerve cells, muscle cells, blood cells and so on. They
become ordered into, first the germ layers, ecto- meso- and endo-derm. From
these layers or leaves are developed the tissues of the body. They are archetypally
two-dimensional and repeat a vegetative form, though as we have seen elsewhere,
the nerve tissue becomes linear, one-dimensional like the fungi. Nevertheless the
nervous system originates from the folding of the planar ectoderm, but in it the
cellular element comes to dominate. In the development of the carcinomata from
epithelium arising from ecto- or endo-derm the planar character of this epithelium
becomes distorted and begins to invade and becomes three-dimensional rather
than two-dimensional. Organs arise out of the interweaving of the tissues and are
morphologically three-dimensional. They are normally well-ordered into characteristic anatomical forms and sizes. Tumours again break down the ordered form
of organs. So all that has come about in embryogenesis in the forming of the
specialized cells, tissues and organs becomes to a great extent undone in tumour
formation.

We can describe the process as a regression, taking over an idea from psychoanalytic theory as proposed by Ferenczi as long ago as 1923. In the benign tumour
the organ-forming has become misplaced, a pseudo-organ form comes into existence but with normal tissues and cells. In pre-cancerous or pre-invasive stages of
cancer formation, the tissues are also deformed and then in fully developed cancer
the cells regress to primitive embryonal forms. What is progressively or rather
regressively destroyed by this metamorphic process is the form of the organism.
And so the question arises, from where do the normal form-producing forces arise
in embryogenesis which result in a baby rather than a tumour?

The embryo comes to lie in the amniotic fluid within the uterus; in a similar
manner the brain floats in the cerebro-spinal fluid within the skull. The brain is a
synthesis of the organs of the body. We can also see how the embryo looks like
an ear. It seems to be listening with its whole being. Does it perchance hearken
to the music of the spheres before 'this muddy vesture of decay doth grossly close

it in'? Are not tones and music the origins of form? We dance to music and make visible in form the inner quality of sound. In the phenomena of Chladni's figures, when powder on a sheet is vibrated by a bow drawn over it, forms of immense variety arise in the powder. We can imagine the human embryo responding to the cosmic music and unfolding the human form as microcosmic image of the macrocosm. We can also imagine that animal embryos respond only to partial aspects of the cosmos, not to the whole zodiac (animal circle). Tumours are even more partial than animals and seem to be the expression of noise rather than music.

We can now approach one of the indications about cancer given by Steiner to doctors. He suggested that we could begin to understand cancer as a misplaced sense organ, more particularly as a misplaced ear. In the head, the realm of the sense organs, the ear and eye constitute a polarity comparable with the female and male genital organs in the pelvic reproductive realm. Whether we try to understand the tumour as a sort of monstrous pregnancy or as a misplaced ear formation it is really saying much the same. In Michelangelo's portrayals in the Sistine Chapel of the creation of Adam and Eve, it is clear that Adam awakes to the vision of the divine whilst Eve is called from the embrace to go forward to pregnancy. In artistic portrayals of the Annunciation the attitude of the Virgin is one of hearkening.

Now if the tendency comes about for ear formation to be displaced, or we might say for the tendency to develop consciousness in the unconscious metabolic organs, to want to know in the sense of the conscious head pole rather than to do, then a tumour may come about.

If this happens we might anticipate that in the nervous system itself certain pathological processes could result. The nervous system and senses are polar to the metabolic and reproductive organs. If then a displacement of ear formation comes about or an awakening in the metabolic organs, then corresponding disturbances might be expected in the nervous organs. Of recent decades much attention has been given to certain paramalignant syndromes. These are a varied group of conditions occurring in relation to malignant tumours but not directly caused by them. Of particular interest are the group of neuromyopathies which may mimic almost any disease of the nervous system and varied muscular disorders. These conditions may arise years before any sign of an actual tumour or cancer comes about. Can we therefore regard them as secondary phenomena to the cancer? Must we not begin to consider them as amongst the primary archetypal phenomena? They probably occur in over 80% of cases of cancer when carefully looked for. It could be that the identification of cancer with the appearance of the tumour mistakes the final stage of the disease with the disease itself.

One further idea relating to the development of cancer needs our attention. It was also suggested to doctors by Steiner. He tried to indicate how forces which in infancy and childhood are mainly occupied with growth and building the bodily organism become, from the time of the change of teeth onwards, so to speak surplus to requirements. What becomes or should become of these surplus forces? It is a matter of concern to doctors and teachers. Our customary ideas of metamorphosis are confined to phenomena in the physical world. We observe the metamorphosis in plants of the leaf into blossoms and fruit. Likewise we observe animal metamorphoses such as the butterfly which emerges after the successive metamorphoses of egg into caterpillar, chrysalis and then into butterfly. Tadpoles become frogs and foetuses undergo striking metamorphosis at birth when the baby opens its lungs and begins to take nourishment. Now we are faced with an extension of the concept of metamorphosis so that we can look for the transformation of forces manifesting on the organic level into forces of thinking, memory and imagination. We think and form mental images with the same forces as earlier were used in growth and body forming. Hegel himself recognized that his mode of thinking was a continuation and extension of the mode of observation used by Goethe in his studies of metamorphosis in nature.

The task of education after the change of teeth is to lead over these forces from the sphere of organic life into the soul realm as thinking and imagination. This metamorphosis calls for methods more artistic than intellectual in style. Intellectual methods fail to lead over these forces and then some of them remain behind in the organic depths as islands of untransformed growth forces. If these forces are unable to find their way, through inadequate educational methods, into progressive upward metamorphosis then we can be sure they will not stay still but will regress, atavistically. In this way islands of regressed forces are formed in the organism to become nuclei of potential tumour formation.

It is not difficult to see that in the prevailing hyper-intellectualized climate of our times many of the more delicate and imaginative thoughts trying to come to consciousness are simply rejected. If Darwinism was the expression of the *laissez-faire* liberal capitalism of the last century, it has now itself become the stimulus to the hyper-competitiveness prevailing in all walks of life. The ego-centric will to be top-dog is seen as justified by the adage, the Devil take the hindmost. And all moral restraints on the will are seen as soft sentimentality. A ferocious unbridled will activity aimed only at supremacy and power at all costs has become the order of the day. The far more valid ideas of Peter Kropotkin in *Mutual Aid* are scarcely mentioned. An image of these unbridled forces, antisocial and utterly self-interested, faces us in the cell life in a malignant tumour. All social restraints needed for the welfare of the whole organism are rejected by the cells.

Gerhardt Booth was able to show how the psyche of cancer patients revealed certain compulsive, obsessional traits which in the jargon of psychoanalysis revealed to him anal-erotic character. The predominant social cultural values from the last decades of the nineteenth century onward have had the same features. The cancer psyche in his view is equally the dominant psyche of this period of history. The cancer psyche is the 'normal' psyche of the last hundred years when the impulse to possess and dominate has reached its acme. Contrasted with this character he found the psyche of tuberculous patients to be idealistic and romantic and to correspond with the prevailing social and cultural values of the earlier one or two centuries. In the psychoanalytic jargon he characterized these as genital erotic. It was during that earlier phase that the life of the feelings emancipated itself from domination by exclusively religious images and that Art became secular. Now in this century the will has become amoral. Everything is permitted to the superior man, as Dostoievsky put into the mouths of some of his characters.

An attempt has been made to approach the riddle of cancer first by seeing it as polar opposite to insanity; then as a distorted pregnancy in which the normal form of development, the miracle of embryogenesis, becomes a regressive destruction of form. This led also to the image of the tumour as a displaced ear formation, a sense organ into which foreign, we might say sub-human forces penetrate rather than the form-producing music of the spheres. Then arose the problem of the metamorphosis of the growth and formative forces from the organic level of action into forces by means of which we think. Through failure of this process many islands of untransformed growth forces are left behind in the organism, where they regress and may become centres of tumour formation. Finally we have noted the coincidence of the cancer psyche or character traits with the prevailing dominant values, the norm, of our times, and that of the tuberculous psyche with the ruling ideals of the previous period. Moreover it seems that from about 1500 onwards it was at first thinking that became emancipated and possessed by the individuality. And to this emancipated thinking the leaders of the time looked as heralding the millennium. Syphilis coincided with this movement; syphilis which as a pandemic destroyed any organ but particularly the very brain.

Syphilis, tuberculosis and cancer are the three great archetypal diseases which during the last 500 years have attacked successively the brain and nervous system, the lung as representative of the rhythmic system and the main organ of the emotional life, and then the metabolic and reproductive organs on which the will is founded. Cancer is a disease in which the tumours destroy the organs of the metabolic and reproductive system. Even when it attacks the lung, it is from the bronchi that it develops and these originate from the alimentary tract. I have the impression that it attacks the lung as a metabolic organ rather than as organ of the rhythmic system. Tumours of the brain do not arise from the nervous elements but from supportive tissues.

Now we have suggested that the epidemic of cancer today, of course linked with more people growing into the cancer-prone period of life, is connected also with the unbridled emancipation of the will. The old moral sanctions no longer have any effectiveness if in fact judging from history they ever did. At the most they seem to have held up an unattainable standard which served to show man up as a sinner, a fallen state. Most moral codes enshrine the will to power of particular tribes, groups, classes, nations. And what is usually called conscience is, as Nietzsche showed, the voice of one's own tribe in oneself. 'Thus conscience doth make cowards of us all'. We have learnt that moral codes are accepted by those in whose interests they work.

So where are we? The cells in the metabolic realm get out of control and multiply, denying the restraining, form-producing, differentiating forces on each level of organization: that of cells, tissues and organs. If however we recall the forces whose failed upward-metamorphosis resulted in atavistic islands, nuclei of tumour formation, then must we not try to imagine what these forces could have become? Could these forces have become or contributed to the capacity for intuition of the good, not some abstract code of goodness but the capacity to grasp the new creative deeds in the particular situations and crises of actual life? These free deeds may indeed arise out of the heart but they need a mobile imaginative thinking to meet them. It is the capacity to grasp what should and could be and the courage to realize it.

The vast upsurge in violence, terrorism, vandalism all over the world point to the failure of the established social values to include into the social order the forces working pathologically in these phenomena. Is it not time to try to understand them as diseases of the social organism? Again and again we are forced to consider whether it is not the very quality of which our civilization is so proud, its intellectual cleverness, that causes these reactions from the unconscious. In this sense we can question whether all this unbridled violence by individuals and gangs does not arise from the same causes as cancerous tumours. Forces vital for the full development of a cultural life through which alone life can attain meaning, are rejected by the intellectualism and materialism of our time, led tragically by a natural science which worships accident, chance and statistics as its Gods.

But these very rejected forces, however atavistic they appear, must contain the seeds of our renewal. One is encouraged to utter such thoughts by the remembrances of many who have died of cancer but who in confronting this illness have been able to unfold healing forces against it which seemed to bring about a wonderful expansion and healing of their being. Inner achievement arose and they and others were able to feel success and life accomplishment before they died. Others who have lived for many years have unfolded quite new faculties and experiences in the new life opening up.

As I have worked for many years with the anthroposophical mistletoe remedy, Iscador, in cancer, I must mention an aspect of its use in addition to its pharmacological cytotoxic and immune stimulating actions. It seems to open up and release the buried forces we have been discussing. It makes it easier for the patients to accept new impulses awakening in them, even if to their customary stereotyped viewpoints these are childish or bizarre. The handicapped children of the soul are most easily accepted in a Christmas atmosphere under the mistletoe, when all divisions of class, race, sex and so on should melt away. In an atmosphere of acceptance and forgiveness the stirrings of a new conscience born in the individual soul may be felt and the inspiration to find the creative novelty, the right thought, word and deed for the unprecedented situations in which we find ourselves. Because our crisis today is unprecedented it cannot be met with conventional moral answers. It is the birth pangs of a new world.

35.   AIDS. Historical perspectives

The whole world is currently gripped by fear of a new disease commonly known as AIDS (acquired immune deficiency syndrome). Already it is facing states in central Africa with overwhelming problems. Between a quarter to a half of hospital beds in some of the towns in this large area are occupied by sufferers from this condition. It is spreading at an alarming speed in all countries of the Western world, and both China and India, which together represent the mass of the world's population, are introducing schemes to screen all foreign students (especially from Africa) for evidence of antibodies to the infecting virus. In the developed countries it has spread up till now mainly by sexual intercourse. That this has been mostly in the homosexual communities has been due to greater promiscuity in some of these circles. The disease has also been conveyed by sharing of needles and syringes amongst drug addicts and by contaminated blood getting into blood banks for transfusion and into special preparations for use in treating haemophilia. The disease can also be transmitted by heterosexual intercourse. In Africa infected blood in transfusions is thought to have been a significant means of spread. It is beyond the technical and financial resources of these countries to introduce adequate screening of blood donors.

How the disease originated is not known. Some have suggested that it arose in Africa where it had existed endemically. Others have suggested that it arose in a laboratory engaged in molecular engineering and escaped. Sir Fred Hoyle the astronomer would probably suggest, as with other new diseases, that it came to earth from the heavens in meteoric or other debris. No one knows. It is understandable that there is panic, and propaganda programmes on an unprecedented scale are being unfurled.

History abounds in the stories and records of devastating epidemics. Thucydides recorded the great plague of Athens during the Peloponesian war. In spite of graphic descriptions no one can agree what the disease was. Some experts think that Rome was devastated by the 'new' diseases of measles and smallpox introduced from the East by the Legions. Leprosy in the Middle Ages assumed gigantic proportions, with strict isolation of cases in leper houses of which 10,000 existed in Europe. Then the Black Death, probably bubonic plague, killed at least a third of the population of Europe. Successive waves of this plague, conveyed by rats, recurred for several centuries. Some historians have estimated that of a population of 150 millions in central and southern America at the time of the Spanish invasion only five million survived a few decades later. The cause was not the might of Spanish arms but again probably measles and smallpox.

More recently at the end of the First World War a pandemic of influenza spread around the world, killing several times as many as were killed in four years of gruesome fighting.

Most of these various plagues were violent, acute conditions liable to kill in a few days. Leprosy was more chronic. There have been in recent centuries widespread epidemics of chronic diseases, and the purpose of this essay is to explore a possible correlation with man's psycho-social development. If we can, then we may also become aware of a meaning in these diseases, however cautious we must be in such matters. We may also be able to approach in an even more tentative way the meaning of AIDS. But first we may remark that these epidemics seem to have come at times of marked changes of consciousness.

The Peloponesian War marked the end of the old city states of Greece and was the prelude to the Macedonian conquests and the Alexandrian campaigns and the Hellenistic culture.

The collapse of Rome marked the collapse of the old Imperial pagan culture and the rising of the new Christian world.

Leprosy came at the transition from the Mediaeval to the Renaissance or more especially perhaps from Romanesque to Gothic, remembering how much the latter was influenced through the Crusades by the Islamic world.

Bubonic plague coming from Asia contributed to the dissolution of the feudal system and consciousness. In England the end of the Plantagenets and the coming of the Tudors can be taken as the beginning of the modern age.

Many of these crises were also connected with periods of racial mixture, most notably in the case of the discovery of America.

If we now turn our attention to the modern age starting in the fifteenth century with the final collapse of the Roman Eastern Empire, the Byzantine, in 1453, we can observe certain waves of chronic diseases following one another. Columbus returned from the Caribbean in 1493. Within a short time of his return the disease syphilis appeared and spread all across Europe. It may or may not have been physically introduced from the New World. Its epidemic growth coincided with this moment. It was the time of Martin Luther, protesting against the sexual and financial corruption of the Catholic world, and in a deeper sense affirming the right of the rising Germanic world to its own judgement and independent thought. It was the time of Paracelsus protesting against the old medical Mediterranean dogmas of Galen and the rest, and demanding observation of nature and fresh unprejudiced learning from nature herself rather than from books. In 1546 came the publication of Copernicus' new model of the solar system, the mechanism or corpse of that system, and of Vesalius' anatomy of the human corpse. The new age was born.

Thinking was becoming emancipated and independent. It was no longer prepared to accept blindly the authority of the Church. Certainly there were martyrs such as Giordano Bruno, and very nearly Galileo as well. But the movement for freedom of thought proceeded. Francis Bacon maintained the right to think freely without disturbing one's religious convictions. Essentially thinking became more abstract, merely intellectual, speculative. Vision of spiritual realities faded into mere ghosts, scientific ideas. In poetry there was the movement of philosophic or metaphysical poetry, complex thoughts woven into poems, and at the same time a tendency to aphoristic expressions, cleverness, wit, a thinking which could be called a thinking thinking, aphoristic, tending towards atomism. Now with this movement towards intellectual autonomy, even anarchy, appeared and flourished the pandemic of syphilis. This disease had a tendency to run a chronic course, through primary, secondary and tertiary stages. It could ruin all systems in the body. It had a particular tendency to destroy the brain and nervous system. It seems to me that it is in its destruction of brain and nerves that we can see its nature in its full flower. The brain, the organ of that mode of thinking then emancipating itself became destroyed by this disease.

One could ask, did this thinking undermine the brain and expose it to this assault? Or, did the disease come to prevent the worst excesses of extreme intellectualism by destroying its organ? Or, some might say, was it a punishment for the arrogance implicit in such thinking? For our present purpose we can content ourselves with noting the appearance of this new mode of natural scientific thinking, prepared to go its own way divorced from both art and the pursuit of beauty, and from religion and moral sanction and the pursuit of goodness. This came about when spiritual vision had vanished and was coincident with an epidemic which destroyed a healthy brain. Fear in particular arose as the emotional companion of this thinking. Fear of syphilis itself is a marked feature; the word syphilophobia was used to denote this. Symptoms of syphilis were often worse at night, the time of fear. At the time when the epidemic was spreading in a most virulent form there was also a veritable obsession with death, with the skeleton. There were dances of death all over Europe, and Hamlet's soliloquy over the skull of Yorick is only an articulate expression of this widespread obsession and fear. Hamlet himself is an excellent example of this emancipated, doubt-filled thinking.

After about two centuries a further movement in emancipation becomes evident. Feelings begin to assert their right to uninhibited expression. In earlier times painting, for instance, had been absorbed in portraying the established religious themes. Emotional life was cultivated in this way, emotions of devotion and so on took precedence. A scale of emotional values was imposed, based not on purely aesthetic values but on religious and moral values. Art was the servant of religion, as thinking had been in scholasticism in its time the servant of religion. Now the demand came to be felt for purely aesthetic values free from religious

279

and philosophical or scientific values. Art and the emotions began to be cultivated for their own sake, a movement culminating in the phrase 'Art for Art's sake'. Music also began to move into the Romantic age. One can also observe how with the early industrial revolution there arose idealistic movements for social reform often sponsored by families such as the Wedgwoods. These movements arose out of feelings, sentiments. In the earlier period of intellectual emancipation its foremost representatives looked to this movement of scientific freedom to create a new and better world. Members of the Royal Society certainly felt a new beginning had come about to replace the old evils. But disillusionment had set in and now Romanticism set about the cultivation of feelings, hoping in this way to reform society. Thinking became more dreamy, idealistic. In place of a 'thinking thinking' there came about a 'feeling thinking'.

What disease now became epidemic, so that every family had one or more members wasting away over years of ill-health, perhaps in sanatoria? Tuberculosis became the white man's scourge. It was not a new disease, but it now became of overwhelming importance. The life of such patients, full of romantic dreamings, is well depicted in Thomas Mann's *The Magic Mountain*.

A psychiatrist in America, G. Booth, undertook psychological Rorschach tests on tuberculous patients. He also came upon sociological studies of the dominant culture-social values in the first half of the nineteenth century. He found the two of them to be nearly identical. The tuberculous psyche corresponded to the 'normal' attitudes dominant at that time.

In which organs did tuberculosis most characteristically develop? Of course it could appear anywhere but typically it destroyed the lungs, the organs with which the feelings are most closely connected. (It has even been suggested that Chopin could not have produced such romantic yearnings in his music had he not had large resonating cavities in his lungs.) The emotions became free and proliferated in formless excess whilst the main organ of these feelings was destroyed.

Again the scene changed. Materialism became dominant. Idealistic movements for social change were overtaken by Marx's dialectic materialism and the 'science' of social revolution. Management, bureaucratic planning and control have taken the place of social idealism. Science has given up the pursuit of Truth, it is concerned only with experiment, aimed at setting the limits to particular theories. Severely pragmatic and practical, it has become the servant of capitalist profit-making or the military ambitions and fears of state governments. Moral restraints have been almost completely abolished as legalized abortion and the experimental interference with conception show. On the other hand experimental interference into the foundations of matter result in nuclear weapons, power stations and so on. Chemistry has led to universal pollution.

The point is that the sphere of the will and action have put off all moral restraint. What you can do, you may do. With this movement we find the compulsive, obsessional attitudes becoming marked. When the will is not informed by ideals and controlled by moral sense these external compulsive and obsessional regulations are regarded as the answer to all evil. The State may intervene, and inwardly the individual develops compulsive and obsessional symptoms. Just as previously we saw thinking and then feeling becoming autonomous so now too the will is emancipated from control.

G. Booth was also able to show that the character revealed in Rorschach tests of cancer patients corresponded with the prevailing social-cultural values of the end of the nineteenth and twentieth centuries. The cancer psyche is the dominant, the normal psyche of this time.

Cancer has become an epidemic and its main assault is on the metabolic and reproductive organs, the organs and functions on which the will is based. Thinking has now become merely practical, technological, concerned only with action, a 'willed thinking' but not inwardly will-filled and enlivened. It is merely the servant of a will which has lost all universal meaning and become utterly egotistic and materialistic. We have reached the point where unless we start to think actively we become thoughtless, unless we actively undertake the culture of our emotions we become inwardly empty and bored, unless we act out of conscious decision we become driven this way and that.

We can see how the three soul functions of thinking, feeling, and willing have become emancipated but at the same time mixed up and confused. Each has lost its way. To try and understand this situation we can help ourselves by looking at another most characteristic feature of our times, the realization that the world and mankind are one whole with the synchronous experience of the individual as an isolated and lonely single.

The world has become in the last hundred years very much a whole, firstly on account of the growth of technology in communications and in the economic life. Modern communications have resulted in the simultaneous reception of the same news and events over the whole planet. Economy has become world economy, all continents and nations are interwoven in the economic process. But secondly the developments in history, geography and anthropology have resulted in knowledge of the different races and cultures of mankind being freely available to everyone. When we look more closely at this vast panorama of mankind presented to us, we find that it also reveals the history of man. Different cultures have arisen at different periods of evolution; to an extraordinary extent they have persisted into our times, to be studied and recorded. Aboriginal peoples in their Australian culture show us a primordial stage of consciousness before agriculture began. Other peoples show us later stages and in the religious heritage of ancient cultures, preserved to some extent, lie treasures of human growth and development. It would of course be the grossest misjudgment to regard any of these as inferior to our own modern civilization. In a similar way we understand that the whole human being is not just the old man or woman but comprises their entire life from conception to grave and even beyond both thresholds as well.

We have before us today a panorama of mankind's evolution and history. At the same time individuals feel more and more isolated, lonely and empty of content. In the past individuals felt themselves embedded in their society, tribe, group. Its content lived in them, its order was their content. They belonged. Today increasingly every individual is bereft and isolated, alienated. The world as a whole appears chaotic, its order is inaccessible to the stock of concepts, accessible to us through our education. The question 'Who am I?' becomes increasingly insistent.

It is obvious that from these two sides we stand today at a crisis point. Popular journalism has of late given much publicity to records of 'near death' experience. At moments of extreme danger many persons near death have recorded the experience of a simultaneous picture of their entire life, confirming the traditional knowledge that at death the individual experiences a panorama of his life. Such knowledge has also been confirmed by those who have developed their inner powers of cognition sufficiently. Can we understand the present condition of human consciousness and its crisis in such terms, as a death experience? It also belongs to 'death experience' or 'crossing the threshold' that thinking, feeling and willing should separate from each other.

In the past these three soul functions worked closely side by side and for some still do. Thoughts give rise naturally to feelings and actions and so on. It belongs to the threshold experience, when this is positively achieved, that the three functions separate. Their harmonizing must then be consciously undertaken by the individuality, the ego. To undertake this task it is understandable that the ego must have found its bearings, its orientation in the realm of wholes, which can also be called the spiritual world. Now it is clear that the ego which during these four or five centuries has been nourished on natural scientific ideas of mechanism and has become really blind to everything which does not have scientific authority, is in no position for such a task. The ego is too weak, and collapses full of doubt and fear and overwhelmed by shame. Thinking, feeling and willing then fall into a muddle instead of developing in distinctiveness. If this is so in the individual, something correlative might be expected on the socio-cultural level.

At this point we must look at the changing order of society in the course of human evolution. We can take it that the archetype of order is to be found in the idea of threefoldness. In the ancient Manu code of India this found expression in the three castes of the Brahmins, the Kshatriyas and the Vaisyas. The Brahmins were the custodians of the realm of spiritual values, the Truth, the Kshatriyas were responsible for government; they were the kings, rulers and warriors; whilst the Vaisyas provided the economic function, as merchants and craftsmen, the providers of material goods. Below these three there was the undifferentiated world of the Sudras, the, so to speak, slaves. Social order depended on these three castes remaining pure. In particular the custodianship of spiritual values had to be free from the responsibilities and privileges of power and rulership and the rulers had to accept the guidance of the Brahmins in respect of principles and truth. At that distant time this primordial pattern of social order was conceived as applying to a particular people and territory.

Many of the essential principles and ruling ideas of this Manu code are contained in Plato's *Republic*. We must remember that this sketch of the ideal State is presented as an enquiry into the nature of justice, *dikaiosune*, or function. It is as much an enquiry into the nature of righteousness in the individual as into order or justice in society. But in one main respect it differs from the Manu code. Plato did not clearly distinguish in his Guardians between the roles of philosopher and king. Was this partial confusion of the two functions of priest and king perhaps inherited from Egypt where the Pharaohs appear to have combined both functions? In any case, we find gradually emerging in the Middle Ages a threefold social order composed of the Church and monasteries which were the repositories of learning and culture; the feudal system of Emperor, Kings, Dukes and so on bound together by oaths of fealty; and the guilds. The latter originating largely in the developing cities comprised the merchants and craftsmen. They also were hierarchically organized on the basis of apprentice, craftsman, and master, probably originating in the ancient craft masonry. In these guilds were also held the secrets of the crafts. All three classes or functions of the social order were hierarchically organized, a principle by no means of universal validity. In the human organism it is the nervous system which is hierarchically organized and brings about differentiation, the digestive metabolic system aims at equality and unity. From this we can see that mankind in the Middle Ages had not yet come fully to earth. All three functions were modelled on the heavenly hierarchies.

During this period of history a great battle raged between the spiritual and temporal powers. In the Eastern Byzantine Empire the emperors always regarded themselves as Christ's representatives on earth and as such supreme in spiritual as well as temporal affairs. The Patriarch was second to the Emperor. In the West the Popes always maintained their primacy in spiritual affairs and tried to extend their power to temporal matters also. The confusion, in principle present in Plato, here dominated centuries of European life.

We must again emphasize that individuals were for the most part wholly contained within their class; one was either a churchman, or within the feudal power structure, or else within the guilds. These functions were not strictly hereditary as they had become in the old caste system, nor were they so conceived in Plato's Republic. Further we can see that the content of the individual was experienced as that of the class to which he belonged and this entity was still felt to be a spiritual entity or at least to have a spiritual content.

This system disintegrated with the end of the Middle Ages. The Reformation destroyed the universal authority of Rome within the Church and at the same time thinking became intellectually emancipated. The growth of the bourgeoisie progressively eroded the old aristocratic feudal system. The old order with its threefold stratification of functions no longer worked. At this point arose the new nation states, in France and England particularly, as well as in Spain. It belongs very much to the 'nation state' that it is regarded as an absolute, responsible to none but itself. It assumes power over the cultural and political life and ultimately tends to regard the economy as also subject to its authority. It is in effect the denial of the idea of order and organism. The threefold archetype is reduced at best to a division between judiciary, legislature and executive. At the same time as socially the nation states began to arise, there began to appear individuals demanding their own sovereignty. And also at this same time the world began to be discovered as a whole. This demanded radical revision of old ideas of order. In a sense, the nation state, territorially based and largely separated from other regions, is the last term of the old order. Its independence was then natural and justified and often had in addition a racial and spiritual basis. The modern nation state tries to act as if it were still in splendid isolation, in spite of the involvement of all peoples today in a world order.

We may be able to throw light on these problems from the field of embryology. We can compare embryogenesis, the coming into being and the development of the individual organism, with anthropogenesis, the coming into being and gradual development of the organism of mankind as a whole. There has been a long controversy in embryology between two theories. The one maintains that everything in the future adult organism is already present in the embryo and fertilized ovum; whilst the other maintains that new forms unfold in the embryonic process that are in no way to be found in the original ovum. The former view is know as preformationism, the latter as epigenesis. For a time it appeared that epigenesis had won the day, but the modern theories of genetics seemed to re-establish preformationism in a much more sophisticated way. It now appears that, whilst the genes provide the basis for a multitude of items in the future adult organisms, the way in which these are woven into the developing form is attributable to epigenesis. We have to imagine the form as the visible 'idea' of the organism. The idea works with the genetic material artistically rather than mechanically, gradually incarnating more and more into full manifestation in the material world. The genetically determined items are progressively woven into the meaningful form of the organism out of an original haphazard chaos.

In man and the higher apes the dividing ovum at first gives rise to the extra-embryonic membranes, the environment in which the future embryo will develop. Only then does the first sketch of the embryo appear in the form of the germ layers or leaves, the ectoderm, mesoderm and endoderm. In addition to these three, which are on the way to becoming specialized and differentiated, there is the mesenchyme. This fourth remains omnipotential and unspecialized. It continues even into the adult in certain components of the blood and lymph system. The three main germ layers give rise to the nervous system, the primitive vertebral axis and the gut respectively. We might expect that they would continue a straight line development into the adult threefold system of nerves and senses, rhythmic, and metabolic limb systems. But they do not. A mixing takes place, so that the metabolic limb system is constituted from endoderm and mesoderm, whilst the rhythmic system arises from both mesoderm and endoderm. The pure threefold image first established becomes confused in the further development. We have suggested something similar in the development of the social order.

Evolution and history reveal a comparable process of anthropogenesis, in the course of which different races and cultures have carried for a time, autonomously, particular functions or missions, before disappearing. Today we stand at what seems to be a decisive point in the birth of mankind as a whole. The nation states and super-powers must sacrifice their claims to absoluteness, and through this sacrifice become able to contribute their own special functional values to the whole.

Two diametrically opposed processes stand in contrast to each other in both embryogenesis and anthropogenesis. On the one hand a primordial unity, really still an 'idea', differentiates and densifies into organs, functions, etc.; on the other hand individual organs arising in relative independence from each other become gradually woven into an organic unity. Could the descent of the primordial unity into differentiation be compared to the Grail, the ascent into organic unity to Prometheus? In Christian Myth and Reality these two become one. We should be able to find a thread to lead us through the labyrinth of immunological phenomena in these pictures even if we can at present take only very small first steps. For the problems are those of self and non-self or of the one and the many.

We may say at once, keeping to the biological field, that this problem of the one and the many or of the self and non-self concerns not only parasites such as bacteria and viruses as well as protozoa and helminths which invade the organism, but includes also the differentiated inner world of the organs, tissues and cells which comprise the body. This differentiated world has a tendency to emancipate from the wholeness of the organism; the cells in a malignant tumour have become autonomous; tissues and organs in the so-called auto-immune diseases become relatively speaking 'non-self' and the organism reacts to them as alien. The ego as the principle of unity has to permeate the organism from birth on. It inherits a body which is not truly individualized but is only a product of heredity. This body is somewhat of a hotch-potch of inherited traits and factors which need to be brought into unity by the incarnating ego, and will disintegrate again into multiplicity at death when soul and spirit leave the body again. Obviously weakness in the ego may allow some of these functions and organs to go their own way. Any thing or process from the outer world must be totally transformed in order to enter wholesomely into the human organism. As Lorenz Oken expressed it at the beginning of the nineteenth century, animal physiology is human pathology. Whatever continues in the human organism as if it were in the outer world is a disease process. The inherited organism is in reality foreign or outer world in relation to the incarnating ego and only gradually can this entity transform the body and build it up as its own. The typical inflammatory diseases of childhood can be seen as an aspect of this process. Through them the ego can achieve a more complete mastery of the organism, can weld the multiplicity more into unity. In this century in the developed world the severity and incidence of these diseases have declined dramatically, even apart from the massive programmes of vaccination and immunization. Perhaps this decline in severity could be understood as a symptom of the weakening of the ego as well as a cause of other diseases which have come increasingly to the fore. Allergic diseases are an example of a range of conditions which do seem to have become far commoner as infectious childhood diseases have declined.

Let us now return to our study of the development of the social order. The nation state reached a certain peak of absoluteness in the France of Louis XIV and then became confronted with the demands for the Rights of Man culminating in the Revolution. Liberty, Equality and Fraternity became the slogans of the day but they were not differentiated as ideals for the three spheres or functions of Society and were only grasped as impotent abstract ideas. In the prevailing intellectualism, the individual man was also reduced to the concept of a citizen, a merely legal abstraction. Consequently the individual became empty of real content, the old spirituality inherent in the traditional social order had vanished, intellectualism failed to provide any real content to take its place. The individuality became impotent and could only find itself in the spurious image of the Great Man, Napoleon, who at his coronation as emperor took the crown from the Pope and placed it on his own head. In the clamour for the Rights of Man the functionally correlative Duties of Man were forgotten.

From then on war between the autonomous nation states has become increasingly destructive. The nation states themselves come to consist of people of different origins, but each group of these seeks to become itself an independent state. As the fact of world unity has become ever more inescapable the inner contradictions grow increasingly critical. Individuals seem to become more than ever impotent to intervene constructively. In place of order we have disorder. We may compare this collapse of order, which is the outer manifestation of the inner weakness of the soul and spirit of society, with that collapse of order in the individual which manifests in the disease AIDS. It is considered that the essential kernel of this disease is the weakening and collapse of the immune system brought about by a specific virus. As a consequence the organism becomes defenceless and subject to other invading disease processes. The most characteristic of these appears to be, first, a rather specific malignant tumour, secondly a very virulent pneumonia and thirdly destruction of the brain. We may note certain correspondences between these conditions and the manifestations of the three archetypal diseases Cancer, Tuberculosis and Syphilis which we considered in the first part of this essay.

286

How can we envisage order being brought about again in society? It becomes obvious that we cannot reinstate the old threefold order simply within the boundaries of the existing states. Nor can the individual be contained within the boundaries of a particular class. The modern individual finds himself facing the whole of mankind, past, present and future, as the great organic, spiritual being which somehow is his content. Every individual finds himself related to this being through various intermediary groupings such as religion, sex, race, nation, state, class or social function. None of these can be considered as absolutes; they are organs of the developing mankind. Each individual is more specifically related to the whole through three aspects of his life. First he is a cultural being, living in the world of values, trying to find his way into the spiritual cultural inheritance of mankind. Secondly he is a social being, living in community with others, and thirdly he is involved in the production, distribution and consumption of material goods; he belongs to the economic life. Whereas in earlier times any particular individual was almost completely contained within his particular class function, today every individual partakes increasingly in all three archetypal functions. Class is transformed into function. Each individual must find himself related in a threefold functional way to society. Is there also an integrating function through which the individual is related to the whole? This question would seem to be closely connected to the problem of the immune system within the individual organism. Earlier we noted that in the early embryo in addition to the three germ layers there is a fourth, the mesenchyme. This enters into the later development of those tissues and cells involved in the immunological processes.

It seems to belong to our time that egotism is expressing itself with unparalleled nakedness. Sensing that its inherent inner self-contradictions are reaching crisis point, egotism asserts itself with ever-increasing violence. Unbridled self-interest, and the pursuit of sensual pleasure are elevated to highest principles. The State, whether called democratic or communist or anything else, pursues its own short-sighted self-interest with total ruthlessness. All states are still pagan, in all of us the egotism of the old Adam is still adamant!

The complexity of the immune processes revealed in modern research gets ever more bewildering and it is not our aim to attempt to elucidate it. But we may use an example to help us in our exploration. Certain white cells in the blood (the B Lymphocytes) normally circulate round and round in a sort of vegetative, almost endless repetition like the nodes up a tall growing plant. But if the lymphocyte meets an antigen, typically a foreign protein, it is converted into a plasma cell, comparable we might say to the metamorphosis of the vegetative leaf into a blossom in the case of a plant. When we relate to the outer world through our senses we create a world of images, which are not substantially real, and bear about the same relation to the real world as our face in a mirror does to ourself. Now, in response to the antigen; the metamorphosed lymphocytes produce antibodies which are, we would say, materialized mirror images. I am suggesting that this process, the production of antibody in response to antigen, is a mixed sensory and metabolic process. That the lymphocyte 'senses' the antigen is obvious, but it responds not just with a mirror image, but with a substantial product, a materialized image. In this respect it is comparable to the digestive metabolic processes in the organism where real substantial processes come about in response to ingested foreign food. The development of antibodies is also intimately bound up with the rhythms of the body, taking different times to unfold according to the character of the response. Can we regard the immune system thus as a mixed system? We observed that it is a feature of the 'threshold' that thinking, feeling and willing separate from each other and that the ego must then hold them in mutual balance. If it fails, they fall back into mutual confusion.

From this point of view, and I agree that it must seem absurd from our customary standpoint, there is something about the system of the immune processes which can only suggest that it is about to break down anyway. It is extraordinary how, today, medical science is bringing about a many-pronged assault on the immune system and at the same time a disease appears which attacks this system. The advances in organ transplantation are dependent on artificially suppressing the immune system. Modern treatments of cancer, whether by surgery, radiation or cytotoxic drugs, all severely suppress the immune responses. Immunization programmes, usually aimed at the infant before it can react fully against the vaccine, introduce foreign proteins or antigens into the circulation. By these means the organic expression of the individuality is undermined. Until modern times, as we have indicated, the individuality was still dreaming and slumbering within the protective womb of group existence, in which instinctive or spiritual wisdom exercised protective sway. Only today has the individual become free from the traditional guiding reins. The ego has not been able to hold the balance in the threefold organism of nerve-sense processes, rhythmic processes and metabolic processes, and consequently strains have been forced on the immune system with which it cannot cope. From this viewpoint the question of the virus is secondary.

When we regard disease processes concretely and not abstractly, all these 'causes', bacterial, viral etc., have to be relegated to the status of symptoms. If there was not already disorder in the organism then these secondary invaders could not flourish. Even the genetic code, in which some aspects of heredity are inscribed and which our geneticist philologists are so painstakingly unravelling, cannot be regarded as causative. It is not causative any more than the works of Shakespeare are caused by the twenty-six letters in which they are coded. Shakespeare was the cause of the way these letters are combined. But an actor can read this code to recreate a copy of Shakespeare's meaning. Only a living person could originally cause the letters to carry a meaning and only another person can with the help of these letters read, interpret and reproduce that meaning. Only a living organism can use a genetic code to reproduce a copy of the ancestors.

We have seen how it has become necessary in dealing with social life to transform the old idea of separate classes or castes into the idea of separate functions into which each individual can enter according to his capacities. Must we not undertake a similar transformation of ideas about the organism? In earlier times different soul functions were located in different organs or regions of the body. The phrenic mind was located by Aristotle in the diaphragmatic region, the Pythagorean Alcmaeon located thinking in the brain. Descartes in totally separating the mechanical body from the waif-like soul left a point of contact in the pineal gland. Lavater the pioneer of a scientific physiognomy saw the human face divided into three regions, an upper, middle and lower. The intellectual capacities were expressed in the forehead, the emotional in the nose and cheeks and the volitional in the jaws. These three obviously relate to the three great body cavities, the cranium containing the brain, the chest containing the lungs and heart, and the abdomen the gut and metabolic organs. Such a way of looking at the problem still belongs to the class system. We can however follow Steiner and begin to think in terms of processes rather than anatomically conceived organs and regions. Then we can relate thinking to the all-pervading nerve processes, emotions and feelings to the all-pervading rhythmic processes and will to the all-pervading metabolic processes.

The ordering of these three functions in their mutual relationships falls more and more to the conscious ego, as we have seen. Today the ego feels enormously insecure, inferior and bereft of that support from God or a spiritual world which a younger mankind felt. Psychologically this shows itself in over-compensation, as exemplified in all the arrogant self-assertion, male chauvinism or feminism of our time. The individual retreats into his castle and puts up an important show of force. The organic expression of this seems to be an ever greater dependence on the whole immune system, until it begins to break down.

The great physiologist Gaskell tried to show the metamorphosis from invertebrate into vertebrate in a way which can illustrate these points. He showed how the primitive vertebrate, the lamprey, passes through a larval stage morphologically similar to the king-crab. In its metamorphosis it turns so to speak inside out. The protective outer skeleton of the invertebrate arthropod has to be replaced by the internal spinal system. Instead of a hard outer protection there comes about an internal spine and a soft exterior is presented to the world. It is as if a similar metamorphosis in our soul life is impending. In place of all our psychological defences with which we confront the world we need an inner spiritual spine and the courage to be vulnerable to the world.

Metamorphosis is one of the most important phenomena to help us with these problems. On the one hand we have to acknowledge a remarkable conservation of form by living creatures. Over countless millennia many species have maintained a seemingly unchanged form in spite of immense changes in the environment. A spectacular example came to light from the depths of the Indian Ocean only a few decades ago. The coelocanth, an antique fish, thought to have become extinct in distant ages, was suddenly caught in the nets of fishermen, unchanged from primordial times. Life in fact is characterized by the maintenance of form against force and inertia or mass. These two are the concepts with which we seek to explain the inorganic world. Force shatters form, inertia resists form. But observation of living creatures shows that they undergo great changes, such as the metamorphosis of caterpillar into chrysalis and into butterfly. And the cycle is repeated so that our idea of the butterfly has to include egg, caterpillar, chrysalis and the butterfly in the whole 'form'. In the case of humans we are all aware of the immense metamorphosis at birth and again at puberty. Study reveals other important moments when the relationship of body and soul unfolds and undergoes metamorphosis. Menopause today has attracted much attention. Shakespeare's Seven Ages of Man are well known. Now diseases are often related to definite ages. Tuberculosis had a connection with adolescence; cancer seems to have a connection with menopause. Of course these things are not rigidly related, but are rather characteristic. It is as though, if a metamorphosis is not properly accomplished in its right time, then a disease may manifest.

We have been trying to see how our present time points to a crisis in every walk of life. Nature herself, the living earth, is changing, growing old. Our waking consciousness is born of the death processes in our brains and our natural science, a product of this awake thinking, carries death everywhere into nature. If our industrial economy is to go on for every expanding then the life of the planet will be destroyed. Our sovereign states have reached the limit of their innate absurdity. Our materialistic culture has produced meaninglessness. In our total crisis we must also accept that our human nature itself must undergo a radical metamorphosis, it cannot continue as it is. And this metamorphosis cannot be just a mental or soul change. It will have to, judging from the vast irreversible changes in the natural kingdoms that have been avalanching upon us, extend also right into the organism itself. It is possible that over the centuries great changes in the human organic functioning have taken place. Usually we think of the ancients having bodies just like ours but with less knowledge and different prejudices. It is easier to accept that our bodies change during our individual lives, but this should show us that the whole of mankind also changes organically and is growing older.

The trend of these considerations is leading towards a very tentative position. The habitual ego-experience, which has in the past been intimately bound up with race, class, culture and so on, and is still closely connected with age and sex, is becoming weak and uncertain. The immune system is, in so far as it is the expression of this ego, on the defensive. The old ego is at the end of its tether and it would seem that only a radical renewal, a birth of the whole in the single can help. We have to find our relationship to the whole of mankind and all the old partial loyalties, absolute in their time, will have to be revalued in their functional significances, relative to the whole. Will a reborn, renewed ego still express itself defiantly, through the immune system? Will it possibly seek in the organic realms to harmonize and balance the functions inwardly, and is there a system through which this function could possibly be exercised? Could the endocrine system taken as a whole, in the manner sketched by Karl König, become the instrument of such a higher function? What we are imagining is of course not within the scope of current empirical investigation. We are trying to see our present troubles and crises as birth pangs of mankind rising from the preparatory stages of evolution and anthropogenesis to the achievement of free and self-guided individuals.

Both the immune system and the endocrine system belong as organs to the blood system. This blood system, coursing through the whole organism and undergoing continuous metamorphosis in the process, can be understood as the instrument of the ego, the expression of the wholeness as such. The immune system is involved in the defence of the individuality as against the outer world. The endocrine system is involved in maintaining the inner wholeness throughout changes in life epochs. Sir Arthur Keith, many years ago, suggested how the different glands came to expression in the different races. These races, belonging really to the evolutionary past, can be understood as metamorphoses of the human archetype. The different periods of individual life can also be regarded as metamorphoses of the developing individuality. We are suggesting that this system, in addition to the actions empirically researched today, has the function of maintaining the wholeness throughout the life-development by means of balancing and ordering the metamorphoses of body and soul.

At the end of the eighteenth century, during the French Revolution, Goethe and Schiller were engaged in discussion about the nature of freedom. Schiller wrote his *Letters on the Aesthetic Education of Mankind* and Goethe wrote *The Fairy Tale of the Green Snake and the Beautiful Lily* which Thomas Carlyle translated into English. In this complex tale there are four kings, a golden, a silver and a bronze king and in the fourth gold, silver and bronze are mixed. The golden, silver and bronze kings are the power-holders respectively of the thinking, feeling and willing functions. Only at the climax of the tale, with the marriage of the young man and the beautiful lily, and the achievement of freedom, and 'when the time has come', does the mixed king collapse leaving the three kings to rise up into their pure functions.

One matter remains to consider: the role of sexuality in the causation of AIDS. We have been trying to consider this disease as a symptom of the weakness and collapse of the ego. We can only regard the behavioural problems leading to the spread of AIDS as symptoms of this collapse. Vladimir Solovyov in *The Meaning of Love* spoke of human sexuality as concerned not only with generation but also with regeneration. Pointing out that human sexuality is greater than animal sexuality but that human reproduction is less, he showed that the meaning of human sex cannot be fully explained as residing solely in reproduction. It serves the needs of reproduction in so far as man belongs to Nature but its greater potentiality is to serve as a force towards human individual rebirth. He points out that the power of natural human egotism is so overwhelming that we could not overcome it if there were not another power equally great. Sex love can be transformed into the power that is strong enough to balance egotism and lead to the possibility of individual rebirth. The ego which uses power and sex for its egotistical satisfaction is not the ego which can undertake the ordering of our soul life and of our cultural spiritual life. The whole mankind is spread out as a panorama before us and we must work towards this wholeness becoming alive and awake in the individual hearts and minds.

PART IV

36.   Healing as art

In the plant kingdom we can delight in the manifestation of beauty. Nature's works here lift our hearts into joy and peace. Nature herself appears to us as an artist. We can indeed find even within the lifeless mineral kingdom objects of surpassing beauty. The plain black carbon in the coal can become transfigured by light into the brilliance of the diamond. Solovyov drew our attention to the way in which the beauty of the diamond arises not from the substance of which it is made, mere carbon, nor from light itself which is invisible. The beauty arises from the union of substance and light without 'division or confusion'. The diamond shows us light-bearing matter and embodied light, illumined coal and petrified rainbow. We can see here beauty arising in the transfiguration of matter through the incarnation in it of another, a supra-material principle. In the play of the shining brilliance of the colours we are no longer aware of the surpassing hardness of its matter. We become aware of the light's activity which would otherwise remain invisible. But the crystal structure is uniform and fixed and the immaterial, ideal element, light, finds only a limited possibility for its transforming activity. This light element is known more directly to us in the light of our consciousness, in our thinking we live in the element of light and with it seek to penetrate the dark depths of nature.

In the plant world, light becomes life and the plant reveals to us an ever-changing metamorphosis of form. The matter in the plant is for a time lifted up into the sphere of life. We do not see the matter in the plant but it enables us to see with our eyes the immaterial plant form. Nor do we see the carbon in the play of colour in the diamond. The free play of the ideal element in the plant is, however, limited; the plant is rooted, not free to move; it is held within the seasonal rhythms of the surrounding world and it expresses the outer laws of the cosmos, not its own inner impulses. This gives to the plant kingdom its pure and innocent quality. Gazing upon the beauty of the blossoming nature, we for a moment forget the decaying ugliness from which it burst forth. In itself the plant as it grows and unfolds presents an image of the self-metamorphosing world of ideas and on its own level can reach a supreme expression of beauty. The element of beauty is in itself useless but that it is objective and not merely subjective, in the eye of the beholder, is exhibited on all sides. Solovyov defined beauty as 'the transfiguration of matter through the incarnation in it of another super-material principle'. The transfiguration of the matter in the plant reaches its height in the blossom and its fragrance. But it is this which has least vitality, least survival value. The plant typically does not need the blossom for producing new plants.

All parts of the plant can in principle give rise again to a new example of the species. Here we come on another of the limitations of the appearance of beauty in the plants. The highest ideal is 'the greatest possible independence of parts combined with the greatest possible unity of the whole'. In the plant the different parts and organs are not so differentiated that they cannot give rise to all the others. It is more differentiated than the mineral but less so than the animal.

The animal organization is on a higher level than the vegetable. Its differentiation into organs and tissues is carried further and its unification into a whole is stronger so that it is free to move in response to the unfolding, within, of instinctive, emotional impulses, an inner world of desire. The deeper more intense penetration of the material by the ideal calls forth in reaction compulsive drives which in the first place are ugly. The animal organism in comparison with the plant is ugly. But the cosmic artist proceeds to adorn this creation with beauty. The scraggy carcass of the peacock becomes adorned in all the splendid coloured forms of its plumage which serve no purpose but to attract the female through an unconscious aesthetic sense. The owl becomes the symbol of wisdom, Athena's bird, not by its miserable plucked skin and bones, but by its majestic feathered form. A slug is hardly an image of beauty but its cousin the snail secretes a shell of infinitely beautiful colours and spiral forms. Some of the higher animals, the mammals, also appear to us moving and clothed with beauty. One thinks of the varied members of the cat family, lions, tigers, leopards and the rest, as also of the deer and gazelles. Skinned, they are ugly. Nature conceals their essential ugliness under their 'hides'. In fact they have hides rather than skins.

The songs of songbirds show us in another way how the crude instincts of animals can be transformed. The reproductive instinct of the animal world is not usually beautiful. The caterwauling of cats is not particularly aesthetic, whereas a blackbird or nightingale or lark can enchant us and inspire poets and musicians. Here the crude expression of the reproductive process becomes transfigured by love into beauty.

And yet, the animal is not free, it is under the compulsion of instinct implanted in its organism. It cannot escape the determinism of its inherited obsessions. Our wonder awakens to the wisdom embodied in the animal world but it is not an individual wisdom but a group one.

The animal forms moreover are all specialized in one direction or another. The

294

birds hardly come to earth, their legs for instance are a mere system of levers, they fly off and are equivalent to our heads alone. Contrasted to the birds we find the cattle and herbivora, bound to the earth with enormously developed digestive systems. In chewing the cud their heads even become subordinated to the digestive system: additional stomachs. The bull is indeed belly through and through. Between these polarically contrasted forms are the carnivora crowned by the lion. In these we see the middle rhythmic chest system assuming the dominance.

Nowhere in the animals do we find a harmoniously balanced expression of the three archetypal functions which are centred in head, and heart and abdomen. Only in Man do we find this perfection and, even if individually we deviate from the human ideal to a greater or lesser degree, we can yet discern the ideal human form as the perfectly balanced harmony of these three. None of them dominates the others; the human is the expression, the incarnation, of the idea of the threefold, the Trinity. This idea realizes 'the greatest possible independence of parts combined with the greatest possible unity of the whole'. Its appearance in the world of sense phenomena is therefore supreme beauty and has become the ideal of artists throughout the ages.

Now at birth the human form is still mostly head, the body and limbs append-ages. The soul enters into this body with the first breath, until then, in embryo and foetus, the soul is still, as it were, hovering around in the realms of the foetal membranes. The soul as individual entity enters into a body borrowed from the parents. The body is determined by hereditary forces and must present an obstacle to the soul seeking expression in this world. This body is not yet the creation and expression of the individuality seeking to embody itself therein. Steiner has drawn attention to the way in which, up until the change of teeth, this soul spirit entity is building its own body using the inherited body as a model, rather as an artist may use another picture as one for his own creation. From this point of view we can envisage that a strong individuality will be able to transform the inherited traits for its own use in building the bodily instrument for its life-work. Even inherited handicaps can be used as obstacles to call forth further creative activity and in a deeper sense may even have been chosen for such a purpose. Their very opposition can become a stimulus. A weaker individuality may not be so able to work upon these hindrances and may have to bear them. We can moreover see that the human form in its threefoldness can become the vehicle for the embodiment of an individuality which can awake not only to consciousness but to self-consciousness. In nature, as we have seen, the spiritual ideal element does indeed progressively become embodied in and transform the inertia of the material but it does not awake to self-consciousness. In man, in awaking to self-consciousness the possibility arises for a free participation in the continuation of the work of creation. The free interpenetration and co-operation of self-conscious persons is a higher achievement than the instinctive herd-togetherness of the natural, whether in animal or man.

During infancy and childhood the typical diseases are the infectious epidemic diseases, even though in our time these have for various known and unknown reasons become much less important than they used to be. The four most characteristic ones are scarlet fever, whooping cough, measles and diphtheria. Inflammatory diseases are characterised by warmth, pain, swelling and redness. They arise in response to foreign substances or organisms or in response to some organ tissue or cell falling out of the organic wholeness. They seek through a sort of digestive process to overcome and revitalize and integrate that which is foreign or is becoming foreign. During childhood the inherited body is felt by the incarnating individuality as foreign or borrowed. In the task of building its own body, this borrowed one must be digested by inflammatory processes. This task may proceed smoothly or through feverish illnesses. The four features of inflammation, *calor, dolor, tumor and rubor*, to give them their traditional Latin names, relate to the four principles of the human organization. Warmth or *calor* is related to the ego, pain or *dolor* indicates a soul element also related to the airy element, Swelling or *tumor* points to the watery and vital processes and redness or *rubor* shows a penetration into the physical and earthy element. We then find the four elements of the ancients turning up in a surprising manner when we thought we had given them up. The four diseases mentioned are related each to one of these elements in particular. Scarlet fever is marked by warmth, fever violent in onset and degree, but also by redness. Whooping cough entails a battle with air which has to be utterly expelled in the paroxysm. In measles the fluid element rises up in catarrhs and threatens to drown the victim whilst in diphtheria earthy deposits form in and obstruct the air passages. Are not these illnesses like echoes of ancient rites of initiation, trials by fire and water as in Mozart's *Magic Flute*?

As we grow up, we have further challenges to meet. At puberty all sorts of emotional and religious-philosophical problems arise. Gradually we have to overcome mere group involvements and excesses and work through these powerful and seductive forces until they come to be instruments of, not masters of, ourselves. It seems likely that tuberculosis for instance can be best understood in relation to this crisis in development.

Later we have to find our way into career, job, profession. Again we meet in these 'ways of life' something which can dominate and drown our essential individuality. Great effort is needed to permeate such objective discipline as a profession entails, with that unique idiom which is the mark of personality.

At every stage we have to overcome and transform these impersonal factors. Merely to dominate and master them to serve one's egotistical aims would be to fall slave to one's own egotism. Only an artistic permeation by our individuality can succeed in winning these capacities over so that they become personal capacities and attributions.

It is easier to approach an understanding of the meaning of acute illnesses, mostly inflammatory in nature and with an inherent tendency to get better, than that of chronic illnesses. We have tried to glance at these acute illnesses as concerned with the course of the incarnation of the individual into an inherited body and into those social, cultural and linguistic bodies into which we have to incarnate in the course of our education and life. These are all part of the 'non-self' reminding us of the successive peelings of the onion in Peer Gynt. These childhood, acute, inflammatory illnesses arise in the course of our largely unconscious efforts to permeate and transform these bodies with our individuality. But in this process we become identified with these elements or bodies; our egotism becomes powerfully increased as we come to think of ourselves as the owner of wealth, knowledge, skill, fame, social, sexual, and national or racial attributes and privileges. On the one hand we do work towards transforming these essentially material elements, spiritualizing them, but on the other we come to think of our essential validity as based on them and become imprisoned in them. The second half of life finds its meaning no longer in becoming a specialist but in the effort to become universal, whole. Obviously this does not mean becoming a specialist at everything; a jigsaw puzzle does not become again a whole picture. Again, it is mostly in relation to these problems that cancer arises.

The diseases of the second half of life are mostly hardening processes. As we grow older all our tissues lose some of their elasticity. It is natural in the head-pole of our organism for these hardening and death processes to dominate the picture. The head is to a large extent bone and nerve. Nerves, as we have frequently mentioned, are representatives of a dying process. As we grow up we already excarnate to a great extent from the brain. We use it then as a mirror in which to reflect our thinking. As we grow older and our bodies become harder they begin to approach the way things are in the head. We begin to excarnate from our bodies. Our limbs are no longer so immediately responsive; we have to use them more as external instruments, rather clumsily. When we die, it is as if our whole body becomes head.

Can we draw any pointers from this as to the problems of healing these diseases? In the head certain forces which up till about the time of the change of teeth are still involved in forming and structuring the brain, begin to become free. In the course of education these same formative forces are led over or metamorphosed into the forces used in thinking and memory. We can surmise that, as, in growing older, the body becomes more like a head, further forces are also potentially liberated for conscious soul activities. But it also appears that the cultivation and development of these forces is greatly dependent on our own inner self-motivated activity. Most of our ordinary everyday activities take their course almost automatically, motivated by desires or self-interest. It does seem that the motives of the inner activity to which we are trying to point are of a different order.

We have sketched how in nature and man we can see the progressive penetration of the material by the ideal spiritual so that we can venture to see as the goal of man's evolutionary development, the full embodiment of the ideal and the full transfiguration of and overcoming of the inertia and heaviness of the material. Here we come up against the fact of death which dogs our life on earth and to which it seems the course of chronic diseases inevitably leads. We cannot fully penetrate the physical body and enlighten its gravity; in the end we have to discard it. Our individuality is not or not yet strong enough to conquer the opaqueness of the material, radically to transform its evil.

There does however stand in the centre of our earth history the figure of Christ and the indications are that he did in entering into the body of Jesus utterly spiritualize or transform this body. The mysterious body of the resurrection cannot have been a mere spectre but a fully metamorphosed physical body in which the death processes have been fully won over to serve the sphere of light and consciousness. Therefore we can at least begin to understand that in him the fullness of truth dwelt bodily. In mankind in general and particular we can perhaps say that we are on the way. We must understand and assimilate the meaning and reality of death.

Not enough recognition is given to the way in which our awake consciousness is based on the destructive death processes rather than on the constructive life processes. It is in our heads that we wake up. We owe to the death we carry round with us in our brains our fully awake consciousness. At present we are normally awake only in our thinking which is reflected in the 'mirror' of the brain; it is a thinking which has become, over the centuries, abstract and grasps only the mechanism in everything. Life escapes its understanding; only the mechanism, the corpse, within the living is accessible to this form of knowledge. We have however achieved our wide-awake consciousness by virtue of this abstract modern thinking. In earlier times we grasped the world with more mobile living thoughts but in a more dreamlike state. Today our consciousness has become sharpened with no surrounding shade, like the laser beam it has contrived, in which the light is imprisoned.

We have suggested that in infancy and childhood the incarnating individuality coming from non-spatial existence into space refashions the inherited body, borrowed from the parents. If this were not so there would be no possibility of human freedom; we should be utterly determined by the inherited destiny as are the animals. Now the recent technological achievements in so-called genetic and molecular biology do indeed indicate a place of determinism, of destiny in human life. But this is only one limiting pole of human reality. It offers the necessary resistance against which the ideal-spiritual individuality can awaken and in freedom begin to work with the ever-potential infinite realm of Providence. The realizing within the limiting frame of the material and sensory of the ideal, the purely spiritual, is essentially the function of art. We commence this work unconsciously in infancy and childhood; in maturity we can co-operate in freedom with the cosmic artist in the work of transforming the dark, meaningless chaos of matter, where mere statistical accident rules. If providence and the spiritual are the realm of the infinite; and destiny and matter the realm of the finite; man and his free-will are the realm of the indefinite.

There is another sphere of human bodily life where we can take up these immense riddles of human existence. In the intake and digestion of food, a transformation takes place of absolute significance. Steiner with great courage indicated that matter must be entirely destroyed from the physical plane in the digestive process. It is then in the instant re-created within the organism. We know from physiology that food is broken down in the digestion, is thoroughly denatured, its livingness stripped from it, but Steiner goes further in affirming the utter elimination of the substance before its reappearance. If the substance, even in mineral state, were simply transferred into the organism, it would determine our existence. Our freedom is based on this destruction of matter in our digestive-metabolic activities. It seems possible, of course, that not all the food we take in is so utterly destroyed. Substances like alcohol and 'poisons' and medicines enter more directly and act as foreign entities within us; then our thinking is not our own free activity but the substance thinking in us.

Human life on earth takes place within definite finite limits and yet we know our inmost being as belonging to the infinite. Our life unfolds in the activity which, to a greater or lesser extent, incorporates the potentiality of the infinite into the limitation of the finite. Essentially this is an artistic activity and a human life must then be viewed as a work of art in which freedom becomes effective. In biography we seek to unveil the work of art that an individual life is. In works of art, crises develop and are resolved. In Shakespeare's last dramas the great crises which in the tragedies end catastrophically are resolved and healed. In human life accidents, illnesses, chance events come to oppose the idealistic dreams of our childhood and youth. We inevitably blot our copy-books, commit mistakes and crimes. The healing or reintegration of these manifestations demands an enhancement, an enlargement of our consciousness so that within a wider vision of the whole they find their place. Without the death processes we should never achieve our true status as man but this then must lead into our free co-operation with the providential infinity to sow the seeds of the future.

Our modern culture which has come about under the chaotic guidance of our materialistic natural science, does not help the individual to unfold the fullness of soul life. So little of the full potential within each individual can today come to conscious acceptance and expression. Our diseases are unconscious shadow expressions or caricatures of our yet to be unfolded genius. We are so to speak pregnant with our own future development and even within the course of a single life we can, not seldom, see a profound and wonderful unfolding proceed during what we call an illness.

Art as we have known it has served to keep alive a vision of the spiritual and infinite as a world of semblance. In the future should not art enter into the self-creation of Man, into the work of bringing to manifestation the infinite within the limits of individual finiteness and destiny? Our life itself must become art and the Healing Art must find how to co-operate in this creative work. Medicine in its origins was religious or spiritual in its character, then it entered into a scientific phase. This has achieved a tremendous knowledge of death and disease and also spread death and disintegration in and around us. Now should begin the age of making all things new, the art of renewal and healing, of conferring meaning on the meaningless.

Bibliography

Adams, George, 'Potentization and the Peripheral Forces of Nature,' *British Homoeopathic Journal*. 1961 (50. 226).

Adams, George & Olive Whicher, *The Living Plant — the Science of Physical and Ethereal Space*, Goethean Science Foundation, Stourbridge 1949.

——, *The Plant between Sun and Earth*, 2 ed. Steiner Press, London 1980.

Arber, Agnes, *Goethe's Botany*, Chronica Botany,Waltham, Mass. 1946.

Bahnson, G. B. and M. B. Bahnson, 'Cancer as an Alternative to Psychosis,' in *Psychosomatic Aspects of Neoplastic Disease*, Pitman Medical, London, 1964.

Barfield, Owen, *The Case for Anthroposophy*, Steiner Press, London 1970.

——, *What Coleridge Thought*, Wesleyan University Press, Conn. 1971.

——, 'Historical Perspectives in the Development of Science,' in *A New Image of Man in Medicine*, Vol. 1, Futura, New York 1979.

Bates, J. A. V. 'Can Voluntary Movement be Localised in the Cerebral Cortex?' *British Association*, Oxford Sep 1954.

——, 'Observations on the Excitable Cortex in Man,' *Lectures on the Scientific Basis of Medicine*, Vol. 5, 1955–56.

Bergson, Henri, *Creative Evolution*, Macmillan, London 1928.

——, *Matter and Memory*, George Allen, London 1913.

Bernard, H. M. *Some Neglected Factors in Evolution*, Putnam, London 1911.

Bhagavan Das, *The Science of Social Organisation or the Laws of Manu*, Theosophical Publishing, Madras 1932.

——, *The Science of Emotions*, Madras 1953.

Bjerre, Paul, *The History and Practice of Psychoanalysis*, Gorham, Boston, & Phillips, London 1920.

Blond, Kasper, *The Liver and Cancer*, Wright, Bristol 1955.

Blond, Kasper, and D. Haler, *The Liver: Porta Malorum*, Wright, Bristol 1950.

Booth, G. 'Cancer and Humanism', in *Psychosomatic Aspects of Neoplastic Disease*, Pitman Medical, London 1964.

Bott, Victor, *Authroposophical Medicine*, Steiner Press, London 1978.

Brieger, J. 'Calcarea carbonica or Ostrea odulis?' *British Homoeopathic Journal*, 1960 (49. 41).

——, 'Cramps and Wheezes,' *British Homoeopathic Journal*, 1964 (53. 248).

Bunning, E. *The Physiological Clock*, Springer, Berlin 1963.

Burke, J. Butler, *The Emergence of Life*, Oxford University Press, 1931.

Burrow, Trigant, *The Social Basis of Consciousness*, Kegan Paul, London 1927.

——, *The Structure of Insanity*, Kegan Paul, London 1932.

Burnett, J. Compton, *Curability of Tumours in Medicine*, Homoeopathic Publishing, London 1898.

Castiglioni, Arturo, *A History of Medicine*, Alfred Knopf, New York 1941.

Cawadias, A. P. 'Constitutional Medicine and Endrocrinology' *British Homoeopathic Journal*, 1939 (29. 42).

Chamberlain, H. S. *Immanuel Kant*, Bodley Head, London 1914.

Clarke, John H. *A Dictionary of Practical Materia Medica*, Homoeopathic Publishing, London 1900.

'Condylomata Acuminata'. *British Medical Journal*, 22 April 1972.

Dale Green, Patricia, *Dog*, Hart-Davies, London 1966.

——, 'The Healing Lick and Rabid Bite,' *British Homoeopathic Journal*, 1964 (53. 51).

Defries, A. *The Interpreter Geddes*, Kegan Paul, London 1933.

Douch, G. 'The Heart as an Organ of Balance,' *British Homoeopathic Journal*, 1978 (67. 100).

Ellenberger, Henri, *The Discovery of the Unconscious*, Allen Lane, London 1970.

Engel, H. H. 'Snakes — an Essay in Interpretation,' *British Homoeopathic Journal*, 1959 (48. 221).

Faculty of Homoeopathy, Scottish Branch, 'Discussion on Rheumatoid Arthritis,' *British Homoeopathic Journal*, 1958 (48. 42).

Ferenczi, Sandor, 'Thalassa. A Theory of Genitality,' *Psychoanalytical Quarterly*, New York 1938.

Fisher, P. 'New Toxology,' *British Homoeopathic Journal*, 1980 (70. 1).

Forsgren, E. *Über die Rhythmik der Leberfunktion, des Stoffwechsels und des Schlafes*, Stockholm 1935.

Forsyth, A. A. *British Poisonous Plants*, HMSO, London 1954.

Foubister, D. M. 'Notes on *Helleborus niger*,' *British Homoeopathic Journal*, 1970 (59. 102)

Fyfe, Agnes, *Moon and Plant. Capillary Dynamic Studies*, Society for Cancer Research, Arlesheim 1967.

——, 'The Mistletoe in the Cycle of the Seasons,' *British Homoeopathic Journal*, 1969 (58. 227).

Goethe, J. W. *The Fairy Tale of the green Snake and the Beautiful Lily*, Floris, Edinburgh 1979.

Grant Watson, E. L. *Wonders of Natural History*, Pleiades Books, London 1947.

Green, Patricia Dale, *see* Dale Green.

Groddeck, G. *The Book of the It*, Vision, London 1950.

——, *Exploring the Unconscious*, Vision, London 1950.

——, *The Unknown Self*, Vision, London 1951.

——, *The World of Man*, Vision, London 1951.

Grohman, Gerbert, *Die Pflanze*, Vol. 2. Freies Geistesleben, Stuttgart 1959.

——, *The Plant*, Steiner Press, London 1974.

Guirdham, Arthur, *Obsession*, Spearman, London 1972.

——, *The Theory of Disease*, Allen & Unwin, London 1957.

Gutman, William, *Homoeopathy*, Homoeopathic Medical, Bombay 1978.

——, '*Aconitum napellus*,' *British Homoeopathic Journal*, 1959 (48. 271).

——, '*Pulsatilla* — the Plant and the Personality,' *British Homoeopathic Journal*, 1973 (62. 182).

Hahnemann, S. *Organon of Medicine*, 6 ed. Boericke & Tafel, Philadelphia 1922.

Harling, M. 'The Snake under the Skin,' *British Homoeopathic Journal*, 1958 (47. 182).

Hauschka, R. *The Nature of Substance*, Vincent Stuart, London 1966.

Hughes, R. *A Manual of Pharmacodynamics*, 7 ed. Ringer, Calcutta 1931.

Husemann, F. *Das Bild des Menschen als Grundlage der Heilkunst*, Freies Geistesleben, Stuttgart 1951.

Husemann, F., O. Wolff, (editors) *The Anthroposphical Approach to Medicine*, Anthroposophic Press, New York 1981–87.

Inman, W. S. 'Emotion and Rodent Ulcer' in *Psychosomatic Aspects of Neoplastic Disease*, Pitman Medical, London 1964.

Jacobi, J. *Paracelsus: Selected Writings*, Routledge & Kegan Paul, London 1951.

Jaworski, Hélan, *Après Darwin (l'arbre biologique)*, Baillière, Paris 1933.

——, 'The Biological Plan,' *British Homoeopathic Journal*, 1959 (48. 33).

——, *La découverte du monde*, Michel, Paris 1927.

——, *Les étapes de l'histoire*, Maloine, Paris 1918.

——, 'The Molluscs — their Significance,' *British Homoeopathic Journal*, 1960 (49. 30).

Jung, Carl G. *Answer to Job*, Routledge & Kegan Paul, London 1954.

——, *Psychological Types*, Kegan Paul, London 1933.

——, *Psychology and Alchemy*, Routledge & Kegan Paul, London 1953.

Kennedy, C. Oliver, 'Rheumatoid Arthritis,' *British Homoeopathic Journal*, 1975 (64. 42).

Kerenyi, C. *Asklepios*, Thames & Hudson, London 1960.

——, *The Gods of the Greeks*, Thames & Hudson, London 1951.

——, *Prometheus*, Thames & Hudson, London 1963.

Kingsbury, J. M. *Deadly Harvest*, Allen & Unwin, London 1967.

König, Karl, *Earth and Man*, Bio-Dynamic Literature, Rhode Island, 1982.

——, 'At Four o'Clock in the Morning,' *British Homoeopathic Journal*, 1958 (47. 33).

——, 'Convallaria majalis,' *British Homoeopathic Journal*, 1958 (48. 254).

——, 'Einige Geisteswissenschaftliche Betrachtungen über die Eihüllen und die erste Anlage des Menschenkeimes,' *Natura*, 1927 (1).

——, 'Embryology and World Evolution,' *British Homoeopathic Journal*, 1968–69 (57. 1, 2, 3, 4; 58. 1 & 2).

——, 'The Indian Summer, the Autumn Crocus and Colchicine,' *British Homoeopathic Journal*, 1958 (47. 102).

——, 'Meditations on the Endocrine Glands, *Golden Blade*, 1952

——, 'Sepia' *British Homoeopathic Journal*, 1960 (49. 89).

——, 'The Signature of the Christmas Rose (*Helleborus niger*),' *British Homoeopathic Journal*, 1959 (48. 262).

——, 'Versuch einer Darstellung der Jüngsten menschlichen Embryonalentwicklung,' *Gäa Sophia*, 1927 (2).

Kropotkin, P. *Mutual Aid*, Pelikan, London 1939.

Lavater, J. C. *Essays on Physiognomy*, Stockdale, London 1810.

Leeser, Otto, 'The Molluscs. Murex and Sepia,' *British Homoeopathic Journal*, 1960 (49. 16).

Lehrs, Ernst, *Man or Matter*, Faber, London 1958.

LeShan, L. 'An Emotional Life-History Pattern Associated with Neoplastic Disease,' *Annals of the New York Academy of Sciences*, 1966 (125. 780).

Manteuffel-Szoege, L. 'On the Movement of the Blood,' *British Homoeopathic Journal*, 1969 (58. 195 & 218).

Mees, L. F. C. *Geheimen van het Skelet Vorm en Metamorfose*, Vrij Geestesleven, Zeist 1981.

——, *Living Metals*, Regency, London 1974.

Morten, Lange, *Mushrooms and Toadstools*, Collins, London 1978.

North, P. *Poisonous Plants and Fungi*, Blandford, London 1967.

Oken, Lorenz, *Elements of Physiophilosophy*, Ray Society, London 1847.

Otto, W. F. *Dionysus Myth and Cult*, Indiana University Press, 1965.

——, *The Homeric Gods*, Thames & Hudson, London 1954.

Paterson, J. 'The Bowel Nosodes,' *British Homoeopathic Journal*, 1950 (40. 195).

Pelikan, Wilhelm, *The Secrets of Metals*, Anthroposophic, New York 1974.

——, 'The Cactaceae,' *British Homoeopathic Journal*, 1976 (65. 2).

——, 'The Lichens — Their Place in Nature as Remedies,' *British Homoeopathic Journal*, 1970 (59. 103).

——, 'The Liliaceae,' *Journal of Anthroposophic Medicine*, 2 & 3.

——, 'The Ranunculaceae,' *British Homoeopathic Journal*, 1976 (65. 240).

Phillips, E. D. *Greek Medicine*, Thames & Hudson, London 1973.

Poppelbaum, H. *Man and Animal*, Anthroposophical Publishing, London 1960.

——, *Man's Eternal Biography*, Adonis, New York 1945.

——, *A New Zoology*, Philosophic-Anthroposophic, Dornach 1961.

Raeside, J. R. 'A Proving of Hirudo Medicine,' *British Homoeopathic Journal*, 1964 (53. 22).

Rassidakis, N. C. et al, 'Malignant Neoplasms as a Cause of Death among Psychiatric Patients,' *International Mental Health Research Newsletter*, 1971–73 (13. 2; 14. 2; 14. 3).

Roberts, M. *Bio-politics*. Dent, London 1938.

Schaefer, Karl, E. H. Hensel, Ronald Brady (editors), 'Historical Perspectives in the Development of Science,' in *Towards a Man-Centred Medical Science*, Futura, New York 1977.

Schad, Wolfgang, *Man and Animals. Towards a biology of form*, Waldorf, New York 1977.

Schwenk, Theodor, *Sensitive Chaos*, Steiner Press, London 1965.

Selawry, A. 'Gestufte Eisentherapie des Gelenkrheumatismus,' *Beiträge zu einer Erweiterung der Heilkunst*, 1972 (25. 126).

Seltman, C. *The Twelve Olympians*, Pan, London 1952.

Sigerist, Henry H. *Great Doctors*, Allen & Unwin, London 1933.

——, *A History of Medicine*, Oxford University Press, 1961.

Smuts, J. C. *Holism and Evolution*, Macmillan, London 1926.

Solovyov, Vladimir, *An Anthology*, SCM Press, London 1950.

——, *The Meaning of Love*, Floris, Edinburgh 1985.

Steiner, Rudolf, *Knowledge of Higher Worlds*, 6 ed. Steiner Press, London 1976.

——, *The Origins of Natural Science*, Steiner Press, London 1985.

——, *Spiritual Science and Medicine*, Steiner Publishing, London 1948.

——, *The Study of Man*, 2 ed. Steiner Press, London 1975.

——, *Theosophy*, 4 ed. Steiner Press, London 1973.

——, *Truth and Knowledge*, Steiner Publications, New York 1981.

Templeton, W. L. 'Psychological Aspects of Rheumatoid Arthritis,' *British Homoeopathic Journal*, 1942 (32. 128).

Treichler, R. *Vom Wesen der Naturkrankheiten und ihrer Behandlung*, Arbeitsgem. anthr. Ärzte, Stuttgart 1956.

——, Chapter on psychiatry in *The Anthroposophical Approach to Medicine*, (F. Husemann, O. Wolff, editors) Anthroposophic Press, New York 1981–87.

Twentyman, Jean M. G. *The Organic Vision of Hélan Jaworski*, New Atlantis, Ditchling 1971.

Twentyman, L. R. 'Peyronie's Disease treated with Hirudo Medicinals,' *British Homoeopathic Journal*, 1972 (61. 164).

Urwick, F. J. *The Message of Plato*, Methuen, London 1920.

Wachsmuth, Günther, *The Etheric Formative Forces in Cosmos, Earth and Man*, Anthroposophical Publishing, London 1932.

Watson, E. L. Grant, *see* Grant Watson

Weihs, Thomas, *Embryogenesis in Myth and Science*, Floris, Edinburgh 1986.

Whaley, Keith and W. Carson Dick, 'Rheumatoid Arthritis: Aetiological and Pathogenic Considerations,' *British Journal of Hospital Medicine*, 1969 (2. 1916).

White, Victor, *God and the Unconcious*, Harvill, London 1952.

——, *Soul and Psyche*, Collins & Harvill, London 1960.

Whitmont, Edward, *Psyche and Substance*, North Atlantic, Berkeley, Calif. 1980.

——, 'An Analysis of a Dynamic Totality: Sepia,' *British Homoeopathic Journal*, 1950 (40. 163).

——, 'Psycho-physiological Reflections on Lachesis,' *British Homoeopathic Journal*, 1975 (64. 14).

Wilkinson, J. J. G. *The Human Body and its Connexion with Man*, New-Church Press, London 1918.

Index

INDEX